T0263476

Migraine and Other Primary Headaches

Guest Editor

RANDOLPH W. EVANS, MD

NEUROLOGIC CLINICS

www.neurologic.theclinics.com

Consulting Editor

RANDOLPH W. EVANS, MD

May 2009 • Volume 27 • Number 2

SAUNDERS an imprint of ELSEVIER, Inc.

W.B. SAUNDERS COMPANY
A Division of Elsevier Inc.

1600 John F. Kennedy Boulevard ● Suite 1800 ● Philadelphia, Pennsylvania 19103-2899

http://www.theclinics.com

NEUROLOGIC CLINICS Volume 27, Number 2
May 2009 ISSN 0733-8619, ISBN-13: 978-1-4377-0505-8, ISBN-10: 1-4377-0505-7

Editor: Donald Mumford

Neurologic Clinics (ISSN 0733-8619) is published quarterly by Elsevier Inc., 360 Park Avenue South, New York, NY 10010–171. Months of issue are February, May, August, and November. Business and editorial offices: 1600 John F. Kennedy Blvd., Suite 1800, Philadelphia, PA 19103-2899. Customer Service Office: 11830 Westline Industrial Drive, St. Louis, MO 63146. Accounting and circulation offices: 11830 Westline Industrial Drive, St. Louis, MO 63146. Periodicals postage paid at New York, NY, and additional mailing offices. Subscription prices are $235.00 per year for US individuals, $378.00 per year for US institutions, $118.00 per year for US students, $295.00 per year for Canadian individuals, $454.00 per year for Canadian institutions, $328.00 per year for international individuals, $454.00 per year for international institutions, and $167.00 for Canadian and foreign students/residents. To receive student/resident rate, orders must be accompanied by name of affiliated institution, date of term, and the *signature* of program/residency coordinator on institution letterhead. Orders will be billed at individual rate until proof of status is received. Foreign air speed delivery is included in all *Clinics* subscription prices. All prices are subject to change without notice. **POSTMASTER:** Send address changes to *Neurologic Clinics*, Elsevier Periodicals Customer Service, 11830 Westline Industrial Drive, St. Louis, MO 63146. **Customer Service: 1-800-654-2452 (US). From outside of the US, call 314-453-7041. Fax: 314-453-5170. E-mail: JournalsCustomerService-usa@elsevier.com (for print support); JournalsOnlineSupport-usa@elsevier.com (for online support).**

Reprints. For copies of 100 or more of articles in this publication, please contact the Commercial Reprints Department, Elsevier Inc., 360 Park Avenue South, New York, New York, 10010-1710; Tel.: (+1) 212-633-3812; Fax: (+1) 212-462-1935, and E-mail: reprints@elsevier.com.

Neurologic Clinics is also published in Spanish by Nueva Editorial Interamericana S.A., Mexico City, Mexico.

Neurologic Clinics is covered in *Current Contents/Clinical Medicine, MEDLINE/PubMed (Index Medicus), EMBASE/Excerpta Medica, and PsycINFO, and ISI/BIOMED.*

Printed and bound in the United Kingdom
Transferred to Digital Print 2011

Cover image: Joseph Jules François Félix Babinski, Illustration of scintillating scotoma drawn by an artist, 1890.

Contributors

CONSULTING EDITOR

RANDOLPH W. EVANS, MD
Clinical Professor, Department of Neurology, Baylor College of Medicine, Houston, Texas

GUEST EDITOR

RANDOLPH W. EVANS, MD
Clinical Professor, Department of Neurology, Baylor College of Medicine, Houston, Texas

AUTHORS

FRANK ANDRASIK, PhD
Distinguished University Professor, Department of Psychology, University of West Florida, Pensacola, Florida

LARS BENDTSEN, MD, PhD
Danish Headache Center, Department of Neurology, University of Copenhagen, Glostrup Hospital, Glostrup, Denmark

MARCELO E. BIGAL, MD, PhD
Global Director for Scientific Affairs, Merck Research Laboratories, Whitehouse Station, New Jersey; Department of Neurology, Albert Einstein College of Medicine, Bronx, New York

SUSAN W. BRONER, MD
The Headache Institute, St. Luke's-Roosevelt Hospital Center, New York, New York

DAWN C. BUSE, PhD
Assistant Professor, Department of Neurology, Albert Einstein College of Medicine of Yeshiva University, New York; Assistant Professor, Clinical Health Psychology Doctoral Program, Ferkauf Graduate School of Psychology of Yeshiva University, New York; Director of Psychology, Montefiore Headache Center, Bronx, New York

F. MICHAEL CUTRER, MD
Associate Professor, Department of Neurology, Mayo Clinic, Rochester, Minnesota

DAVID W. DODICK, MD
Professor, Department of Neurology, Mayo Clinic Arizona, Phoenix, Arizona

RANDOLPH W. EVANS, MD
Clinical Professor, Department of Neurology, Baylor College of Medicine, Houston, Texas

ROD FOROOZAN, MD
Assistant Professor, Department of Ophthalmology, Baylor College of Medicine, Cullen Eye Institute, Houston, Texas

PETER J. GOADSBY, MD, PhD, DSc, FRACP, FRCP
Professor, Headache Group, Department of Neurology, University of California San
Francisco, San Francisco, California

RIGMOR JENSEN, MD, PhD
Professor, Danish Headache Center, Department of Neurology, University
of Copenhagen, Glostrup Hospital, Glostrup, Denmark

CHRISTINE L. LAY, MD
Director, Centre for Headache, Women's College Hospital, Toronto, Ontario, Canada

THOMAS LEMPERT, MD
Vestibular Research Group, Charité, Berlin; Professor of Medicine, Director, Department
of Neurology, Neurologische Abteilung, Schlosspark-Klinik, Heubnerweg, Berlin,
Germany

DONALD W. LEWIS, MD
Professor and Chairman, Department of Pediatrics, Children's Hospital of The King's
Daughters, Eastern Virginia Medical School, Norfolk, Virginia

RICHARD B. LIPTON, MD
Department of Neurology, Albert Einstein College of Medicine, Bronx, New York;
Department of Epidemiology and Population Health, Albert Einstein College of Medicine,
Bronx, New York; The Montefiore Headache Center, Bronx, New York

HANNELORE NEUHAUSER, MD, MPH
Neurologist, Senior Epidemiologist, Department of Epidemiology, Robert Koch Institut,
Berlin; Vestibular Research Group, Charité, Berlin, Germany

JULIO PASCUAL, MD, PhD
Service of Neurology, University Hospital Marqués de Valdecilla, Santander, Spain

TODD D. ROZEN, MD
Michigan Head-Pain and Neurological Institute, Ann Arbor, Michigan; Clinical Associate
Professor, Wayne State University, Detroit, Michigan

TODD J. SCHWEDT, MD
Assistant Professor of Neurology and Anesthesiology, Director, Washington University
Headache Center, Washington University School of Medicine, St. Louis, Missouri

STEPHEN D. SILBERSTEIN, MD
Professor, Department of Neurology, Director, Jefferson Headache Center, Thomas
Jefferson University Hospital, Pennsylvania, Philadelphia

RODERICK C. SPEARS, MD
Center for Headache and Pain, Neurological Institute, Cleveland Clinic, Cleveland, Ohio

STEWART J. TEPPER, MD
Director of Research, Center for Headache and Pain, Neurological Institute, Cleveland
Clinic, Cleveland, Ohio

BERT B. VARGAS, MD
Center for Neurosciences, Tucson, Arizona

Contents

We describe the epidemiology and comorbidities of migraine, which affects 12% of adults in occidental countries. Prevalence is three times higher in women, but 6% of men are affected, making it the most prevalent neurologic disorder in men. Although migraine is a remarkably common cause of temporary disability, many migraineurs have never consulted a physician for the problem. Many disorders are comorbid with migraine. For some such as depression, the association has been well described, but for others, the relationship has been recently suggested, such as in the case of clinical and subclinical vascular brain lesions and coronary heart disease.

Migraine is a common, disabling disorder of the central nervous system. The disorder has three key features. The tendency is largely inherited, the sufferer is sensitive to exogenous and endogenous triggers that very often involve challenges to normal homeostatic biology, and the attack phenotype, when severe, is the stereotypical migraine attack. The attack itself consists of an abnormal perception of otherwise normal circumstances, such as pain without evidence of primary nociceptive activation, and light and sound sensitivity without change in ambient stimuli. The disturbance in the brain is of the subcortical aminergic sensory modulatory systems, and probably includes brainstem, hypothalamic, and thalamic changes that produce the rich clinical presentation seen in practice.

Neurologic symptoms are a prominent and often disturbing component of the migraine syndrome in many patients. Collectively termed "aura," migraine-related neurologic symptoms include visual, sensory, language, and motor disturbance. They occur in about one quarter of migraine patients, are classically transient, and are thought to occur as the result of cortical phenomena. Recently, motor symptoms previously included as a type of migraine aura have been reclassified as a component of hemiplegic migraine—a distinct migraine subtype. The tendency to aura is likely to be influenced by complex genetic and perhaps epigenetic factors.

Vestibular migraine (VM) designates recurrent attacks of vertigo that are caused by migraine. VM presents with attacks of spontaneous or positional vertigo, lasting seconds to days, accompanied by migrainous symptoms. Because headache is often absent during acute attacks, other migrainous features have to be identified by thorough history taking. In contrast, vestibular testing serves mainly for the exclusion of other diagnoses. Treatment is targeted at the underlying migraine.

Most primary headaches can be diagnosed using the history and examination. Judicious use of neuroimaging and other testing, however, is indicated to distinguish primary headaches from the many secondary causes that may share similar features. This article evaluates the reasons for diagnostic testing and the use of neuroimaging, electroencephalography, lumbar puncture, and blood testing. The use of diagnostic testing in adults and children who have headaches and a normal neurologic examination, migraine, trigeminal autonomic cephalalgias, hemicrania continua, and new daily persistent headache are reviewed.

The goals of acute treatment of migraine are cost-effective rapid relief, consistent reduction of disability, and reduced use of rescue medications. Key to acute treatment is matching medication to disability as a surrogate marker for disease severity with a stratified care approach. In the absence of vascular contraindications, triptans are first-line acute treatments for disabling migraine. Acute treatment success can be assessed with use of the paper tool, Migraine-ACT. Opioids and butalbital should be avoided in acute migraine treatment. Triptan type can be selected for patients by differences in speed or effect, formulation, and formulary tier.

The pharmacologic treatment of migraine may be acute (abortive) or preventive (prophylactic), and patients with frequent severe headaches often require both approaches. Preventive therapy is used to try to reduce the frequency, duration, or severity of attacks. The preventive medications with the best-documented efficacy are amitriptyline, divalproex, topiramate, and the beta-blockers. Choice is made based on a drug's proven efficacy, the physician's informed belief about medications not yet evaluated in controlled trials, the drug's adverse events, the patient's preferences and headache profile, and the presence or absence of coexisting disorders. Because comorbid medical and psychologic illnesses are prevalent in patients who have migraine, one must consider comorbidity when choosing preventive drugs. Drug therapy may be beneficial for both disorders; however, it is also a potential confounder of optimal treatment of either.

and acute and preventative pharmacologic measures. A growing body of controlled pediatric data is beginning to emerge regarding migraine treatment in children, lessening our dependence on extrapolated adult data.

Of the nearly 32 million Americans with migraine, 24 million are women. It is a disorder affecting women throughout their lifetimes, from childhood and puberty through the postmenopausal years. In childhood, before puberty girls are afflicted with migraine at approximately the same rate as boys, but after puberty, there is an emerging female predominance. Estrogen plays a key role in this epidemiologic variation but is not the only factor. There are numerous times when hormonal influences have an impact on migraine and its pattern, including menarche, oral contraceptive use, pregnancy, perimenopause, and menopause. Hence practitioners treating women with migraine need to have a clear understanding of these special considerations.

Migraine is positively associated with cardio- and cerebrovascular disorders and with structural heart anomalies. Migraine is more prevalent among people with right-to-left shunt by means of patent foramen ovale, atrial septal defects, and pulmonary arteriovenous malformations and among those with altered cardiac anatomy, such as mitral valve prolapse, atrial septal aneurysm, and congenital heart disease. Meanwhile, migraine increases the risk for cardiovascular disease and stroke. Although several hypotheses exist, explanation for these associations is lacking. This article reviews data supporting the association of migraine with right-to-left shunt, structural heart anomalies, cardiovascular disease, and ischemic stroke.

The substantial societal and individual burdens associated with tension-type headache (TTH) constitute a previously overlooked major public health issue. TTH is prevalent, affecting up to 78% of the general population, and 3% suffer from chronic TTH. Pericranial myofascial nociception probably is important for the pathophysiology of episodic TTH, whereas sensitization of central nociceptive pathways seems responsible for the conversion of episodic to chronic TTH. Headache-related disability usually can be reduced by identification of trigger factors combined with nonpharmacologic and pharmacologic treatments, but effective treatment modalities are lacking. Benefits can be gained by development of specific and effective treatment strategies.

The trigeminal autonomic cephalalgias (TACs) are a group of primary headache syndromes all marked by headache and associated autonomic features. The TACs include cluster headache, paroxysmal hemicrania, hemicrania continua, and short-lasting unilateral neuralgiform headache attacks with conjunctival injection and tearing syndrome. Diagnosis is made after looking at headache frequency, duration, and accompanying symptoms. Each TAC has its own unique treatment modality, which is discussed in depth.

This article reviews "other primary headaches," a classification of the International Headache Society that includes primary stabbing headaches, primary cough headache, primary exertional headache, primary headache associated with sexual activity, hypnic headache, primary thunderclap headache, and new daily persistent headache. Clinicians should be aware that these headaches may be symptomatic to structural lesions and therefore usually require careful neuroimaging evaluation.

FORTHCOMING ISSUES

August 2009
Movement Disorders
Joseph Jankovic, MD, *Guest Editor*

November 2009
Epilepsy
Steven Schachter, MD, *Guest Editor*

February 2010
Neurology and Systemic Disease
Alireza Minagar, MD, *Guest Editor*

RECENT ISSUES

February 2009
Neuroimaging
Laszlo Mechtler, MD, *Guest Editor*

November 2008
Stroke
Sean D. Ruland, DO and
Philip B. Gorelick, MD, MPH, FACP,
Guest Editors

August 2008
Current Issues in Clinical Neurovirology:
Pathogenesis, Diagnosis and Treatment
Christopher Power, MD and
Richard T. Johnson, MD, *Guest Editors*

RELATED INTEREST

Neuroimaging Clinics of North America May 2008
Cranial Nerves
Jan Casselman, MD, PhD, *Guest Editor*

THE CLINICS ARE NOW AVAILABLE ONLINE!

Access your subscription at:
www.theclinics.com

Preface

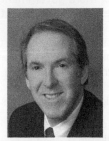

Randolph W. Evans, MD
Guest Editor

This issue of *Neurologic Clinics* reviews migraine and other primary headaches, one of the most common disorders seen by neurologists (accounting for about 20% of the general neurologist's practice), which affects 90% of the population and is the cause of 90% of all headaches. Secondary headache disorders were reviewed in *Neurologic Clinics* in 2004. Primary headache manifestations vary from the most mundane to among the most interesting in all of neurology. Migraine and tension-type headaches affect huge portions of the population, at times with significant impairment, with about 35 million persons yearly having attacks in the United States. Tension-type headaches have a lifetime prevalence of up to 78%. Neurologists may be particularly interested in migraine as over 50% of neurologists themselves are migraineurs.

Many of the neurologist's patients (and often the bane of their practice) are the 4-5% of the population with chronic daily headache and 0.5% with severe daily headaches who may be unresponsive to treatment in perhaps 30% of cases. Among the trigeminal autonomic cephalalgias, headaches can range from the uncommon, such as cluster headache with a prevalence only as high as 2 out of 1000 people, to the extremely rare short-lasting unilateral neuralgiform headache attacks with conjunctival injection and tearing. Other uncommon primary headaches are equally fascinating such as stabbing, cough, exertional, sexual, thunderclap, hypnic, and new daily persistent headaches.

This issue reviews the following topics: the epidemiology, burden and comorbidities of migraine; pathophysiology of migraine; transient neurologic dysfunction in migraine; vestibular migraine; diagnostic testing for migraine and other primary headaches; acute treatment of migraine; preventive migraine treatment; behavioral medicine for migraine; chronic migraine; pediatric migraine; women and migraine; the migraine association with cardiac anomalies, cardiovascular disease and stroke; tension-type headache; trigeminal autonomic cephalalgias; and other primary headaches. I hope this issue will update your knowledge of this exciting and rapidly expanding field and further your interest in headaches (and the subspecialty of headache medicine for which you can now gain subspecialty certification through the United Council for Neurologic Subspecialties).

Neurol Clin 27 (2009) xi–xii
doi:10.1016/j.ncl.2009.01.004
0733-8619/09/$ – see front matter © 2009 Elsevier Inc. All rights reserved.

neurologic.theclinics.com

Although the pathophysiology of primary headaches is poorly understood, effective treatments may often be available, but better treatments are clearly needed. Neurologists, people with headaches, and their families should lobby for more government funding for headache research as annual funding for migraine research is only about $13 million in the United States and €6 million in Europe.

I thank our distinguished contributors for their outstanding articles. I also thank Don Mumford, senior developmental editor, and the Elsevier production team for an excellent job. Finally, I am grateful for the support of my wife, Marilyn, and our children, Elliott, Rochelle, and Jonathan.

Competing interests: my wife, my three children, and I are all migraineurs (but that's not why I became a neurologist).

Randolph W. Evans, MD
Baylor College of Medicine
1200 Binz #1370
Houston, TX 77004, USA

E-mail address:
rwevans@pol.net (R.W. Evans)

The Epidemiology, Burden, and Comorbidities of Migraine

Marcelo E. Bigal, MD, PhD[a,b,*], Richard B. Lipton, MD[b,c,d]

KEYWORDS

- Migraine • Prevalence • Epidemiology
- Comorbidities • Chronic daily headaches

Migraine is one of the most burdensome of the primary headache disorders.[1-3] Epidemiologic data can be used to describe this burden as well as its scope and distribution[4] Understanding sociodemographic, genetic, and environmental risk factors for migraine helps identify groups at highest risk for migraine and may provide clues to treatment strategies or disease mechanisms.

Because migraine is common and disabling, it is a significant public health problem impacting individual sufferers, their families, and, more broadly, society. Quantifying the burden of migraine is a prelude to measuring the benefits of treatment and planning health care interventions designed to minimize the burden of illness. Finally, epidemiologic studies have identified a number of conditions that are comorbid with migraine; these conditions occur with migraine at a higher frequency than would be expected by chance.[5,6] Comorbidity must be considered in formulating treatment plans and may provide insights into the mechanisms of disease.[7]

In this article, we review the epidemiology and burden of migraines. We also discuss the comorbidities of migraine, focusing on established comorbidities (eg, depression) as well as newly identified associations (eg, cardiovascular disease).

THE EPIDEMIOLOGY OF MIGRAINE

The epidemiology of migraine has been extensively studied and reviewed.[8] Herein, instead of compiling all the studies, we discuss in a little more details a few representative studies.

---

[a] Merck Research Laboratories, 1 Merck Drive, Whitehouse Station, NJ 08889, USA
[b] Department of Neurology, Albert Einstein College of Medicine, Bronx, NY, USA
[c] Department of Epidemiology and Population Health, Albert Einstein College of Medicine, Bronx, NY, USA
[d] The Montefiore Headache Center, Bronx, NY, USA
* Corresponding author. Merck Research Laboratories, 1 Merck Drive, Whitehouse Station, NJ 08889, USA.
E-mail address: marcelo_bigal@merck.com (M.E. Bigal).

Neurol Clin 27 (2009) 321–334
doi:10.1016/j.ncl.2008.11.011
0733-8619/08/$ – see front matter © 2009 Elsevier Inc. All rights reserved.

neurologic.theclinics.com

The Incidence of Migraine

The incidence of migraine has been investigated in a limited number of studies. Using the reported age of migraine onset from a prevalence study, Stewart and colleagues[9] found that, in females, the incidence of migraine with aura peaked between ages 12 and 13 (14.1/1000 person-years); migraine without aura peaked between ages 14 and 17 (18.9/1000 person-years). In males, migraine with aura peaked in incidence several years earlier, around 5 years of age at 6.6/1000 person-years; the peak for migraine without aura was 10/1000 person-years between 10 and 11 years. New cases of migraine were uncommon in men in their twenties (**Fig. 1**). Similar findings were seen in Europe. In the Danish population, the annual incidence of migraine in those aged 25 to 64 years was of 8/1,000, being 15/1,000 in males and 3/1,000 in females. Prevalence peaked in younger women (20/1,000).[10] The gap between peak incidence in adolescence and peak prevalence in middle life indicates that migraine is a condition of long duration.

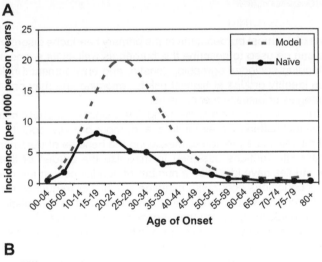

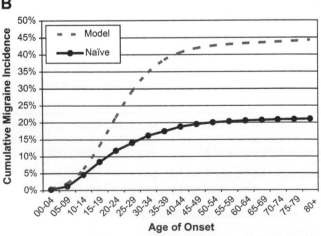

Fig.1. Estimates of age-specific incidence of migraine (A) and of cumulative incidence (B) in females using the naïve and model-based estimating procedures.

More recently, Stewart and colleagues[11] used age of onset of migraine, derived from the American Migraine Prevalence and Prevention Study (AMPP, n = 193,477) to estimate migraine incidence. Two methods were used to estimate age-specific incidence. First, the "naïve method" is based on the assumptions that there is no systematic bias in reporting age of onset or errors in underreporting among inactive cases. The second method assumes that these errors occur and used a statistical model to adjust for their effect on estimates. This method assumes that the probability of error depends on how long ago the event occurred and makes use of patterns in the data by current age and reported duration of time with migraine. The median age of onset using the naïve method was 19 for males and 20 for females (**Fig. 2**). The cumulative lifetime incidence was 7.4% for males and 21% for females. In contrast, the median age of onset for migraine in the model-based estimates is 23.0 for males and 25.3 for females. The cumulative incidence of migraine by age 85 is 18.5% in males and 44.3% in females (**Fig. 1**). Based on these findings, it was suggested that migraine is a dynamic state with high rates of both onset and remission.

THE PREVALENCE OF MIGRAINE

The published estimates of migraine prevalence have varied broadly, probably because of differences in study methodology. Before puberty, migraine prevalence is higher in boys than in girls. As adolescence approaches, incidence and prevalence increase more rapidly in girls than in boys. The prevalence increases throughout childhood and early adult life until approximately age 40, after which it declines (**Fig. 2**). Overall, prevalence is highest from 25 to 55, the peak years from economic productivity.[8–12]

In the United States, three very large studies assessed the epidemiology of migraine in adults. The American Migraine Study-1 (AMS-1), collected information from 15,000 households representative of the US population in 1989.[10] AMS-II, used virtually identical methodology 10 years later.[11] Finally, the American Migraine Prevention and Prevalence study (AMPP) replicated, in its first research phase, the methods of AMS-I and AMS-II.[12] In these three very large studies, the prevalence of migraine was about 18% in women and 6% in men (**Fig. 3**).

PREVALENCE OF MIGRAINE IN CHILDREN

The prevalence of headache in children, has been investigated in a number of school- and population-based studies.[12–14] By age 3, headache occurs in 3% to 8% of children. At age 5, 19.5% have headache, and by age 7, 37 to 51.5% have headaches. In 7 to 15 year olds, headache prevalence ranges from 57% to 82%. The prevalence

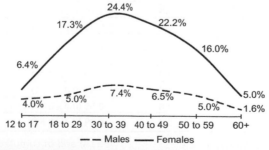

Fig. 2. One year period prevalence of migraine by age and sex adjusted for demographics.

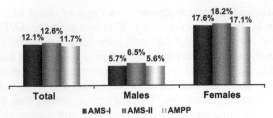

Fig. 3. Prevalence of migraine in the American Migraine Study (AMS)-1, AMS-2, and AMPP for total sample and by sex.

increases from ages 3 to 11 in both boys and girls with higher headache prevalence in 3- to 5-year-old boys than in 3- to 5-year-old girls. Thus, the overall prevalence of headache increases from preschool age children to mid adolescence when examined using various cross-sectional studies.[15]

In the AMPP, the 1-year prevalence for migraine at this age range was 6.3%. The prevalence in boys was 5.0%; in girls it was 7.7%. **Table 1** displays the crude and adjusted prevalence ratios for several demographic features, stratifying by sex. The adjusted prevalence in boys was remarkably stable, ranging from 2.9% to 4.1%. It did not significantly differ in any age. In girls, compared with the age of 12, the prevalence was significantly higher in those at older ages. For both sexes, the prevalence was significantly higher in whites than African Americans.[16]

Table 1
Sex-specific migraine prevalence and prevalence ratios in adolescents. Results from the AMPP study

—	Adjusted Prevalence		Adjusted Prevalence Ratio[b]	
	Male	Female	Male	Female
Race				
White[a]	5.1	7.5	1	1
Black	2.6	4.4	0.51 (0.34–0.76)	0.59 (0.44–0.78)
Age				
12[a]	3.4	3.2	1	1
13	3.6	4.4	1.07 (0.73–1.55)	1.39 (0.95–2.02)
14	4.0	4.6	1.17 (0.82–1.69)	1.45 (1.00–2.09)
15	3.9	6.0	1.16 (0.81–1.67)	1.88 (1.32–2.68)
16	2.9	6.2	0.85 (0.55–1.26)	1.94 (1.37–2.78)
17	4.1	9.8	1.20 (0.83–1.73)	3.09 (2.23–4.26)
18	3.9	7.8	1.16 (0.81–1.67)	2.45 (1.75–3.42)
19	3.2	6.3	0.93 (0.63–1.36)	1.99 (1.40–2.81)
Household Income				
Under $22,500[a]	5.8	8.1	1	1
$22,500–$39,999	3.5	5.9	0.60 (0.45–0.79)	0.72 (0.57–0.91)
$40,000–$59,999	3.1	6.2	0.53 (0.40–0.72)	0.76 (0.61–0.95)
$60,000–$89,999	3.4	4.8	0.59 (0.45–0.77)	0.59 (0.47–0.75)
$90,000 and Over	2.8	4.4	0.49 (0.36–0.65)	0.54 (0.43–0.67)

[a] Reference group for Odds Ratio.
[b] Adjusted by age, sex, and sociodemographic features.

Prevalence by Race and Geographic Region

Migraine prevalence varies by race and geographic region. In the United States, the lowest prevalence is observed among Asian-Americans, intermediate estimates are reported in African Americans, and the highest prevalence estimates are observed among whites, before and after adjusting for demographic covariates.[17] A meta-analysis confirmed these findings: prevalence was lowest in Africa and Asia, and higher in Europe and Central/South America. The highest estimates were found in North America.[18]

Because migraine prevalence is low in Africa and Asia, and remains low among African Americans and Asians in the United States, it has been hypothesized that there are race-related differences in genetic susceptibility to migraine.[19] However, because prevalence in Asia is even lower than in the United States, other variables such as environmental risk factors or culturally determined differences in symptom reporting may further explain the international variation.

Prevalence by Socioeconomic Status

In the United States, three very large population-based studies found that in the community, migraine prevalence is inversely related to household income.[20–22] As income or education increased, migraine prevalence declined. This inverse relationship may be explained by two alternative hypotheses. According to the social causation hypothesis, factors associated with low socioeconomic status act to increase disease prevalence. The opposing social selection hypothesis suggests that disease-related dysfunction interferes with educational and occupational functioning, which in turn would lead to low income. The alternative hypotheses were tested in an adolescent population study (because adolescents make a modest contribution to the family income).[16] In adolescents with family history of migraine, household income did not have a significant effect, probably because of the higher biological predisposition or because of a common stressor event. In those without a strong predisposition, household income was associated with prevalence. This suggests the social causation hypothesis rather than the social selection hypothesis, highlighting the need for exploration of environmental risk factors related to low income and migraine and the search for specific comorbidities and stressors in this group.[16]

THE BURDENS OF MIGRAINE
The Burden of Migraine to the Individual

Migraine is a public health problem of enormous scope that has an impact on both the individual sufferer and on society.[8,23,24] The AMPP, conducted in 2005, estimated that 35 million US residents had migraine headaches, meaning that nearly one in four US households had someone with migraine.[25] Twenty-five percent of women in the United States who had migraine experienced four or more severe attacks a month; 35% experienced one to four severe attacks a month; 38% experience one or less than one severe attack a month. Similar frequency patterns were observed for men. Around 37% of the migraineurs had five or more headache days per month. During migraine attacks, most migraineurs reported severe impairment or the need for bed rest (53.7%); just 7.2% reported no attack-related impairment. Over a 3-month period, 35.1% of the migraineurs had at least 1 day of activity restriction related to headache.[22]

The Burden of Migraine to the Family

Because migraine affects women more often than men and is most prevalent between the ages of 25 and 55, the years of child rearing, a substantial impact on family life might be expected. A Canadian study reported that 90% of people with migraine reported postponing their household work because of headaches, 30% had canceled family and social activities during their last migraine attack, and two-thirds feared letting others down because of their headaches.[26] Other studies[27,28] found that migraine attacks brought significant disruption to family life, with impact on spouses, children, and friends.

In an epidemiologic study conducted in the United Kingdom and the United States, the impact of migraine on family life was assessed both from the perspective of those with migraine and from the perspective of their partners.[29] Of people with migraine living with a household partner, 85% reported substantial reductions in their ability to do household work and chores, 45% missed family social and leisure activities, and 32% avoided making plans for fear of cancellation because of headaches. One half believed that, because of their migraine, they were more likely to argue with their partners (50%) and children (52%), whereas majorities (52%–73%) reported other adverse consequences for their relationships with their partner and children and at work. A third (36%) believed they would be better partners but for their headaches. Participating partners partly confirmed these findings: 29% felt that arguments were more common because of headaches and 20% to 60% reported other negative effects on relationships at home. Compared with subjects who did not have migraine regarding their work performance, a significantly higher proportion of migraine partners were unsatisfied with work demands placed on them ($P = .02$), with their level or responsibilities and duties ($P = .02$), and with their ability to perform ($P = .001$). These results suggest that the impact of migraine extends to household partners and other family members.[29]

Societal Impact of Migraine

Migraine has an enormous impact on society. Studies have evaluated both the indirect costs of migraine as well as the direct costs.[1,30–32] Indirect costs include the aggregate effects of migraine on productivity at work (paid employment), for household work, and in other roles. This includes both the cost of absenteeism (missed work) and reduced productivity while at work. Hu and colleagues[30] estimated that productivity losses caused by migraine cost American employers 13 billion dollars per year. These issues have been reviewed recently in more detail elsewhere.[31,33–35]

Migraine's impact on health care use is marked as well. The National Ambulatory Medical Care Survey, conducted from 1976 to 1977, found that 4% of all visits to physicians' offices (more than 10 million visits a year) were for headache.[30] Migraine also results in major use of emergency rooms and urgent care centers.[35] Vast amounts of prescription and over-the-counter (OTC) medications are taken for headache disorders. OTC sales of pain medication (for all conditions) were estimated to be 3.2 billion dollars in 1999 (US) and headache accounts for about one third of OTC analgesic use. (Consumer Health care Products Association. OTC Sales Statistics - 1995–1999. AC Neilsen, April 2000).

In a very recent study, Stewart and colleagues mailed a questionnaire to 193,477 participants in the American Migraine Prevalence and Prevention study. Lost Productive Time (LPT) was the sum of missed hours plus reduced productivity hour equivalents. The mean LPT per week was 1.8 hours for headache and 2.8 for all health-related causes; 76.5% of the headache-related LPT was explained by reduced performance (ie, presenteeism). The 29% of migraine cases with 11+ headache-d/mo accounted for 49% of overall LPT; the 19% of those with pain score of 9 to 10 on a 0 to 10 scale accounted for 33% of the overall LPT.[36]

The Comorbidities of Migraine

The term "comorbidity," coined by Feinstein,[37] is now widely used to refer to the greater than coincidental association of two conditions in the same individual. Migraine has been noted to be comorbid with a number of other illnesses in specialty care and in population samples (**Box 1**) (for review see.[38,39]) Failure to classify and analyze comorbid diseases can create misleading medical statistics and may cause spurious comparisons during the evaluation and treatment planning for patients. Here we briefly discuss the comorbidity of migraine with psychiatric, pain, and vascular disorders.

Psychiatric Disorders

Cross-sectional associations and bidirectional associations between migraine and a variety of psychiatric and somatic conditions have been reported in the literature.

Box 1
Conditions comorbid with migraine

Psychiatric

    Depression

    Anxiety

    Panic disorder

    Bipolar

Neurologic

    Epilepsy

    Tourette's[a]

Vascular

    Raynaud's phenomenon

    Blood pressure (inconsistent)

    Ischemic stroke, sub-clinical stroke, white matter abnormalities

Heart

    Patent foramen ovale[a]

    Mitral valve prolapse[a]

    Atrial septal aneurysm[a]

Other

    Snoring/sleep apnea[a]

    Asthma/allergy

    Systemic lupus erythematosus[a]

    Non-headache pain

[a] *Data from* clinical samples only.

Patel and colleagues[40] assessed the prevalence of major depression in individuals with migraine, probable migraine (a subtype of migraine missing just one migraine feature), and controls. Participants were identified from members of a mixed model health maintenance organization. The overall prevalence of major depression was 28.1% for migraine 19.5% for probable migraine, 23.9% for migraine and probable migraine polled together, and 10.3% for the control group. The prevalence of major depression was elevated in all migraine groups compared with controls on both crude and adjusted (by age, sex, education) prevalence ratios.

Breslau and Colleagues.[39] measured the bidirectional associations of migraine, severe nonmigraine headache, and depression in a population-based cohort from the Detroit metropolitan area. A cross-sectional study of more than 50,000 adults by Zwart and colleagues[41] (the Nord-Trøndelag Health Study) measured the co-occurrence of headache and depression or anxiety disorders. Participants were age 20 or older, and the study included headache diagnosis, a medical examination, and administration of the Hospital Anxiety and Depression scale. Overall, the individuals with migraine headache were more likely to have depression (odds ratio [OR] = 2.7 [2.3–3.2]) or anxiety disorders (OR = 3.2 [2.8–3.6]) than the nonheadache controls. Similar associations were seen for nonmigraine headache and depression (OR = 2.2 [2.0–2.5]) or anxiety disorders (OR = 2.7 [2.4–3.0]). There was a linear trend associated with headache frequency. Thus, for migraine headache less than 7 days per month, 7–14 days per month, 15+ days per month, respectively, the association with depression was OR = 2.0 (1.6–2.5), OR = 4.2 (3.2–5.6), and OR = 6.4 (4.4–9.3). A similar trend was seen for anxiety disorders and for nonmigraine headache with depression or anxiety disorders.

It is of interest to what extent chronic pain conditions other than migraine are associated with depression and anxiety. A study by McWilliams and colleagues[42] used data from an adult US population (the Midlife Development in the United States Survey) to look at the cross-sectional associations between three pain conditions (migraine, arthritis, back pain) and three psychiatric disorders (depression, generalized anxiety disorder, panic attacks). The associations between the three psychiatric disorders were roughly similar for the three pain conditions (ie, the association between migraine and depression was roughly similar to the association between back pain and depression). However, the investigators noted that the association between pain and anxiety was generally stronger than the association between pain and depression.

Comorbid pain

Migraine has been reported to be comorbid with other chronic pain conditions in cross-sectional and prospective studies of children or young adults. In a study by El-Metwally and colleagues,[43] of 1756 third and fifth grade schoolchildren in Finland, children were examined for the presence of nontraumatic musculoskeletal pain symptoms and were tested for hypermobility. They were re-evaluated after 14 years to determine factors related to the prognosis of musculoskeletal pain. Baseline headache once or more a week (not characterized by type) was found to be a negative prognostic factor—that is, the children with comorbid headache were more likely to have persistent musculoskeletal pain at follow-up compared with the children without comorbid headache.

Hestbaek and colleagues studied more than 9,000 adolescents and young adults in a cross-sectional population-based study with the purpose of describing conditions comorbid with low back pain. Headache (not characterized by type) was associated with LBP ≤30 days per year (OR = 2.1 [1.8–2.5]) and with LBP greater than 30 days per year (OR = 3.4 [2.3–5.0]). Both LBP and headache were associated with asthma in this sample.[44,45]

Hagen and Colleagues.[46] from the Nord-Trøndelag Health Study measured the co-occurrence of headache and musculoskeletal symptoms, defined as musculoskeletal pain or stiffness in muscles and joints lasting continuously for at least 3 months. In this study, individuals with headache were roughly twice as likely to report musculoskeletal symptoms as those without headache. The elevated risk was similar in those with nonmigrainous (OR = 1.8 [1.8–1.9]) and migrainous (OR = 1.9 [1.8–2.0]) headaches. However, headache frequency was a stronger predictor of comorbid musculoskeletal symptoms than headache type. Thus, for headache less than 7 days per month, 7 to 14 days per month, or 15+ days per month, respectively, the association with musculoskeletal symptoms was OR = 1.5 (1.4–1.6), OR = 3.2 (2.9–3.5), and OR = 5.3 (4.4–6.5) for women and OR = 1.7 (1.6–1.8), OR = 3.2 (2.8–3.8), and OR = 3.6 (2.9–4.5) for men.

A population-based study by Von Korff and colleagues[47] studied the comorbidity of chronic back and neck pain with other physical and mental disorders. Data are from the National Comorbidity Survey Replication (NCS-R), a nationally representative face-to-face household survey of adults 18 years of age and older. Chronic spinal pain was defined as self-reported "chronic back or neck problems." Comorbid mental disorders were based on DSM-IV criteria and included mood disorders, anxiety disorders, and substance use disorders. Results showed that chronic spinal pain was associated with mood disorders (OR = 2.5 [1.9–3.2]), anxiety disorders (OR = 2.3 [1.9–2.7]), and substance use disorders (primarily alcohol abuse or dependence) (1.6 [1.2–2.2]). In addition, chronic spinal pain was associated with other chronic pain (OR = 4.8 [3.9–5.8]), which included arthritis (OR = 3.9 [3.2–4.7]), migraine (5.2 [4.1–6.4]), other headache (OR = 4.0 [2.9–5.3]), and other chronic pain (OR = 3.7 [2.9–4.7]).

Vascular disorders

Migraine and stroke The association between migraine and ischemic stroke is well known and has been demonstrated in case-control studies as well as cross-sectional studies in patients selected from specialty care settings, registries, and from the general population. A meta-analysis of 11 case-control studies and three cohort studies published before 2004 showed that, relative to individuals without migraine, the risk of stroke was increased in migraineurs (pooled relative risk [RR] = 2.16, 95% confidence interval [CI] = 1.9–2.5).[48] This risk was nominally higher for migraine with aura (MA), (RR = 2.27; 95% CI, 1.61–3.19) but was also apparent in patients with migraine without aura (MO), (RR = 1.83; 95% CI, 1.06–3.15).

More recently, two large longitudinal studies added to the evidence linking migraine and ischemic stroke. As a part of the Women's Health Study, the relationship between migraine and stroke was assessed, using a large cohort and data prospectively gathered over an average of more than 10 years.[49] Compared with nonmigraineurs, participants who reported any history of migraine or migraine without aura had no increased risk of any stroke type. Participants who reported migraine with aura had increased adjusted hazards ratios (HRs) of 1.53 (95% CI, 1.02–2.31) for total stroke and 1.71 (95% CI, 1.11–2.66) for ischemic stroke but no increased risk for hemorrhagic stroke. The increased risk for ischemic stroke was further magnified (HR = 2.25; 95% CI, 1.30 to 3.91) for the youngest age group in this cohort (45–54 years). The associations remained significant after adjusting for cardiovascular risk factors and were not apparent for nonmigraine headache.

The second prospective study used data from the Atherosclerosis Risk in Communities Study and included more than 12,000 men and women aged 55 and older.[50] Compared with participants without migraine or other headache, migraineurs had a 1.8-fold increased risk of ischemic stroke (RR = 1.84; 95% CI, 0.89–3.82). The fact that the risk estimates did not reach statistical significance may be because of migraine classification, because the category of "other headache with aura" showed a significant increased risk of ischemic stroke (RR = 2.91; 95% CI, 1.39–6.11). Similarly, in the Stroke Prevention in Young Women study, women with MA had 1.5 greater odds of ischemic stroke (95% CI, 1.1–2.0).[51]

Migraine and coronary heart disease Because of the association between MA and ischemic stroke, it is of interest whether migraine is similarly associated with coronary heart disease as well. Although some studies yielded negative or conflicting results for overall migraine,[52] case reports and large-scale cohort studies found an association between migraine and chest pain, and in some cases migraine was associated with documented ischemic electrocardiographic changes.[48]

Three population studies supported the relationship between migraine, specially MA, and coronary disease. In the first, Rose and colleagues[53] looked at the association between headaches lasting 4 or more hours (including migraine and nonmigraine headache) and Rose angina. Participants were age 45 to 64 at baseline and were from the Atherosclerosis Risk in Communities study. The headache group was roughly twice as likely to have a history of Rose angina, with the risk most elevated in the headache group with aura.

In the Women's Health Study, MA but not MO approximately doubled the relative risk of major cardiovascular disease (ischemic stroke, myocardial infarction, coronary revascularization procedures, angina, as well as death related to ischemic cardiovascular events). These associations remained significant after adjusting for many cardiovascular risk factors.[54]

As part of the Physician's Health Study, men with migraine (with or without aura) were at increased risk for major CVD (HR = 1.24; 95% CI, 1.06–1.46), a finding that was driven by a 42% increased risk of myocardial infarction.[55]

MIGRAINE AND MARKERS OF SUBCLINICAL VASCULAR DISEASE
Subclinical Brain Lesions

Deep brain lesions, found incidentally in neuroimaging examinations, have long been reported as happening more frequently in migraineurs, although most studies lacked a contemporaneous control group.[56] In a well-designed population-based study from the Netherlands, Kruit and colleagues[57] randomly selected approximately 150 individuals from each of three groups for neuroimaging (MA, MO, and nonmigraine controls). They excluded individuals with a history of stroke, transient ischemic attack (TIA), or with abnormal neurologic examination. This study included blinded evaluation of magnetic resonance imaging by a neuro-radiologist, and aura classification was performed under the supervision of expert headache diagnosticians without knowledge of the magnetic resonance imaging results. Overall, there were no differences in the prevalence of clinically relevant infarcts between migraineurs and controls. This may be explained by the exclusion of prior history of TIA and stroke (which would also exclude those with clinically relevant infarcts). However, those with MA had significant increase of subclinical infarcts in the cerebellar region of the posterior circulation. The highest risk for these lesions was seen in those with MA and more than one headache attack per month (OR = 15.8; 95% CI, 1.8–140). In addition, women with migraine were about twice as likely to have deep white matter lesions as the nonmigraineurs (OR = 2.1; 95% CI, 1.0–4.1). Consistent with the earlier studies on clinical stroke and white matter abnormalities, these findings were independent of the presence of some traditional cardiovascular risk factors.[58]

Migraine and Patent Foramen Ovale

Initial studies indicate an increased prevalence of patent foramen ovale (PFO) in migraineurs with aura and an increased prevalence of migraine and migraine with aura in persons with PFO.[59,60] In a quantitative systematic review of articles on migraine and PFO, the estimated strength of association between PFO and migraine, reflected by summary ORs, was 5.13 (95% CI, 4.67–5.59], and between PFO and migraine with aura the OR was 3.21 (95% CI, 2.38–4.17). The grade of evidence was low. The association between migraine and PFO was OR 2.54 (95% CI, 2.01–3.08). The grade of evidence was low to moderate.[61]

SUMMARY

In this chapter, we reviewed the epidemiology of migraine including recent data on incidence, prevalence, and comorbidities. In particular, we highlighted emerging evidence linking migraine with aura to ischemic stroke and myocardial infarction. We also reviewed data on the economic impact of migraine. In aggregate, these data show that migraine is extremely burdensome and worthy of treatment.

REFERENCES

1. Ferrari MD. The economic burden of migraine to society. Pharmacoeconomics 1998;13(6):667–76.
2. Hamelsky SW, Lipton RB, Stewart WF, et al. An assessment of the burden of migraine using the willingness to pay model. Cephalalgia 2005;25(2):87–100.
3. Lipton RB, Stewart WF, Von Korff M, et al. The burden of migraine. A review of cost to society. Pharmacoeconomics 1994;6(3):215–21.
4. Lipton RB, Bigal ME. The epidemiology of migraine. Am J Med 2005;118(Suppl 1): 3S–10S.
5. Breslau N. Psychiatric comorbidity in migraine. Cephalalgia 1998;18(Suppl 22): 56–8 [discussion: 58–61].
6. Scher AI, Stewart WF, Lipton RB, et al. The comorbidity of headache with other pain syndromes. Headache 2006;46(9):1416–23.
7. Solomon GD, Price KL. Burden of migraine. A review of its socioeconomic impact. Pharmacoeconomics 1997;11(Suppl 1):1–10.
8. Stovner L, Hagen K, Jensen R, et al. The global burden of headache: a documentation of headache prevalence and disability worldwide. Cephalalgia 2007;27(3): 193–210.
9. Stewart WF, Linet MS, Celentano DD, et al. Age- and sex-specific incidence rates of migraine with and without visual aura. Am J Epidemiol 1991;134(10):1111–20.
10. Lyngberg AC, Rasmussen BK, Jorgensen T, et al. Incidence of primary headache: a Danish epidemiologic follow-up study. Am J Epidemiol 2005;161(11): 1066–73.
11. Stewart WF, Bigal ME, Lipton RB, et al. Lifetime migraine incidence. Results from the American Migraine Prevalence and Prevention study. Headache 2005;46:52.
12. Abu-Arefeh I, Russell G. Prevalence of headache and migraine in schoolchildren. BMJ 1994;309(6957):765–9.
13. Bille B. Migraine and tension-type headache in children and adolescents. Cephalalgia 1996;16(2):78.
14. Bille B. A 40-year follow-up of school children with migraine. Cephalalgia 1997; 17(4):488–91 [discussion: 487].

15. Bigal ME, Liberman JN, Lipton RB, et al. Age-dependent prevalence and clinical features of migraine. Neurology 2006;67(2):246–51.
16. Bigal ME, Lipton RB, Winner P, et al. Migraine in adolescents: association with socioeconomic status and family history. Neurology 2007;69(1):16–25.
17. Stewart WF, Lipton RB, Celentano DD, et al. Prevalence of migraine headache in the United States. Relation to age, income, race, and other sociodemographic factors. J Am Med Assoc 1992;267(1):64–9.
18. Stewart WF, Simon D, Schechter A, et al. Population variation in migraine prevalence: a meta-analysis. J Clin Epidemiol 1995;48(2):269–80.
19. Stewart WF, Lipton RB, Liberman J, et al. Variation in migraine prevalence by race. Neurology 1996;47(1):52–9.
20. Lipton RB, Diamond S, Reed M, et al. Migraine diagnosis and treatment: results from the American Migraine Study II. Headache 2001;41(7):638–45.
21. Lipton RB, Stewart WF, Simon D, et al. Medical consultation for migraine: results from the American Migraine Study. Headache 1998;38(2):87–96.
22. Lipton RB, Bigal ME, Diamond M, et al. Migraine prevalence, disease burden, and the need for preventive therapy. Neurology 2007;68(5):343–9.
23. Steiner TJ, Scher AI, Stewart WF, et al. The prevalence and disability burden of adult migraine in England and their relationships to age, gender and ethnicity. Cephalalgia 2003;23(7):519–27.
24. Dahlof CG, Solomon GD. The burden of migraine to the individual sufferer: a review. Eur J Neurol 1998;5(6):525–33.
25. Diamond S, Bigal ME, Silberstein S, et al. Patterns of diagnosis and acute and preventive treatment for migraine in the United States: results from the American migraine prevalence and prevention study. Headache 2007;47(3): 355–63.
26. MacGregor EA, Brandes J, Eikermann A, et al. Impact of migraine on patients and their families: the Migraine And Zolmitriptan Evaluation (MAZE) survey–Phase III. Curr Med Res Opin 2004;20(7):1143–50.
27. Stang PE, Crown WH, Bizier R, et al. The family impact and costs of migraine. Am J Manag Care 2004;10(5):313–20.
28. Evans RW, Lipton RB, Ritz KA, et al. A survey of neurologists on self-treatment and treatment of their families. Headache 2007;47(1):58–64.
29. Lipton RB, Bigal ME, Kolodner K, et al. The family impact of migraine: population-based studies in the USA and UK. Cephalalgia 2003;23(6):429–40.
30. Hu XH, Markson LE, Lipton RB, et al. Burden of migraine in the United States: disability and economic costs. Arch Intern Med 1999;159(8):813–8.
31. Lipton RB, Stewart WF, Von Korff M, et al. Burden of migraine: societal costs and therapeutic opportunities. Neurology 1997;48(3 Suppl 3):S4–9.
32. Burton WN, Conti DJ, Chen CY, et al. The economic burden of lost productivity due to migraine headache: a specific worksite analysis. J Occup Environ Med 2002;44(6):523–9.
33. Elston Lafata J, Moon C, Leotta C, et al. The medical care utilization and costs associated with migraine headache. J Gen Intern Med 2004;19(10):1005–12.
34. Edmeads J, Mackell JA. The economic impact of migraine: an analysis of direct and indirect costs. Headache 2002;42(6):501–9.
35. Osterhaus JT, Gutterman DL, Plachetka JR, et al. Healthcare resource and lost labour costs of migraine headache in the US. Pharmacoeconomics 1992;2(1): 67–76.
36. Stewart WF, Wood GC, Razzaghi H, et al. Work Impact of migraine headaches. J Occup Environ Med 2008;50(7):736–45.

37. Feinstein AR. The basic elements of clinical science. J Chronic Dis 1963;16: 1125–33.
38. Scher AI, Bigal ME, Lipton RB, et al. Comorbidity of migraine. Curr Opin Neurol 2005;18(3):305–10.
39. Breslau N, Lipton RB, Stewart WF, et al. Comorbidity of migraine and depression: investigating potential etiology and prognosis. Neurology 2003;60(8):1308–12.
40. Patel NV, Bigal ME, Kolodner KB, et al. Prevalence and impact of migraine and probable migraine in a health plan. Neurology 2004;63(8):1432–8.
41. Zwart JA, Dyb G, Hagen K, et al. Depression and anxiety disorders associated with headache frequency. The Nord-Trondelag Health Study. Eur J Neurol 2003;10(2):147–52.
42. McWilliams LA, Goodwin RD, Cox BJ, et al. Depression and anxiety associated with three pain conditions: results from a nationally representative sample. Pain 2004;111(1–2):77–83.
43. El-Metwally A, Salminen JJ, Auvinen A, et al. Prognosis of non-specific musculo-skeletal pain in preadolescents: a prospective 4-year follow-up study till adoles-cence. Pain 2004;110(3):550–9.
44. Hestbaek L, Leboeuf-Yde C, Kyvik KO, et al. Is comorbidity in adolescence a predictor for adult low back pain? A prospective study of a young population. BMC Musculoskelet Disord 2006;7:29.
45. Hestbaek L, Leboeuf-Yde C, Kyvik KO, et al. Comorbidity with low back pain: a cross-sectional population-based survey of 12- to 22-year-olds. Spine 2004; 29(13):1483–91 [discussion: 1492].
46. Hagen K, Einarsen C, Zwart JA, et al. The co-occurrence of headache and musculoskeletal symptoms amongst 51 050 adults in Norway. Eur J Neurol 2002;9(5):527–33.
47. Von Korff M, Crane P, Lane M, et al. Chronic spinal pain and physical-mental co-morbidity in the United States: results from the national comorbidity survey repli-cation. Pain 2005;113(3):331–9.
48. Etminan M, Takkouche B, Isorna FC, et al. Risk of ischaemic stroke in people with migraine: systematic review and meta-analysis of observational studies. BMJ 2005;330(7482):63.
49. Kurth T, Slomke MA, Kase CS, et al. Migraine, headache, and the risk of stroke in women: a prospective study. Neurology 2005;64(6):1020–6.
50. Stang PE, Carson AP, Rose KM, et al. Headache, cerebrovascular symptoms, and stroke: the atherosclerosis risk in communities study. Neurology 2005; 64(9):1573–7.
51. MacClellan LR, Mitchell BD, Cole JW, et al. Familial aggregation of ischemic stroke in young women: the stroke prevention in young women study. Genet Epi-demiol 2006;30(7):602–8.
52. Rosamond W. Are migraine and coronary heart disease associated? An epidemi-ologic review. Headache 2004;44(Suppl 1):S5–12.
53. Rose KM, Carson AP, Sanford CP, et al. Migraine and other headaches: associ-ations with Rose angina and coronary heart disease. Neurology 2004;63(12): 2233–9.
54. Kurth T, Gaziano JM, Cook NR, et al. Migraine and risk of cardiovascular disease in women. J Am Med Assoc 2006;296(3):283–91.
55. Kurth T, Gaziano JM, Cook NR, et al. Migraine and risk of cardiovascular disease in men. Arch Intern Med 2007;167(8):795–801.
56. Porter A, Gladstone JP, Dodick DW, et al. Migraine and white matter hyperinten-sities. Curr Pain Headache Rep 2005;9(4):289–93.

57. Kruit MC, Van Buchem MA, Hofman PA, et al. Migraine as a risk factor for subclinical brain lesions. J Am Med Assoc 2004;291(4):427–34.
58. Kruit MC, Launer LJ, Ferrari MD, et al. Brain stem and cerebellar hyperintense lesions in migraine. Stroke 2006;37(4):1109–12.
59. Diener HC, Kurth T, Dodick D, et al. Patent foramen ovale and migraine. Curr Pain Headache Rep 2007;11(3):236–40.
60. Diener HC, Kurth T, Dodick D, et al. Patent foramen ovale, stroke, and cardiovascular disease in migraine. Curr Opin Neurol 2007;20(3):310–9.
61. Schwedt TJ, Demaerschalk BM, Dodick DW. Patent foramen ovale and migraine: a quantitative systematic review. Cephalalgia 2008;28(5):531–40.

Pathophysiology of Migraine

Peter J. Goadsby, MD, PhD, DSc, FRACP, FRCP

KEYWORDS

• Migraine • Brainstem • Pain • Sensory processing

An understanding of the pathophysiology of migraine should be based upon the anatomy and physiology of the pain-producing structures of the cranium integrated with knowledge of central nervous system (CNS) modulation of these pathways. Headache in general, and in particular migraine[1] and cluster headache,[2] is understood better now than it has been the case for the last four millennia.[3,4] Here current views concerning migraine are reviewed and lead to the conclusion that the disorder is a disturbance in the brain of the subcortical aminergic sensory modulatory systems, and probably includes brainstem, hypothalamic, and thalamic structures among those key to the expression of the problem.

MIGRAINE- EXPLAINING THE CLINICAL FEATURES

Migraine is in essence a familial episodic disorder whose key marker is headache with certain associated features (**Box 1**). These features give clues to its pathophysiology and ultimately provide insights leading to new treatments. The essential elements to be considered are:

Genetics of migraine
Physiologic basis for the aura
Anatomy of head pain, particularly that of the trigeminovascular system
Physiology and pharmacology of activation of the peripheral branches of ophthalmic branch of the trigeminal nerve
Physiology and pharmacology of the trigeminal nucleus, in particular its caudal-most part, the trigeminocervical complex
Brainstem and diencephalic modulatory systems that influence trigeminal pain transmission and other sensory modality processing

Migraine is a form of sensory processing disturbance with wide ramifications for CNS function, and although pain is used as the exemplar symptom, a brain-centered explanation provides a likely way to provide a generic explanation for the condition's manifestations.

Headache Group, Department of Neurology, University of California, San Francisco, 1635 Divisadero Street, San Francisco, CA 94115, USA
E-mail address: pgoadsby@headache.ucsf.edu

Neurol Clin 27 (2009) 335–360
doi:10.1016/j.ncl.2008.11.012
0733-8619/08/$ – see front matter © 2009 Elsevier Inc. All rights reserved.

neurologic.theclinics.com

Box 1
International Headache Society features of migraine

Repeated episodic headache (4 to 72 hours) with the following features:

Any two of:

    Unilateral

    Throbbing

    Worsened by movement

    Moderate or severe

Any one of:

    Nausea/vomiting

    Photophobia and phonophobia

Data from Headache Classification Committee of The International Headache Society. The International classification of headache disorders (second edition). Cephalalgia 2004;24(Suppl 1): 1–160.[5]

GENETICS OF MIGRAINE

One of the most important aspects of the pathophysiology of migraine is the inherited nature of the disorder.[6] It is clear from clinical practice that many patients have first-degree relatives who also suffer from migraine.[3,7] Transmission of migraine from parents to children has been reported as early as the 17th century,[8] and numerous published studies have reported a positive family history.[9]

Genetic Epidemiology

Studies of twin pairs are the classical method to investigate the relative importance of genetic and environmental factors. A Danish study included 1013 monozygotic and 1667 dizygotic twin pairs of the same gender, obtained from a population-based twin register.[10] The pairwise concordance rate was significantly higher among monozygotic than dizygotic twin pairs ($P<.05$). Several studies have attempted to analyze the possible mode of inheritance in migraine families, and conflicting results have been obtained.[11–13] Both twin studies and population-based epidemiologic surveys strongly suggest that migraine without aura is a multifactorial disorder, caused by a combination of genetic and environmental factors. An unexplained but epidemiologically well-established predisposition relates to methyltetrahydrofolate reductase gene mutation C677 T that is over-represented in migraine with aura.[14] The presence of aura seems to be associated, in rarer inherited cases such as CADASIL (cerebral autosomal dominant arteriopathy with subcortical infarcts and leukoencephalopathy[15]) or autosomal dominant retinal vasculopathy with cerebral leukodystrophy,[16] with structural protein dysfunction and perhaps with an embryonic syndrome that includes patent foramen ovale.[17] Such a view makes the small excess stroke risk for young migraineurs unsurprising,[18] and suggests common genetics as opposed to a pathophysiological link for migraine pain.

Familial Hemiplegic Migraine

In approximately 50% of the reported families, familial hemiplegic migraine (FHM) has been assigned to chromosome 19p13.[19,20] Few clinical differences have been found between chromosome 19-linked and unlinked FHM families. Indeed, the clinical phenotype does not associate particularly with the known mutations.[21] The most striking exception is cerebellar ataxia, which occurs in approximately 50% of the chromosome 19-linked, but in none of the unlinked families.[19,20,22–24] Another less striking difference includes the fact that patients from chromosome 19-linked families are more likely to have attacks that can be triggered by minor head trauma or are that associated with coma.[25]

The biologic basis for the linkage to chromosome 19 is mutations[26] involving the $Ca_v2.1$ (P/Q) type voltage-gated calcium channel[27] CACNA1A gene. Now known as FHM-I, this mutation is responsible for about 50% of identified families. One consequence of this mutation may be enhanced glutamate release. Mutations in the ATP1A2 gene[28,29] have been identified to be responsible for about 20% of FHM families. Interestingly, the phenotype of some FHM-II involves epilepsy.[30,31] The gene codes for a Na^+/K^+ ATPase, and the mutation results in a smaller electrochemical gradient for Na^+. One effect of this change is to reduce or inactivate astrocytic glutamate transporters leading to a build-up of synaptic glutamate. It also has been suggested that alternating hemiplegia of childhood can be caused by ATP1A2 mutations.[32] The latter cases are most unconvincing for migraine. Dichgans and colleagues[33] reported a missense mutation (Q1489 K) in SCN1A in three German families, thus characterizing the genetic defect of what now is known as FHM-III. This mutation affects a highly conserved amino acid in a part of the channel that contributes to its rapid closure after opening in response to membrane depolarization (fast inactivation). This represents a gain of function: instead of the channel rapidly closing, allowing the membrane to repolarize fully after an action potential, the mutated channel allows a persistent sodium influx.

Taken together, the known mutations suggest that migraines, or at least the neurologic manifestations currently called the aura, are ionopathies.[6,34] Linking the channel disturbance for the first time to the aura process has demonstrated that human mutations expressed in a knock-in mouse produce a reduced threshold for cortical spreading depression (CSD),[35] which has some interesting implications for understanding that process.[36]

MIGRAINE AURA

Migraine aura is defined as a focal neurologic disturbance manifested as visual, sensory, or motor symptoms.[5] It is seen in about 30% of patients,[37] and it is neurally driven.[38,39] The case for the aura being the human equivalent of the CSD of Leao[40,41] has been made.[42] In people, visual aura has been described as affecting the visual field, suggesting the visual cortex, and it starts at the center of the visual field, propagating to the periphery at a speed of 3 mm/min.[43] This is very similar to spreading depression described in rabbits.[40] Blood flow studies in patients also have shown that a focal hyperemia tends to precede the spreading oligemia,[44] and again this is similar to what would be expected with spreading depression. After this passage of oligemia, the cerebrovascular response to hypercapnia in patients is blunted, while autoregulation remains intact.[45–47] Again this pattern is repeated with experimental spreading depression.[48–50] An interesting recent study suggested that female mice are more susceptible generally to CSD than male mice,[51] which would be consistent with the excess risk of migraine in females after menarche that is still with them, on a population basis, into menopause and afterwards. Human observations have rendered the arguments reasonably sound that human aura has as its equivalent in animals CSD.[52] An area of controversy surrounds whether aura in fact triggers the rest of the attack, and is indeed painful.[53] Based on the available experimental and clinical data, this author is not convinced that aura is painful,[54] but this does not diminish its interest or the importance of understanding it. Indeed therapeutic developments may shed even further light on these relationships.

Therapeutic Manipulation of Aura

Tonabersat is a CSD inhibitor that has entered clinical trials in migraine.[55] Tonabersat (SB-220,453) inhibits CSD, CSD-induced nitric oxide (NO) release, and cerebral vasodilation.[56,57] Tonabersat does not constrict isolated human blood vessels,[58] but does inhibit trigeminally induced craniovascular effects.[59] Remarkably topiramate, a proven preventive agent in migraine,[60–62] also inhibits CSD in cat and rat,[63] and in the rat with prolonged dosing.[64] Tonabersat is inactive in the human NO model of migraine,[65] as is propranolol,[66] although valproate showed some activity in that model.[67] Topiramate inhibits trigeminal neurons activated by nociceptive intracranial afferents,[68] but not by a mechanism local to the trigeminocervical complex,[69] and thus CSD inhibition may be a model system to contribute to the development of preventive medicines. The model predicts that agents interacting with Na^+-based mechanisms might be effective,[70] as would glutamate- α-amino-3-hydroxy-5-methylisoxazole-4-propionate (AMPA) receptor mechanisms, but not γ-aminobutyric acid (GABA)ergic mechanisms, at least directly.[71] Glutamate, N-methyl-D-aspartate (NMDA)-mediate effects have been reported to important in CSD[48] and in an open label study in migraine aura.[72] These may suggest some way forward for the management of at least the most disabled group with persistent or prolonged aura.

HEADACHE—ANATOMY
The Trigeminal Innervation of Pain-Producing Intracranial Structures

Surrounding the large cerebral vessels, pial vessels, large venous sinuses, and dura mater is a plexus of largely unmyelinated fibers that arise from the ophthalmic division of the trigeminal ganglion[73] and in the posterior fossa from the upper cervical dorsal roots.[74] Trigeminal fibers innervating cerebral vessels arise from neurons in the trigeminal ganglion that contain substance P and calcitonin gene-related peptide (CGRP),[75] both of which can be released when the trigeminal ganglion is stimulated in people or cats.[76] Stimulation of the cranial vessels, such as the superior sagittal sinus (SSS), is certainly painful in people.[77,78] Human dural nerves that innervate the cranial vessels largely consist of small-diameter myelinated and unmyelinated fibers[79] that almost certainly subserve a nociceptive function.

HEADACHE PHYSIOLOGY—PERIPHERAL CONNECTIONS
Plasma Protein Extravasation

A series of laboratory experiments in the 1990s suggested that migraine pain may be caused by a sterile neurogenically driven inflammation of the dura mater.[80] Neurogenic plasma extravasation can be seen during electrical stimulation of the trigeminal ganglion in the rat.[81] Plasma extravasation can be blocked by ergot alkaloids, indomethacin, acetylsalicylic acid, and the serotonin-$5HT_{1B/1D}$ agonist sumatriptan.[82] Furthermore, preclinical studies have suggested CSD may be a sufficient stimulus to activate trigeminal neurons,[83] although this has been a controversial area.[54,84–87] In addition, there are structural changes in the dura mater that are observed after trigeminal ganglion stimulation. These include mast cell degranulation and changes in postcapillary venules including platelet aggregation.[00,00] Although it generally is accepted that such changes, and particularly the initiation of a sterile inflammatory response, would cause pain,[90,91] it is not clear whether this is sufficient of itself, or requires other stimulators, or promoters. Preclinical studies suggest that CSD may be a sufficient stimulus to activate trigeminal neurons,[83] although this has been a controversial area.[54,84–87] Neurogenic dural plasma extravasation fails to predict medicines effective in either the acute or preventive treatment of migraine.[92]

Although plasma extravasation in the retina, which is blocked by sumatriptan, can be seen after trigeminal ganglion stimulation in experimental animals, no changes are seen with retinal angiography during acute attacks of migraine or cluster headache.[93] A limitation of the experimental component of this study was the probable sampling of both retina and choroidal elements in rats, given that choroidal vessels have fenestrated capillaries.[94] Clearly, however, blockade of neurogenic plasma protein extravasation is not completely predictive of antimigraine efficacy in people,[92] as evidenced by the failure in clinical trials of substance P, neurokinin-1 antagonists,[95–98] specific plasma protein extravasation (PPE) blockers, CP122,288,[99] and 4991w93,[100] an endothelin antagonist[101] and a neurosteriod.[102]

The most recent development in this area has been the testing of blockade of inducible NO synthase (NOS), which is expressed in the dura mater in the context again of an inflammatory response.[103] Inducible NOS (iNOS) inhibition with GW274150 has analgesic properties in rat models.[104] NOS inhibition is attractive as a target in some respects, because NOS inhibition using a nonselective inhibitor has been shown in a small study to abort acute migraine.[105] GW274150, a potent, selective iNOS inhibitor with good oral bioavailability,[106] has been studied as an acute attack treatment[107] using an adaptive design[108] and in a preventive study.[109] In both studies, the iNOS inhibition approach failed. Importantly, the authors took blood samples and could determine that at the maximum doses used there was at least 80% iNOS inhibition in the patients. This approach does not seem viable and provides further data to support a view that inflammatory pain mechanisms are not important in either the initiation or maintenance of a migraine attack.

Sensitization and migraine

Although it is highly doubtful that there is a significant sterile inflammatory response in the dura mater during migraine, it is clear that some form of sensitization takes place during migraine, because allodynia is common. About two thirds of patients complain of pain from non-noxious stimuli, allodynia.[110–113] A particularly interesting aspect is the demonstration of allodynia in the upper limbs ipsilateral and contralateral to the pain. This finding is consistent with at least third-order neuronal sensitization, such as sensitization of thalamic neurons, and firmly places the pathophysiololgy within the CNS. Sensitization in migraine may be peripheral with local release of inflammatory markers, which certainly would activate trigeminal nociceptors.[91] More likely in migraine there is a form of central sensitization, which may be classical central sensitization,[90] or a form of disinhibitory sensitization with dysfunction of descending modulatory pathways.[114] Interestingly, the presence or absence of allodynia does not predict outcome from acute therapy in randomized controlled trials.[115,116]

Just as dihydroergotamine (DHE) can block trigeminovascular nociceptive transmission,[117] probably at least by a local effect in the trigeminocervical complex;[118,119] DHE can block central sensitization associated with dural stimulation by an inflammatory soup.[120] Indeed localization of DHE binding in the midbrain dorsal raphe nucleus and periaqueductal gray matter (PAG),[121] and the antinociceptive effect of naratriptan when injected locally into PAG[122] or sensory thalamus,[123] offer challenges to the orthodoxy that acute antimigraine medicines are simply inhibitors of the trigeminovascular system.

Neuropeptide Studies

Electrical stimulation of the trigeminal ganglion in people and cats leads to increases in extracerebral blood flow and local release of both CGRP and SP.[76] In the cat, trigeminal ganglion stimulation also increases cerebral blood flow by a pathway traversing the greater superficial petrosal branch of the facial nerve,[124] again releasing a powerful vasodilator peptide, vasoactive intestinal polypeptide (VIP).[125,126] Interestingly, the VIP-ergic innervation of the cerebral vessels is predominantly anterior rather than posterior,[127] and this may contribute to this regions vulnerability to spreading depression, explaining why the aura so very often is seen to commence posteriorly. Stimulation of the more specifically pain-producing superior sagittal sinus[78] increases cerebral blood flow[128] and jugular vein CGRP levels.[129] Human evidence that CGRP is elevated in the headache phase of severe migraine,[130,131] although not less severe attacks,[132] cluster headache,[133,134] and chronic paroxysmal hemicrania,[135] supports the view that the trigeminovascular system may be activated in a protective role in these conditions. Moreover, NO-donor triggered migraine, which is in essence typical migraine,[136,137] also results in increases in CGRP[138] that are blocked by sumatriptan,[139] just as in spontaneous migraine.[140] It is of interest in this regard that compounds that have not shown activity in migraine,[100,141] notably the conformationally restricted analog of sumatriptan, CP122,288,[142] and the conformationally restricted analog of zolmitriptan, 4991w93,[143] were both ineffective inhibitors of CGRP release after superior sagittal sinus in the cat. The development of nonpeptide highly specific CGRP antagonists[144,145] and the announcement of positive studies with CGRP antagonists in acute migraine[146–148] firmly establish this as a novel and important new emerging principle for acute migraine, although it may not be useful as a disease marker.[132] At the same time, the lack of any effect of CGRP blockers on plasma protein extravasation[149] explains in some part why that model has proved inadequate at translation into human therapeutic approaches.

HEADACHE PHYSIOLOGY—CENTRAL CONNECTIONS
The Trigeminocervical Complex

Fos immunohistochemistry is a method for looking at activated cells by plotting the expression of Fos protein.[150] After meningeal irritation with blood Fos expression is noted in the trigeminal nucleus caudalis,[151] while after stimulation of the superior sagittal sinus Fos-like immunoreactivity is seen in the trigeminal nucleus caudalis and in the dorsal horn at the C_1 and C_2 levels in the cat[152] and monkey.[153,154] These latter findings are in accord with similar data using 2-deoxyglucose measurements with superior sagittal sinus stimulation.[155] Similarly, stimulation of a branch of C_2, the greater occipital nerve, increases metabolic activity in the same regions (ie, trigeminal nucleus caudalis and $C_{1/2}$ dorsal horn).[156] In experimental animals, one can record directly from trigeminal neurons with both supratentorial trigeminal input and input from the greater occipital nerve, a branch of the C_2 dorsal root.[157] Stimulation of the greater occipital nerve for 5 minutes results in substantial increases in responses to supratentorial dural stimulation, which can last for over an hour.[157] Conversely, stimulation of the middle meningeal artery dura mater with the C-fiber irritant mustard oil sensitizes responses to occipital muscle stimulation.[158] It can be shown, again using the Fos method, that this interaction is likely to involve at least activation of NMDA-subtype glutamate receptors.[159] Taken together, these data suggest convergence of cervical and ophthalmic inputs at the level of the second-order neuron. Moreover, stimulation of a lateralised structure, the middle meningeal artery, produces Fos expression bilaterally in both cat and monkey brain.[154] This group of neurons from the superficial laminae of trigeminal nucleus caudalis and $C_{1/2}$ dorsal horns should be regarded functionally as the trigeminocervical complex.

These data demonstrate that trigeminovascular nociceptive information comes by way of the most caudal cells. This concept provides an anatomic explanation for the referral of pain to the back of the head in migraine. Moreover, experimental pharmacologic evidence suggests that abortive antimigraine drugs (eg, ergot derivatives,[117,118] acetylsalicylic acid,[160] sumatriptan,[161,162] eletriptan,[163,164] naratriptan,[165,166] rizatriptan[167] and zolmitriptan,[168] and the novel approach of CGRP receptor antagonists)[169] can have actions at these second-order neurons that reduce cell activity and suggest a further possible site for therapeutic intervention in migraine. The triptan action can be dissected out to involve each of the $5\text{-}HT_{1B}$, $5\text{-}HT_{1D}$, and $5\text{-}HT_{1F}$ receptor subtypes,[170] and are consistent with the localization of these receptors on peptidergic nociceptors.[171] Interestingly, triptans also influence the CGRP promoter,[172] regulate CGRP secretion from neurons in culture,[173] and may not access their receptors until the trigeminovascular system is activated.[174] Furthermore, the demonstration that some part of this action is postsynaptic with either $5\text{-}HT_{1B}$ or $5\text{-}HT_{1D}$ receptors located nonpresynatically[175,176] offers a prospect of highly anatomically localized targets for treatment. Certainly the triptan $5\text{-}HT_{1B/1D/1F}$ receptors are not highly localized, because they can be identified at every level of the peripheral sensory inputs from the trigeminal ganglion through the cervical, thoracic, lumbar, and sacral dorsal root ganglia.[177]

Serotonin–5-HT$_{1F}$ receptor agonists and migraine

Some, but not all, of the triptans are $5\text{-}HT_{1B/1D}$ receptor agonists are also potent $5\text{-}HT_{1F}$ receptor agonists.[178] A notable example is naratriptan, which is highly potent by the injectable route.[179] With the same second messenger activity as the $5HT_{1B}$ and $5\text{-}HT_{1D}$ receptors, adenylate cyclase inhibition,[180] and no contractile effects on blood vessels so far identified,[181–183] it is a good novel neural target for migraine treatment. It can be shown that $5\text{-}HT_{1F}$ activation inhibits trigeminal nucleus Fos activation[184] and neuronal firing in response to dural stimulation, the latter without cranial vascular effects.[170] One early compound was found to be effective in clinic[185] but had toxicologic problems unrelated to the mechanism, and another COL-144 has been shown to be an effective acute antimigraine treatment in a randomized controlled trial.[186] These data add further to the concept that vascular mechanisms are not necessary for acute migraine treatments.[187]

Glutamatergic transmission in the trigeminocervical complex

A potential target for antimigraine drugs is the family of glutamate receptors (GluRs), which consist of the ionotropic (iGluRs): NMDA, AMPA, kainate; and the metabotropic glutamate receptors (mGluRs) 1 through 8. NMDA receptor channel blockers have been shown reduce nociceptive trigeminovascular transmission in vivo.[188–192] The AMPA/kainate antagonists 6-cyano-7-nitroquinoxaline-2,3-dione (CNQX) and 2,3-Dioxo-6-nitro-1,2,3,4-tetrahydrobenzoquinoxaline-7-sulfonamide reduced c-fos expression after activation of structures involved in nociceptive pathways,[193] and direct application of CNQX in the trigeminocervical complex attenuated neurons with nociceptive trigeminovascular inputs.[194] Regarding the group 3 mGluR receptor the agonist L-(+)-2-Amino-4-phosphonobutyric acid decreased c-fos expression in an animal model of trigeminovascular nociceptive processing.[193] It is also notable that the group 1 mGluR5 modulator ADX10059[195] has been reported to be effective in the acute treatment of migraine.[196]

Kainate receptors are constituted by the low-affinity iGluR5, iGluR6, iGluR7, and the high-affinity KA1 and KA2 subunits, which form different homo- or heteromeric assemblies, giving rise to functional receptors. The presence of iGluR5 subunits in the trigeminal ganglion neurons[197] and at the presynaptic sites of primary afferents[198,199] indicates a possible role of kainate receptors in trigeminovascular physiology. Most recently, it was shown that activation of the iGluR5 kainate receptors with the selective agonist iodowillardiine is able to inhibit neurogenic dural vasodilation,[200] probably by inhibition of prejunctional release of CGRP from trigeminal afferents.[201] Furthermore, in a double-blinded randomized placebo-controlled study in acute migraine, LY466195, an iGluR5 kainate receptor antagonist, was effective at the 2-hour pain-free endpoint.[202] In a separate small study of acute migraine, intravenous application of the decahydroisoquinoline AMPA/iGluR5 antagonist LY293558 improved headache pain in two thirds of migraineurs and relieved the associated symptoms of the attack.[203] Taken together, these studies suggest a strong basis to pursue glutamate targets, with some care to considering how to do this without attracting unwanted adverse effects.

Higher-Order Processing

Following transmission in the caudal brain stem and high cervical spinal cord, information is relayed rostrally.

Thalamus

Processing of vascular nociceptive signals in the thalamus occurs in the ventroposteromedial (VPM) thalamus, medial nucleus of the posterior complex, and intralaminar thalamus.[204] Zagami[205] has shown by application of capsaicin to the superior sagittal sinus that trigeminal projections with a high degree of nociceptive input are processed in neurons, particularly in the VPM thalamus and in its ventral periphery. These neurons in the VPM can be modulated by activation of $GABA_A$ inhibitory receptors,[206] and perhaps of more direct clinical relevance by propranolol through a β_1-adrenoceptor mechanism.[207] Remarkably, triptans, through 5-HT$_{1B/1D}$ mechanisms, also can inhibit VPM neurons locally, as demonstrated by microiontophoretic application,[123] suggesting a hitherto unconsidered locus of action for triptans in acute migraine. Importantly, human imaging studies have confirmed activation of thalamus contralateral to pain in acute migraine,[208,209] cluster headache,[210] SUNCT (short-lasting unilateral neuralgiform headache with conjunctival injection and tearing),[211,212] and hemicrania contniua.[213]

Activation of modulatory regions

Stimulation of nociceptive afferents in the superior sagittal sinus in the cat activates neurons in the ventrolateral PAG.[214] PAG activation in turn feeds back to the trigeminocervical complex with an inhibitory influence.[215,216] PAG clearly is included in the area of activation seen in positron emission tomography (PET) studies in migraineurs,[217] and may have a more generic antinociceptive role.[218] This typical negative feedback system will be considered further as a possible mechanism for the symptomatic manifestations of migraine (**Table 1**).

Another potential modulatory region activated by stimulation of nociceptive trigeminovascular input is the posterior hypothalamic gray.[219] This area is crucially involved in several primary headaches, notably cluster headache,[2] Short-lasting unilateral neuralgiform headache attacks with SUNCT,[211] paroxysmal hemicrania,[220] and hemicrania continua.[213] Moreover, the clinical features of the premonitory phase[221–223] and other features of the disorder[224,225] suggest dopamine neuron involvement. It can be shown

Table 1 Neuroanatomical processing of vascular head pain		
	Structure	Comments
Target innervation: • Cranial vessels • Dura mater	Ophthalmic branch of trigeminal nerve	—
1st	Trigeminal ganglion	Middle cranial fossa
2nd	Trigeminal nucleus (quintothalamic tract)	Trigeminal n. caudalis & C_1/C_2 dorsal horns
3rd	Thalamus	Ventrobasal complex Medial nucleus of posterior group Intralaminar complex
Modulatory	Midbrain Hypothalamus	Periaqueductal gray matter Orexinergic mechanisms
Final	Cortex	• Insulae • Frontal cortex • Anterior cingulate cortex • Basal ganglia

in the experimental animal that D_2 family receptors are seen more often in rat trigeminocervical neurons than D_1 family receptors and that dopamine locally iontophoresed into the trigeminocervical complex, but not administered intravenously, inhibits trigeminovascular nociceptive transmission.[226] Moreover, it seems plausible that this effect, at least in part, emanates from the dopamine-containing A11 neurons,[227] which inhibit trigeminovascular nociceptive transmission through a D_2 receptor-mediated mechanism,[228] and after lesioning of this region, trigeminal nociceptive transmission is facilitated.[229] Orexinergic neurons in the posterior hypothalamus can have both pro- and antinociceptive down-stream effects[230] and are activated when trigeminovascular nociceptive afferents are stimulated.[231] Orexin A activation of the OX_1 receptor can modulate dural–vascular responses to trigeminal afferent activation[232] and inhibit second-order trigeminovascular neurons in the trigeminocervical complex.[233] Orexinergic mechanisms may be an attractive component to the central matrix of neuronal systems that are dysfunctional in migraine.[234]

THE VASCULAR HYPOTHESIS: A GOOD STORY RUINED BY THE FACTS

For much of the later part of the 20th century, a rather straightforward concept dominated thinking about migraine.[235] First, proposed in some part by Willis[236] and best articulated by Wolff,[78] the theory explained the pain of migraine to be caused by dilation of cranial vessels. By the later part of the 19th century, neuronal theories had been articulated,[237] and indeed Gowers[238] seemed happy with that concept. It is now clear that the vascular hypothesis is untenable as an explanation for migraine pathophysiology and some of the data behind this view are covered here.

Recently, it was shown that pituitary adenylate cyclase activating peptide (PACAP-38) infusion could produce cranial vasodilation and trigger a delayed migraine in sufferers but not in controls, and not in migraineurs when infused with placebo.[239] The same group using the same methods has shown VIP another member, with PACAP, of the secretin/glucagon peptide superfamily, can induce an equal craniovascular vasodilation but does not trigger migraine.[240] So it is not the dilation but the receptor site activated. Put simply, the vasodilation is an epiphenomenon neither sufficient nor necessary. Another lynch pin of the vascular argument came from the behavior of cranial vessels in migraine sufferers. It had been shown that ergotamine could produce vasoconstriction in line with its efficacy in migraine.[241] When more closely examined it was shown that vascular changes were unrelated to the phase of the attack; indeed blood flow could be reduced or normal during the pain phase.[38] Most recently, using high-resolution 3 T magnetic resonance angiography, it was reported that migraine triggered by nitroglycerin occurs without any continuing change in intracranial or extracranial vessels.[242] An important result is that the neuronal–vascular acute treatment debate[243] is now full circle in favor of a neuronal approach. Triptans, serotonin 5-HT$_{1B/1D}$ receptor agonists, which are extremely effective treatments,[1] and were developed initially as cranial vasoconstrictors,[244] for some time described have been to have effects on neuronal transmission in the brain.[161] The most recent studies demonstrate that calcitonin gene-related peptide (CGRP) receptor antagonists, developed based on the elevation of CGRP in acute, severe migraine[130] and its normalization with treatment,[130] such as olcegepant (BIBN4096BS)[146] and telcagepant (MK0974),[147,148] are both effective, and without vascular effects.[245] Similarly, purely neurally acting 5-HT$_{1F}$ receptor agonists are effective and devoid of vasoconstrictor actions.[186] Taken together, be it triggering, measuring or inducing vascular change with therapies, vascular change is neither necessary, sufficient, nor needed in migraine, in short an epiphenomenon of the neural substrates that are activated by the underlying pathophysiology of the disorder.

CENTRAL MODULATION OF TRIGEMINAL PAIN
Brain Imaging in Humans

Functional brain imaging with PET has demonstrated activation of the dorsal midbrain, including the PAG, and in the dorsal pons, near the locus coeruleus, in studies during migraine without aura.[217] Dorsolateral pontine activation is seen with PET in spontaneous episodic[209,246,247] and chronic migraine,[248] and with nitrogylcerin-triggered attacks.[208,249] These areas are active immediately after successful treatment of the headache but are not active interictally. The activation corresponds with the brain region that Raskin[250] initially reported, and Veloso confirmed,[251] to cause migraine-like headache when stimulated in patients who have electrodes implanted for pain control. Similarly, Welch and colleagues[252] have noted excess iron in the PAG of patients who have episodic and chronic migraine. Additionally, chronic migraine can develop after a bleed into a cavernoma in the region of the PAG,[253] or with a lesion of the pons.[254] What could dysfunction of these brain areas lead to?

Animal Experimental Studies of Sensory Modulation

It has been shown in the experimental animal that stimulation of nucleus locus coeruleus, the main central noradrenergic nucleus, reduces cerebral blood flow in a frequency-dependent manner[255] through an α_2-adrenoceptor-linked mechanism.[256] This reduction is maximal in the occipital cortex.[257] Although a 25% overall reduction in cerebral blood flow is seen, extracerebral vasodilatation occurs in parallel.[255] In addition, the main serotonin-containing nucleus in the brain stem, the midbrain dorsal raphe nucleus, can increase cerebral blood flow when activated.[258] Furthermore, stimulation of PAG will inhibit sagittal sinus-evoked trigeminal neuronal activity in cats,[215] while blockade of P/Q-type voltage-gated Ca^{2+} channels in the PAG facilitates trigeminovascular nociceptive processing[114] with the local GABAergic system in the PAG still intact.[216]

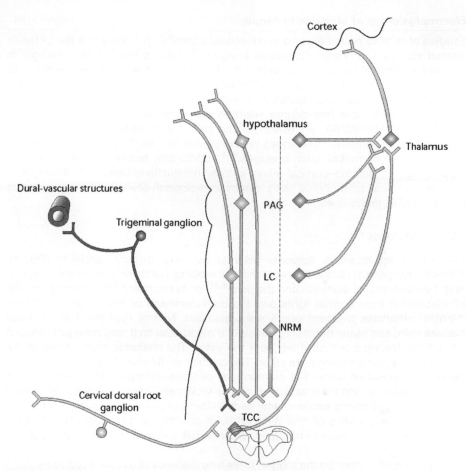

Fig. 1. Pathophysiology of migraine. Diagram of some structures involved in the transmission of trigeminovascular nociceptive input and the modulation of that input that forms the basis of a model of the pathophysiology of migraine.[187] Afferents from dural–vascular structures innervated predominantly by branches of the first (ophthalmic division) of the trigeminal nerve whose cell bodies are found in the trigeminal ganglion (Vg) project to second order neurons in the trigeminocervical complex (TCC). The TCC extends from trigeminal nucleus caudalis to the caudal portion of the dorsal horn of the C_2 spinal cord. Input from cervical structures, such as joints or muscle, project through cell bodes in the upper cervical dorsal root ganglia (DRG) to the TCC. TCC neurons project to ventrobasal thalamus (thalamus) and thence to cortex. Sensory modulation can occur by descending influences onto the TCC that largely respect the midline (*dashed line*), such as those from hypothalamus, midbrain periaqueductal gray (PAG), pontine locus coeruleus (LC), and nucleus raphe magnus (RVM). These influences are cartooned as being direct, but both direct and indirect projections are recognized. In addition, sensory modulation can occur from at least LC, PAG, and hypothalamic projects to thalamus nuclei as ascending systems again that largely respect the midline.

Electrophysiology of Migraine in People

Studies of evoked potentials and event-related potentials provide some link between animal studies and human functional imaging.[259] Authors have shown changes in neurophysiological measures of brain activation, but there is much discussion as to how to interpret such changes.[260] Perhaps the most reliable theme is that the migrainous brain does not habituate to signals in a normal way,[261–264] nor indeed do patients who have first-degree relatives with migraine.[265] Similarly, contingent negative variation (CNV), an event related potential, is abnormal in migraineurs compared with controls.[266] Changes in CNV predict attacks,[267] and preventive therapies alter and normalize such changes.[268] Additionally, recent evidence suggests involvement of thalamo–cortical relays in these habituations deficits.[269] Attempts to correlate clinical phenotypes with electrophysiological changes[270] may enhance further studies in this area.

WHAT IS MIGRAINE?

Migraine is an inherited, episodic disorder involving sensory sensitivity (**Fig. 1**). Patients complain of pain in the head that is throbbing, but there is no reliable relationship between vessel diameter and the pain[38,271] or its treatment.[272] Patients complain of discomfort from normal lights and the unpleasantness of routine sounds. Some mention otherwise pleasant odors are unpleasant. Normal movement of the head causes pain, and many mention a sense of unsteadiness as if they have just stepped off a boat, having been nowhere near the water. The anatomic connections of, for example, the pain pathways are clear. The ophthalmic division of the trigeminal nerve subserves sensation within the cranium and perhaps underpins why the top of the head is headache, and the maxillary division is facial pain. The convergence of cervical and trigeminal afferents explains why neck stiffness or pain is so common in primary headache. The genetics of channelopathies is opening up a plausible way to think about the episodic nature of migraine. Where is the lesion, however; what is actually the pathology?

Migraine aura cannot be the trigger; there is no evidence at all after 4000 years that it occurs in more than 30% of migraine patients. Aura can be experienced without pain at all, and it is seen in the other primary headaches. There is not a photon of extra light that migraine patients receive over others, so for that symptom, and phonophobia and osmophobia, the basis of the problem must be abnormal central processing of a normal signal. Perhaps electrophysiological changes in the brain have been mislabelled as hyperexcitability, whereas dyshabituation might be a simpler explanation. If migraine was basically n sensory attentional problem with changes in cortical synchronisation,[273] hypersynchronisation,[274] all its manifestations could be accounted for in a single overarching pathophysiological hypothesis of a disturbance of subcortical sensory modulation systems.[275] Although it seems likely that the trigeminovascular system, and its cranial autonomic reflex connections, the trigeminal-autonomic reflex,[126] act as a feed-forward system to facilitate the acute attack, the fundamental problem in migraine is in the brain.

REFERENCES

1. Goadsby PJ, Lipton RB, Ferrari MD. Migraine—current understanding and treatment. N Engl J Med 2002;346:257–70.
2. Goadsby PJ. Pathophysiology of cluster headache: a trigeminal autonomic cephalgia. Lancet Neurol 2002;1:37–43.

3. Lance JW, Goadsby PJ. Mechanism and management of headache. 7th edition. New York: Elsevier; 2005.
4. Olesen J, Tfelt-Hansen P, Ramadan N, et al. The headaches. Philadelphia: Lippincott, Williams & Wilkins; 2005.
5. Headache Classification Committee of The International Headache Society. The International classification of headache disorders. Cephalalgia 2004;24(Suppl 1): 1–160.
6. Ferrari MD, Goadsby PJ. Migraine as a cerebral ionopathy with abnormal central sensory processing. In: Gilman S, editor. Neurobiology of disease. New York: Elsevier; 2007. p. 333–48.
7. Silberstein SD, Lipton RB, Goadsby PJ. Headache in clinical practice. 2nd edition. London: Martin Dunitz; 2002.
8. Willis T. Opera Omnia. Amstelaedami: Henricum Wetstenium; 1682.
9. Russell MB. Genetic epidemiology of migraine and cluster headache. Cephalalgia 1997;17:683–701.
10. Ulrich V, Gervil M, Kyvik KO, et al. Evidence of a genetic factor in migraine with aura: a population-based Danish twin study. Ann Neurol 1999;45:242–6.
11. Mochi M, Sangiorgi S, Cortelli P, et al. Testing models for genetic determination in migraine. Cephalalgia 1993;13:389–94.
12. Lalouel JM, Morton NE. Complex segregation analysis with pointers. Hum Hered 1981;31:312–21.
13. Russell MB, Iselius L, Olesen J. Investigation of the inheritance of migraine by complex segregation analysis. Hum Genet 1995;96:726–30.
14. Scher AI, Terwindt GM, Verschuren WM, et al. Migraine and MTHFR C677T genotype in a population-based sample. Ann Neurol 2006;59:372–5.
15. Joutel A, Corpechot C, Ducros A, et al. Notch3 mutations in CADASIL, a hereditary adult-onset condition causing stroke and dementia. Nature 1996;383: 707–10.
16. Richards A, van den Maagdenberg AM, Jen JC, et al. C-terminal truncations in human 3'-5' DNA exonuclease TREX1 cause autosomal dominant retinal vasculopathy with cerebral leukodystrophy. Nat Genet 2007;39:1068–70.
17. Diener HC, Kurth T, Dodick D. Patent foramen ovale and migraine. Curr Pain Headache Rep 2007;11:236–40.
18. Kurth T. Migraine and ischaemic vascular events. Cephalalgia 2007;27:965–75.
19. Joutel A, Ducros A, Vahedi K, et al. Genetic heterogeneity of familial hemiplegic migraine. Am J Hum Genet 1994;55:1166–72.
20. Ophoff RA, Rv Eijk, Sandkuijl LA, et al. Genetic heterogeneity of familial hemiplegic migraine. Genomics 1994;22:21–6.
21. Ducros A, Denier C, Joutel A, et al. The clinical spectrum of familial hemiplegic migraine associated with mutations in a neuronal calcium channel. N Engl J Med 2001;345:17–24.
22. Joutel A, Bousser MG, Biousse V, et al. A gene for familial hemiplegic migraine maps to chromosome 19. Nat Genet 1993;5:40–5.
23. Haan J, Terwindt GM, Bos PL, et al. Familial hemiplegic migraine in the Netherlands. Clin Neurol Neurosurg 1994;96:244–9.
24. Teh BT, Silburn P, Lindblad K, et al. Familial cerebellar periodic ataxia without myokymia maps to a 19-cM region on 19p13. Am J Hum Genet 1995;56: 1443–9.
25. Terwindt GM, Ophoff RA, Haan J, et al. The Dutch Migraine Genetics Research Group. Familial hemiplegic migraine: a clinical comparison of families linked and unlinked to chromosome 19. Cephalalgia 1996;16:153–5.

26. Ophoff RA, Terwindt GM, Vergouwe MN, et al. Familial hemiplegic migraine and episodic ataxia type-2 are caused by mutations in the Ca^{2+} channel gene CACNL1A4. Cell 1996;87:543–52.

27. Ertel EA, Campbell KP, Harpold MM, et al. Nomenclature of voltage-gated calcium channels. Neuron 2000;25(3):533–5.

28. Marconi R, De Fusco M, Aridon P, et al. Familial hemiplegic migraine type 2 is linked to 0.9 Mb region on chromosome 1q23. Ann Neurol 2003;53:376–81.

29. De Fusco M, Marconi R, Silvestri L, et al. Haploinsufficiency of ATP1A2 encoding the Na^+/K^+ pump $\alpha2$ subunit associated with familial hemiplegic migraine type 2. Nat Genet 2003;33:192–6.

30. Vanmolkot KRJ, Kors EE, Hottenga JJ, et al. Novel mutations in the Na^+, K^+-ATPase pump gene ATP1A2 associated with familial hemiplegic migraine and benign familial infantile convulsions. Ann Neurol 2003;54:360–6.

31. Jurkat-Rott K, Freilinger T, Dreier JP, et al. Variability of familial hemiplegic migraine with novel A1A2 Na^+/K^+-ATPase variants. Neurology 2004;62: 1857–61.

32. Swoboda KJ, Kanavakis E, Xaidara A, et al. Alternating hemiplegia of childhood or familial hemiplegic migraine? A novel ATP1A2 mutation. Ann Neurol 2004;55: 884–7.

33. Dichgans M, Freilinger T, Eckstein G, et al. Mutation in the neuronal voltage-gated sodium channel SCN1A causes familial hemiplegic migraine. Lancet 2005;366:371–7.

34. Goadsby PJ, Ferrari MD. Migraine: a multifactorial, episodic neurovascular channelopathy? In: Rose MR, Griggs RC, editors. Channelopaties of the nervous system. Oxford (United Kingdom): Butterworth Heinemann; 2001. p. 274–92.

35. van den Maagdenberg AMJM, Pietrobon D, Pizzorusso T, et al. A Cacna1a knock-in migraine mouse model with increased susceptibility to cortical spreading depression. Neuron 2004;41:701–10.

36. Goadsby PJ. Migraine aura: a knock-in mouse with a knock-out message. Neuron 2004;41:679–80.

37. Rasmussen BK, Olesen J. Migraine with aura and migraine without aura: an epidemiological study. Cephalalgia 1992;12:221–8.

38. Olesen J, Friberg L, Skyhoj-Olsen T, et al. Timing and topography of cerebral blood flow, aura, and headache during migraine attacks. Ann Neurol 1990;28:791–8.

39. Cutrer FM, Sorensen AG, Weisskoff RM, et al. Perfusion-weighted imaging defects during spontaneous migrainous aura. Ann Neurol 1998;43:25–31.

40. Leao AAP. Spreading depression of activity in cerebral cortex. J Neurophysiol 1944;7:359–90.

41. Leao AAP. Pial circulation and spreading activity in the cerebral cortex. J Neurophysiol 1944;7:391–6.

42. Lauritzen M. Pathophysiology of the migraine aura. The spreading depression theory. Brain 1994;117:199–210.

43. Lashley KS. Patterns of cerebral integration indicated by the scotomas of migraine. Arch Neurol Psychiatry 1941;46:331–9.

44. Olesen J, Larsen B, Lauritzen M. Focal hyperemia followed by spreading oligemia and impaired activation of rCBF in classic migraine. Ann Neurol 1981;9:344–52.

45. Sakai F, Meyer JS. Abnormal cerebrovascular reactivity in patients with migraine and cluster headache. Headache 1979;19:257–66.

46. Lauritzen M, Skyhoj-Olsen T, Lassen NA, et al. The changes of regional cerebral blood flow during the course of classical migraine attacks. Ann Neurol 1983;13:633–41.

47. Harer C, Kummer Rv. Cerebrovascular CO_2 reactivity in migraine: assessment by transcranial Doppler ultrasound. J Neurol 1991;238:23–6.
48. Kaube H, Goadsby PJ. Anti-migraine compounds fail to modulate the propagation of cortical spreading depression in the cat. Eur Neurol 1994;34:30–5.
49. Lambert GA, Michalicek J, Storer RJ, et al. Effect of cortical spreading depression on activity of trigeminovascular sensory neurons. Cephalalgia 1999;19:631–8.
50. Kaube H, Knight YE, Storer RJ, et al. Vasodilator agents and supracollicular transection fail to inhibit cortical spreading depression in the cat. Cephalalgia 1999;19:592–7.
51. Brennan KC, Romero-Reyes M, Lopez Valdes HE, et al. Reduced threshold for cortical spreading depression in female mice. Ann Neurol 2007;61:603–6.
52. Hadjikhani N, Sanchez del Rio M, Wu O, et al. Mechanisms of migraine aura revealed by functional MRI in human visual cortex. Proc Natl Acad Sci U S A 2001; 98:4687–92.
53. Moskowitz MA, Bolay H, Dalkara T. Deciphering migraine mechanisms: clues from familial hemiplegic migraine genotypes. Ann Neurol 2004;55:276–80.
54. Goadsby PJ. Migraine, aura, and cortical spreading depression: why are we still talking about it? Ann Neurol 2001;49:4–6.
55. Goadsby PJ, Ferrari MD, Csanyi A, et al. Randomized double-blind, placebo-controlled proof-of-concept study of the cortical spreading depression inhibiting agent tonabersat in migraine prophylaxis. Cephalalgia, 2009;29: in press.
56. Read SJ, Smith MI, Hunter AJ, et al. SB-220453, a potential novel antimigraine compound, inhibits nitric oxide release following induction of cortical spreading depression in the anaesthetized cat. Cephalalgia 1999;20:92–9.
57. Smith MI, Read SJ, Chan WN, et al. Repetitive cortical spreading depression in a gyrencephalic feline brain: inhibition by the novel benzoylamino-benzopyran SB-220453. Cephalalgia 2000;20:546–53.
58. MaassenVanDenBrink A, van den Broek RW, de Vries R, et al. The potential anti-migraine compound SB-220453 does not contract human isolated blood vessels or myocardium; a comparison with sumatriptan. Cephalalgia 2000;20:538–45.
59. Parsons AA, Bingham S, Raval P, et al. Tonabersat (SB-220453) a novel benzopyran with anticonvulsant properties attenuates trigeminal nerve-induced neurovascular reflexes. Br J Pharmacol 2001;132:1549–57.
60. Diener HC, Tfelt-Hansen P, Dahlof C, et al. Topiramate in migraine prophylaxis—results from a placebo-controlled trial with propranolol as an active control. J Neurol 2004;251:943–50.
61. Brandes JL, Saper JR, Diamond M, et al. Topiramate for migraine prevention: a randomized controlled trial. JAMA 2004;291:965–73.
62. Silberstein SD, Neto W, Schmitt J, et al. Topiramate in migraine prevention: results of a large controlled trial. Arch Neurol 2004;61:490–5.
63. Akerman S, Goadsby PJ. Topiramate inhibits cortical spreading depression in rat and cat: a possible contribution to its preventive effect in migraine. Cephalalgia 2004;24:783–4.
64. Ayata C, Jin H, Kudo C, et al. Suppression of cortical spreading depression in migraine prophylaxis. Ann Neurol 2006;59:652–61.
65. Tvedskov JF, Iversen HK, Olesen J. A double-blind study of SB-220453 (Tonerbasat) in the glyceryltrinitrate (GTN) model of migraine. Cephalalgia 2004;24: 875–82.
66. Tvedskov JF, Thomsen LL, Iversen HK, et al. The effect of propranolol on glyceryltrinitrate-induced headache and arterial response. Cephalalgia 2004;24: 1076–87.

67. Tvedskov JF, Thomsen LL, Iversen HK, et al. The prophylactic effect of valproate on glyceryltrinitrate induced migraine. Cephalalgia 2004;24:576–85.
68. Storer RJ, Goadsby PJ. Topiramate inhibits trigeminovascular neurons in the cat. Cephalalgia 2004;24:1049–56.
69. Storer RJ, Goadsby PJ. Topiramate has a locus of action outside of the trigeminocervical complex. Neurology 2005;64(Suppl 1):A150–1.
70. Akerman S, Holland PR, Goadsby PJ. Mechanically induced cortical spreading depression associated regional cerebral blood flow changes are blocked by Na+ ion channel blockade. Brain Res 2008;1229:27–36.
71. Akerman S, Holland PR, Goadsby PJ. Needle-stick induced regional cerebral blood flow change (rCBF) is affected by Na^+ channel blockade, AMPA/kainate antagonism and GABA agonists, but not by voltage-dependent Ca^{2+} channel or ATP-dependent K^+ channel blockade. Cephalalgia 2005;25:871.
72. Kaube H, Herzog J, Kaufer T, et al. Aura in some patients with familial hemiplegic migraine can be stopped by intranasal ketamine. Neurology 2000;55:139–41.
73. Liu-Chen L-Y, Gillespie SA, Norregaard TV, et al. Colocalization of retrogradely transported wheat germ agglutinin and the putative neurotransmitter substance P within trigeminal ganglion cells projecting to cat middle cerebral. J Comp Neurol 1984;225:187–92.
74. Arbab MA-R, Wiklund L, Svendgaard NA. Origin and distribution of cerebral vascular innervation from superior cervical, trigeminal, and spinal ganglia investigated with retrograde and anterograde WGA-HRP tracing in the rat. Neuroscience 1986;19:695–708.
75. Uddman R, Edvinsson L, Ekman R, et al. Innervation of the feline cerebral vasculature by nerve fibers containing calcitonin gene-related peptide: trigeminal origin and coexistence with substance P. Neurosci Lett 1985;62:131–6.
76. Goadsby PJ, Edvinsson L, Ekman R. Release of vasoactive peptides in the extracerebral circulation of man and the cat during activation of the trigeminovascular system. Ann Neurol 1988;23:193–6.
77. Feindel W, Penfield W, McNaughton F. The tentorial nerves and localization of intracranial pain in man. Neurology 1960;10:555–63.
78. Wolff HG. Headache and other head pain. 1st edition. New York: Oxford University Press; 1948.
79. Penfield W, McNaughton FL. Dural headache and the innervation of the dura mater. Arch Neurol Psychiatry 1940;44:43–75.
80. Moskowitz MA. Basic mechanisms in vascular headache. Neurol Clin 1990;8:801–15.
81. Markowitz S, Saito K, Moskowitz MA. Neurogenically mediated leakage of plasma proteins occurs from blood vessels in dura mater but not brain. J Neurosci 1987;7:4129–36.
82. Moskowitz MA, Cutrer FM. SUMATRIPTAN: a receptor-targeted treatment for migraine. Annu Rev Med 1993;44:145–54.
83. Bolay H, Reuter U, Dunn AK, et al. Intrinsic brain activity triggers trigeminal meningeal afferents in a migraine model. Nat Med 2002;8:136–42.
84. Moskowitz MA, Nozaki K, Kraig RP. Neocortical spreading depression provokes the expression of C-fos protein-like immunoreactivity within the trigeminal nucleus caudalis via trigeminovascular mechanisms. J Neurosci 1993;13:1167–77.
85. Ingvardsen BK, Laursen H, Olsen UB, et al. Possible mechanism of c-fos expression in trigeminal nucleus caudalis following spreading depression. Pain 1997;72:407–15.

86. Ingvardsen BK, Laursen H, Olsen UB, et al. Comment on Ingvardsen et al. PAIN, 72 (1997) 407–415—Reply to Moskowitz et al. Pain 1998;76:266–7.
87. Ebersberger A, Schaible H-G, Averbeck B, et al. Is there a correlation between spreading depression, neurogenic inflammation, and nociception that might cause migraine headache? Ann Neurol 2001;41:7–13.
88. Dimitriadou V, Buzzi MG, Moskowitz MA, et al. Trigeminal sensory fiber stimulation induces morphological changes reflecting secretion in rat dura mater mast cells. Neuroscience 1991;44:97–112.
89. Dimitriadou V, Buzzi MG, Theoharides TC, et al. Ultrastructural evidence for neurogenically mediated changes in blood vessels of the rat dura mater and tongue following antidromic trigeminal stimulation. Neuroscience 1992;48:187–203.
90. Burstein R, Yamamura H, Malick A, et al. Chemical stimulation of the intracranial dura induces enhanced responses to facial stimulation in brain stem trigeminal neurons. J Neurophysiol 1998;79:964–82.
91. Strassman AM, Raymond SA, Burstein R. Sensitization of meningeal sensory neurons and the origin of headaches. Nature 1996;384:560–3.
92. Peroutka SJ. Neurogenic inflammation and migraine: implications for therapeutics. Mol Interv 2005;5:306–13.
93. May A, Shepheard S, Wessing A, et al. Retinal plasma extravasation can be evoked by trigeminal stimulation in rat but does not occur during migraine attacks. Brain 1998;121:1231–7.
94. Steuer H, Jaworski A, Stoll D, et al. In vitro model of the outer blood–retina barrier. Brain Res Brain Res Protoc 2004;13:26–36.
95. Diener H-C, The RPR100893 Study Group. RPR100893, a substance-P antagonist, is not effective in the treatment of migraine attacks. Cephalalgia 2003;23:183–5.
96. Goldstein DJ, Wang O, Saper JR, et al. Ineffectiveness of neurokinin-1 antagonist in acute migraine: a crossover study. Cephalalgia 1997;17:785–90.
97. Norman B, Panebianco D, Block GA. A placebo-controlled, in-clinic study to explore the preliminary safety and efficacy of intravenous L-758, 298 (a prodrug of the NK1 receptor antagonist L-754, 030) in the acute treatment of migraine. Cephalalgia 1998;18:407.
98. Connor HE, Bertin L, Gillies S, et al. The GR205171 Clinical Study Group. Clinical evaluation of a novel, potent, CNS-penetrating NK_1 receptor antagonist in the acute treatment of migraine. Cephalalgia 1998;18:392.
99. Roon K, Diener HC, Ellis P, et al. CP-122, 288 blocks neurogenic inflammation, but is not effective in aborting migraine attacks: results of two controlled clinical studies. Cephalalgia 1997;17:245.
100. Earl NL, McDonald SA, Lowy MT, 4991W93 Investigator Group. Efficacy and tolerability of the neurogenic inflammation inhibitor, 4991W93, in the acute treatment of migraine. Cephalalgia 1999;19:357.
101. May A, Gijsman HJ, Wallnoefer A, et al. Endothelin antagonist bosentan blocks neurogenic inflammation, but is not effective in aborting migraine attacks. Pain 1996;67:375–8.
102. Data J, Britch K, Westergaard N, et al. A double-blind study of ganaxolone in the acute treatment of migraine headaches with or without an aura in premenopausal females. Headache 1998;38:380.
103. Reuter U, Bolay H, Jansen-Olesen I, et al. Delayed inflammation in rat meninges: implications for migraine pathophysiology. Brain 2001;124:2490–502.

104. De Alba J, Clayton NM, Collins SD, et al. GW274150, a novel and highly selective inhibitor of the inducible isoform of nitric oxide synthase (iNOS), shows analgesic effects in rat models of inflammatory and neuropathic pain. Pain 2006; 120:170–81.
105. Lassen LH, Ashina M, Christiansen I, et al. Nitric oxide synthesis inhibition in migraine. Lancet 1997;349:401–2.
106. Alderton WK, Angell AD, Craig C, et al. GW274150 and GW273629 are potent and highly selective inhibitors of inducible nitric oxide synthase in vitro and in vivo. Br J Pharmacol 2005;145:301–12.
107. Palmer JE, Guillard FL, Laurijssens BE, et al. A randomised, single-blind, placebo-controlled, adaptive clinical trial of GW274150, a selective iNOS inhibitor, in the treatment of acute migraine. Cephalalgia 2009;29:124.
108. Hall DB, Meier U, Diener HC. A group sequential adaptive treatment assignment design for proof of concept and dose selection in headache trials. Contemp Clin Trials 2000;26:349–64.
109. Hoye K, Laurijssens BE, Harnisch LO, et al. Efficacy and tolerability of the iNOS inhibitor GW274150 administered up to 120 mg daily for 12 weeks in the prophylactic treatment of migraine. Cephalalgia 2009;29:132.
110. Selby G, Lance JW. Observations on 500 cases of migraine and allied vascular headache. J Neurol Neurosurg Psychiatr 1960;23:23–32.
111. Burstein R, Cutrer MF, Yarnitsky D. The development of cutaneous allodynia during a migraine attack. Brain 2000;123:1703–9.
112. Burstein R, Yarnitsky D, Goor-Aryeh I, et al. An association between migraine and cutaneous allodynia. Ann Neurol 2000;47:614–24.
113. Lipton RB, Bigal ME, Ashina S, et al. Cutaneous allodynia in the migraine population. Ann Neurol 2008;63:148–58.
114. Knight YE, Bartsch T, Kaube H, et al. P/Q-type calcium channel blockade in the PAG facilitates trigeminal nociception: a functional genetic link for migraine? J Neurosci 2002;22(RC213):1–6.
115. Cady R, Martin V, Mauskop A, et al. Symptoms of cutaneous sensitivity pretreatment and post-treatment: results from the rizatriptan TAME studies. Cephalalgia 2007;27:1055–60.
116. Goadsby PJ, Zanchin G, Geraud G, et al. Early versus non-early intervention in acute migraine- "Act when Mild- AwM." A double-blind placebo-controlled trial of almotriptan. Cephalalgia 2008;28:383–91.
117. Hoskin KL, Kaube H, Goadsby PJ. Central activation of the trigeminovascular pathway in the cat is inhibited by dihydroergotamine. A c-Fos and electrophysiology study. Brain 1996;119:249–56.
118. Lambert GA, Lowy AJ, Boers P, et al. The spinal cord processing of input from the superior sagittal sinus: pathway and modulation by ergot alkaloids. Brain Res 1992;597:321–30.
119. Storer RJ, Goadsby PJ. Microiontophoretic application of serotonin (5HT)$_{1B/1D}$ agonists inhibits trigeminal cell firing in the cat. Brain 1997;120:2171–7.
120. Pozo-Rosich P, Oshinsky M. Effect of dihydroergotamine (DHE) on central sensitisation of neurons in the trigeminal nucleus caudalis. Neurology 2005; 64(Suppl 1):A151.
121. Goadsby PJ, Gundlach AL. Localization of [^{3}H]-dihydroergotamine binding sites in the cat central nervous system: relevance to migraine. Ann Neurol 1991;29:91–4.
122. Bartsch T, Knight YE, Goadsby PJ. Activation of 5-HT$_{1B/1D}$ receptors in tho periaqueductal grey inhibits meningeal nociception. Ann Neurol 2004;56:371–81.

123. Shields KG, Goadsby PJ. Serotonin receptors modulate trigeminovascular responses in ventroposteromedial nucleus of thalamus: a migraine target? Neurobiol Dis 2006;23:491–501.
124. Goadsby PJ, Duckworth JW. Effect of stimulation of trigeminal ganglion on regional cerebral blood flow in cats. Am J Phys 1987;253:R270–4.
125. Goadsby PJ, Macdonald GJ. Extracranial vasodilatation mediated by VIP (vasoactive intestinal polypeptide). Brain Res 1985;329:285–8.
126. May A, Goadsby PJ. The trigeminovascular system in humans: pathophysiological implications for primary headache syndromes of the neural influences on the cerebral circulation. J Cereb Blood Flow Metab 1999;19:115–27.
127. Matsuyama T, Shiosaka S, Matsumoto M, et al. Overall distribution of vasoactive intestinal polypeptide-containing nerves on the wall of the cerebral arteries: an immunohistochemical study using whole mounts. Neuroscience 1983;10:89–96.
128. Lambert GA, Goadsby PJ, Zagami AS, et al. Comparative effects of stimulation of the trigeminal ganglion and the superior sagittal sinus on cerebral blood flow and evoked potentials in the cat. Brain Res 1988;453:143–9.
129. Zagami AS, Goadsby PJ, Edvinsson L. Stimulation of the superior sagittal sinus in the cat causes release of vasoactive peptides. Neuropeptides 1990;16:69–75.
130. Goadsby PJ, Edvinsson L, Ekman R. Vasoactive peptide release in the extracerebral circulation of humans during migraine headache. Ann Neurol 1990;28:183–7.
131. Gallai V, Sarchielli P, Floridi A, et al. Vasoactive peptides levels in the plasma of young migraine patients with and without aura assessed both interictally and ictally. Cephalalgia 1995;15:384–90.
132. Tvedskov JF, Lipka K, Ashina M, et al. No increase of calcitonin gene-related peptide in jugular blood during migraine. Ann Neurol 2005;58:561–8.
133. Goadsby PJ, Edvinsson L. Human in vivo evidence for trigeminovascular activation in cluster headache. Brain 1994;117:427–34.
134. Fanciullacci M, Alessandri M, Figini M, et al. Increase in plasma calcitonin gene-related peptide from extracerebral circulation during nitroglycerin-induced cluster headache attack. Pain 1995;60:119–23.
135. Goadsby PJ, Edvinsson L. Neuropeptide changes in a case of chronic paroxysmal hemicrania— evidence for trigemino–parasympathetic activation. Cephalalgia 1996;16:448–50.
136. Iversen HK, Olesen J, Tfelt-Hansen P. Intravenous nitroglycerin as an experimental headache model. Basic characteristics. Pain 1989;38:17–24.
137. Afridi S, Kaube H, Goadsby PJ. Glyceryl trinitrate triggers premonitory symptoms in migraineurs. Pain 2004;110:675–80.
138. Juhasz G, Zsombok T, Modos EA, et al. NO-induced migraine attack: strong increase in plasma calcitonin gene-related peptide (CGRP) concentration and negative correlation with platelet serotonin release. Pain 2003;106:461–70.
139. Juhasz G, Zsombok T, Jakab B, et al. Sumatriptan causes parallel decrease in plasma calcitonin gene-related peptide (CGRP) concentration and migraine headache during nitroglycerin-induced migraine attack. Cephalalgia 2005;25:179–83.
140. Goadsby PJ, Edvinsson L. The trigeminovascular system and migraine: studies characterizing cerebrovascular and neuropeptide changes seen in humans and cats. Ann Neurol 1993;33:48–56.
141. Roon KI, Olesen J, Diener HC, et al. No acute antimigraine efficacy of CP-122, 288, a highly potent inhibitor of neurogenic inflammation: results of two randomized double-blind placebo-controlled clinical trials. Ann Neurol 2000;47:238–41.

142. Knight YE, Edvinsson L, Goadsby PJ. Blockade of CGRP release after superior sagittal sinus stimulation in cat: a comparison of avitriptan and CP122, 288. Neuropeptides 1999;33:41–6.

143. Knight YE, Edvinsson L, Goadsby PJ. 4991W93 inhibits release of calcitonin gene-related peptide in the cat but only at doses with $5HT_{1B/1D}$ receptor agonist activity. Neuropharmacology 2001;40:520–5.

144. Doods H, Hallermayer G, Wu D, et al. Pharmacological profile of BIBN4096BS, the first selective small molecule CGRP antagonist. Br J Pharmacol 2000;129:420–3.

145. Williams TM, Stump CA, Nguyen DN, et al. Nonpeptide calcitonin gene-related peptide receptor antagonists from a benzodiazepinone lead. Bioorg Med Chem Lett 2006;16:2595–8.

146. Olesen J, Diener H-C, Husstedt I-W, et al. Calcitonin gene-related peptide (CGRP) receptor antagonist BIBN4096BS is effective in the treatment of migraine attacks. N Engl J Med 2004;350:1104–10.

147. Ho T, Mannix L, Fan X, et al. Randomized controlled trial of an oral CGRP antagonist, MK-0974, in acute treatment of migraine. Neurology 2008;70:1004–12.

148. Ho TW, Ferrari MD, Dodick DW, et al. Efficacy and tolerability of MK-0974 (telcagepant), a new oral antagonist of calcitonin gene-related peptide receptor, compared with zolmitriptan for acute migraine: a randomised, placebo-controlled, parallel treatment trial. Lancet 2009;372:2115–23.

149. Grant AD, Pinter E, Salmon AM, et al. An examination of neurogenic mechanisms involved in mustard oil-induced inflammation in the mouse. Eur J Pharmacol 2005;507:273–80.

150. Morgan JI, Curran T. Stimulus transcription coupling in the nervous system: involvement of the inducible proto-oncogenes Fos and jun. Annu Rev Neurosci 1991;14:421–51.

151. Nozaki K, Boccalini P, Moskowitz MA. Expression of c-fos-like immunoreactivity in brainstem after meningeal irritation by blood in the subarachnoid space. Neuroscience 1992;49:669–80.

152. Kaube H, Keay KA, Hoskin KL, et al. Expression of c-fos-like immunoreactivity in the caudal medulla and upper cervical cord following stimulation of the superior sagittal sinus in the cat. Brain Res 1993;629:95–102.

153. Goadsby PJ, Hoskin KL. The distribution of trigeminovascular afferents in the nonhuman primate brain Macaca nemestrina: a c-fos immunocytochemical study. J Anat 1997;190:367–75.

154. Hoskin KL, Zagami A, Goadsby PJ. Stimulation of the middle meningeal artery leads to Fos expression in the trigeminocervical nucleus: a comparative study of monkey and cat. J Anat 1999;194:579–88.

155. Goadsby PJ, Zagami AS. Stimulation of the superior sagittal sinus increases metabolic activity and blood flow in certain regions of the brainstem and upper cervical spinal cord of the cat. Brain 1991;114:1001–11.

156. Goadsby PJ, Hoskin KL, Knight YE. Stimulation of the greater occipital nerve increases metabolic activity in the trigeminal nucleus caudalis and cervical dorsal horn of the cat. Pain 1997;73:23–8.

157. Bartsch T, Goadsby PJ. Stimulation of the greater occipital nerve induces increased central excitability of dural afferent input. Brain 2002;125:1496–509.

158. Bartsch T, Goadsby PJ. Increased responses in trigeminocervical nociceptive neurones to cervical input after stimulation of the dura mater. Brain 2003;126:1801–13.

159. Le Doare K, Akerman S, Holland PR, et al. Expression of Fos in the trigeminocervical complex of rat following stimulation of occipital afferents. Cephalalgia 2005;25:986–7.

160. Kaube H, Hoskin KL, Goadsby PJ. Intravenous acetylsalicylic acid inhibits central trigeminal neurons in the dorsal horn of the upper cervical spinal cord in the cat. Headache 1993;33:541–50.

161. Kaube H, Hoskin KL, Goadsby PJ. Inhibition by sumatriptan of central trigeminal neurones only after blood–brain barrier disruption. Br J Pharmacol 1993;109: 788–92.

162. Levy D, Jakubowski M, Burstein R. Disruption of communication between peripheral and central trigeminovascular neurons mediates the antimigraine action of 5HT 1B/1D receptor agonists. Proc Natl Acad Sci U S A 2004;101:4274–9.

163. Goadsby PJ, Hoskin KL. Differential effects of low dose CP122, 288 and eletriptan on Fos expression due to stimulation of the superior sagittal sinus in cat. Pain 1999;82:15–22.

164. Lambert GA, Boers PM, Hoskin KL, et al. Suppression by eletriptan of the activation of trigeminovascular sensory neurons by glyceryl trinitrate. Brain Res 2002;953:181–8.

165. Goadsby PJ, Knight YE. Inhibition of trigeminal neurons after intravenous administration of naratriptan through an action at the serotonin (5HT$_{1B/1D}$) receptors. Br J Pharmacol 1997;122:918–22.

166. Cumberbatch MJ, Hill RG, Hargreaves RJ. Differential effects of the 5HT$_{1B/1D}$ receptor agonist naratriptan on trigeminal versus spinal nociceptive responses. Cephalalgia 1998;18:659–64.

167. Cumberbatch MJ, Hill RG, Hargreaves RJ. Rizatriptan has central antinociceptive effects against durally evoked responses. Eur J Pharmacol 1997;328:37–40.

168. Goadsby PJ, Hoskin KL. Inhibition of trigeminal neurons by intravenous administration of the serotonin (5HT)$_{1B/D}$ receptor agonist zolmitriptan (311C90): are brain stem sites a therapeutic target in migraine? Pain 1996;67:355–9.

169. Storer RJ, Akerman S, Goadsby PJ. Calcitonin gene-related peptide (CGRP) modulates nociceptive trigeminovascular transmission in the cat. Br J Pharmacol 2004;142:1171–81.

170. Goadsby PJ, Classey JD. Evidence for 5-HT$_{1B}$, 5-HT$_{1D}$ and 5-HT$_{1F}$ receptor inhibitory effects on trigeminal neurons with craniovascular input. Neuroscience 2003;122:491–8.

171. Potrebic S, Ahn AH, Skinner K, et al. Peptidergic nociceptors of both trigeminal and dorsal root ganglia express serotonin 1D receptors: implications for the selective antimigraine action of triptans. J Neurosci 2003;23:10988–97.

172. Durham PL, Sharma RV, Russo AF. Repression of the calcitonin gene-related peptide promoter by 5-HT$_1$ receptor activation. J Neurosci 1997;17:9545–53.

173. Durham PL, Russo AF. Regulation of calcitonin gene-related peptide secretion by a serotonergic antimigraine drug. J Neurosci 1999;19:3423–9.

174. Ahn AH, Basbaum AI. Tissue injury regulates serotonin 1D receptor expression: implications for the control of migraine and inflammatory pain. J Neurosci 2006; 26:8332–8.

175. Goadsby PJ, Akerman S, Storer RJ. Evidence for postjunctional serotonin (5-HT$_1$) receptors in the trigeminocervical complex. Ann Neurol 2001;50:804–7.

176. Maneesri S, Akerman S, Lasalandra MP, et al. Electron microsopic demonstration of pre- and postsynaptic 5-HT$_{1D}$ and 5-HT$_{1F}$ receptor immunoreactivity (IR) in the rat trigeminocervical complex (TCC): new therapeutic possibilities for the triptans. Cephalalgia 2004;24:148.

177. Classey JD, Bartsch T, Goadsby PJ. Immunohistochemical examination of 5HT$_{1B}$, 5HT$_{1D}$, and 5HT$_{1F}$ receptor expression in rat trigeminal ganglion (TRG) and dorsal root ganglia (DRG) neurons. Cephalalgia 2002;22:595–6.

178. Goadsby PJ. The pharmacology of headache. Prog Neurobiol 2000;62:509–25.
179. Dahlof C, Hogenhuis L, Olesen J, et al. Early clinical experience with subcutaneous naratriptan in the acute treatment of migraine: a dose ranging study. Eur J Neurol 1998;5:469–77.
180. Adham N, Kao H-T, Schechter LE, et al. Cloning of another human serotonin receptor (5-HT$_{1F}$): a fifth 5-HT$_1$ receptor subtype coupled to the inhibition of adenylate cyclase. Proc Natl Acad Sci U S A 1993;90:408–12.
181. Bouchelet I, Case B, Olivier A, et al. No contractile effect for 5-HT$_{1D}$ and 5-HT$_{1F}$ rececptor agonists in human and bovine cerebral arteries: similarity with human coronary artery. Br J Pharmacol 2000;129:501–8.
182. Shepheard S, Edvinsson L, Cumberbatch M, et al. Possible antimigraine mechanisms of action of the 5HT$_{1F}$ receptor agonist LY334370. Cephalalgia 1999;19:851–8.
183. Razzaque Z, Heald MA, Pickard JD, et al. Vasoconstriction in human isolated middle meningeal arteries: determining the contribution of 5-HT$_{1B}$- and 5-HT$_{1F}$-receptor activation. Br J Clin Pharmacol 1999;47(1):75–82.
184. Mitsikostas DD, Sanchez del Rio M, Moskowitz MA, et al. Both 5-HT$_{1B}$ and 5-HT$_{1F}$ receptors modulate c-fos expression within rat trigeminal nucleus caudalis. Eur J Pharmacol 1999;369:271–7.
185. Goldstein DJ, Roon KI, Offen WW, et al. Selective serotonin 1F (5-HT (1F)) receptor agonist LY334370 for acute migraine: a randomised controlled trial. Lancet 2001;358:1230–4.
186. Reuter U, Pilgrim AJ, Diener H-C, et al. COL-144, a selective 5-HT1F agonist, for the treatment of migraine attacks. Cephalalgia 2009;29:122.
187. Goadsby PJ. Can we develop neurally acting drugs for the treatment of migraine? Nat Rev Drug Discov 2005;4:741–50.
188. Classey JD, Knight YE, Goadsby PJ. The NMDA receptor antagonist MK-801 reduces Fos-like immunoreactivity within the trigeminocervical complex following superior sagittal sinus stimulation in the cat. Brain Res 2001;907:117–24.
189. Mitsikostas DD, Sanchez del Rio M, Waeber C, et al. The NMDA receptor antagonist MK-801 reduces capsaicin-induced c-fos expression within rat trigeminal nucleus caudalis. Pain 1998;76:239–48.
190. Storer RJ, Goadsby PJ. Trigeminovascular nociceptive transmission involves N-methyl-D-aspartate and non-N-methyl-D-aspartate glutamate receptors. Neuroscience 1999;90:1371–6.
191. Knyihar-Csillik E, Toldi J, Krisztin-Peva B, et al. Prevention of electrical stimulation-induced increase of c-fos immunoreaction in the caudal trigeminal nucleus by kynurenine combined with probenecid. Neurosci Lett 2007;418:122–6.
192. Peeters M, Gunthorpe MJ, Strijbos PJ, et al. Effects of pan- and subtype-selective N-methyl-D-aspartate receptor antagonists on cortical spreading depression in the rat: therapeutic potential for migraine. J Pharmacol Exp Ther 2007;321:564–72.
193. Mitsikostas DD, Sanchez del Rio M, Waeber C, et al. Non-NMDA glutamate receptors modulate capsaicin induced c-fos expression within trigeminal nucleus caudalis. Br J Pharmacol 1999;127:623–30.
194. Andreou AP, Storer RJ, Holland PR, et al. CNQX inihibits trigeminovascular neurons in the rat: a microiontophoresis study. Cephalalgia 2006;26:1383.
195. Porter RH, Jaeschke G, Spooren W, et al. Fenobam: a clinically validated non-benzodiazepine anxiolytic is a potent, selective, and noncompetitive mGlu5 receptor antagonist with inverse agonist activity. J Pharmacol Exp Ther 2005;315:711–21.

196. Goadsby PJ, Keywood C. Investigation of the role of mGluR5 inhibition in migraine: a proof of concept study of ADX10059 in acute treatment of migraine. Neurology, 2009; in press.

197. Sahara Y, Noro N, Iida Y, et al. Glutamate receptor subunits GluR5 and KA-2 are coexpressed in rat trigeminal ganglion neurons. J Neurosci 1997;17: 6611–20.

198. Hwang SJ, Pagliardini S, Rustioni A, et al. Presynaptic kainate receptors in primary afferents to the superficial laminae of the rat spinal cord. J Comp Neurol 2001;436:275–89.

199. Lucifora S, Willcockson HH, Lu CR, et al. Presynaptic low- and high-affinity kainate receptors in nociceptive spinal afferents. Pain 2006;120:97–105.

200. Williamson DJ, Hargreaves RJ, Hill RG, et al. Sumatriptan inhibits neurogenic vasodilation of dural blood vessels in the anaesthetized rat—intravital micro-scope studies. Cephalalgia 1997;17:525–31.

201. Andreou AP, Holland PR, Goadsby PJ. Activation of GluR5 kainate receptors inhibits neurogenic dural vasodilation in animal model of trigeminovascular acti-vation. Br J Pharmacol, 2009; in press.

202. Johnson KW, Nisenbaum ES, Johnson MP, et al. Innovative drug development for headache disorders: glutamate. In: Olesen J, Ramadan N, editors. Innova-tive drug development for headache disorders. Oxford (United Kingdom): Oxford University Press; 2008. p. 185–94.

203. Sang CN, Ramadan NM, Wallihan RG, et al. LY293558, a novel AMPA/GluR5 antagonist, is efficacious and well-tolerated in acute migraine. Cephalalgia 2004;24:596–602.

204. Zagami AS, Goadsby PJ. Stimulation of the superior sagittal sinus increases meta-bolic activity in cat thalamus. In: Rose FC, editor. New advances in headache research: 2. London: Smith-Gordon and Company Limited; 1991. p. 169–71.

205. Zagami AS, Lambert GA. Craniovascular application of capsaicin activates nociceptive thalamic neurons in the cat. Neurosci Lett 1991;121:187–90.

206. Shields KG, Kaube H, Goadsby PJ. GABA receptors modulate trigeminovascu-lar nociceptive transmission in the ventroposteromedial (VPM) thalamic nucleus of the rat. Cephalalgia 2003;23:728.

207. Shields KG, Goadsby PJ. Propranolol modulates trigeminovascular responses in thalamic ventroposteromedial nucleus: a role in migraine? Brain 2005;128: 86–97.

208. Bahra A, Matharu MS, Buchel C, et al. Brainstem activation specific to migraine headache. Lancet 2001;357:1016–7.

209. Afridi S, Giffin NJ, Kaube H, et al. A PET study in spontaneous migraine. Arch Neurol 2005;62:1270–5.

210. May A, Bahra A, Buchel C, et al. Hypothalamic activation in cluster headache attacks. Lancet 1998;352:275–8.

211. May A, Bahra A, Buchel C, et al. Functional MRI in spontaneous attacks of SUNCT: short-lasting neuralgiform headache with conjunctival injection and tearing. Ann Neurol 1999;46:791–3.

212. Cohen AS, Matharu MS, Kalisch R, et al. Functional MRI in SUNCT shows differ-ential hypothalamic activation with increasing pain. Cephalalgia 2004;24: 1098–9.

213. Matharu MS, Cohen AS, McGonigle DJ, et al. Posterior hypothalamic and brain-stem activation in hemicrania continua. Headache 2004;44:747–61, 462–3.

214. Hoskin KL, Bulmer DCE, Lasalandra M, et al. Fos expression in the midbrain periaqueductal grey after trigeminovascular stimulation. J Anat 2001;197:29–35.

215. Knight YE, Goadsby PJ. The periaqueductal gray matter modulates trigemino-vascular input: a role in migraine? Neuroscience 2001;106:793–800.
216. Knight YE, Bartsch T, Goadsby PJ. Trigeminal antinociception induced by bicu-culline in the periaqueductal grey (PAG) is not affected by PAG P/Q-type calcium channel blockade in rat. Neurosci Lett 2003;336:113–6.
217. Weiller C, May A, Limmroth V, et al. Brain stem activation in spontaneous human migraine attacks. Nat Med 1995;1:658–60.
218. Tracey I, Ploghaus A, Gati JS, et al. Imaging attentional modulation of pain in the periaqueductal gray in humans. J Neurosci 2002;22:2748–52.
219. Benjamin L, Levy MJ, Lasalandra MP, et al. Hypothalamic activation after stim-ulation of the superior sagittal sinus in the cat: a Fos study. Neurobiol Dis 2004; 16:500–5.
220. Matharu MS, Cohen AS, Frackowiak RSJ, et al. Posterior hypothalamic activa-tion in paroxysmal hemicrania. Ann Neurol 2006;59:535–45.
221. Giffin NJ, Ruggiero L, Lipton RB, et al. Premonitory symptoms in migraine: an electronic diary study. Neurology 2003;60:935–40.
222. Kelman L. The premonitory symptoms (prodrome): a tertiary care study of 893 migraineurs. Headache 2004;44:865–72.
223. Schoonman GG, Evers DJ, Terwindt GM, et al. The prevalence of premonitory symptoms in migraine: a questionnaire study in 461 patients. Cephalalgia 2006;26:1209–13.
224. Bes A, Geraud A, Guell A, et al. Dopaminergic hypersensitivity in migraine: a diagnostic test? Nouv Presse Med 1982;11:1475–8.
225. Peroutka SJ. Dopamine and migraine. Neurology 1997;49:650–6.
226. Bergerot A, Storer RJ, Goadsby PJ. Dopamine inhibits trigeminovascular trans-mission in the rat. Ann Neurol 2007;61:251–62.
227. Skagerberg G, Bjorklund A, Lindvall O, et al. Origin and termination of the diencephalo–spinal dopamine system in the rat. Brain Res Bull 1982;9: 237–44.
228. Charbit AR, Bergerot A, Goadsby PJ. Stimulation of dopaminergic A11 cell group inihibits nociceptive transmission in the trigeminal nucleus caudalis. Cephalalgia 2006;26:1383–4.
229. Charbit AR, Holland PR, Goadsby PJ. Stimulation or lesioning of dopaminergic A11 cell group affects neuronal firing in the trigeminal nucleus caudalis. Ceph-alalgia 2007;27:605.
230. Bartsch T, Levy MJ, Knight YE, et al. Differential modulation of nociceptive dural input to [hypocretin] Orexin A and B receptor activation in the posterior hypotha-lamic area. Pain 2004;109:367–78.
231. Holland PR, Akerman S, Lasalandra MP, et al. Hypothalamic neurons that contain orexin A and B express c-fos in response to superior sagittal sinus (SSS) stimulation in the cat. Cephalalgia 2005;25:1194–5.
232. Holland PR, Akerman S, Goadsby PJ. Orexin 1 receptor activation attenuates neurogenic dural vasodilation in an animal model of trigeminovascular nocicep-tion. J Pharmacol Exp Ther 2005;315:1380–5.
233. Holland PR, Akerman S, Goadsby PJ. Modulation of nociceptive dural input to the trigeminal nucleus caudalis via activation of the orexin 1 receptor in the rat. Eur J Neurosci 2006;24:2825–33.
234. Holland PR, Goadsby PJ. The hypothalamic orexinergic system: pain and primary headaches. Headache 2007;47:951–62.
235. Goadsby PJ. The vascular theory of migraine—a great story wrecked by the facts. Brain 2009;132:6–7.

236. Willis T. The anatomy of the brain and nerves. Tercentenary Edition—1964 edition. Montreal: McGill University Press; 1664.
237. Liveing E. On Megrim, sick headache, and some allied disorders. A contribution to the pathology of nerve storms. London: Arts & Boeve Nijmegen; 1873.
238. Gowers WR. A manual of diseases of the nervous system. Philadelphia: P. Blakiston, Son & Company; 1888.
239. Henrik S, Steffen B, Wienecke T, et al. PACAP38 indcues migraine-like attacks and vasodilatation—a causative role in migraine pathogenesis? Brain, 2009;132: in press.
240. Rahmann A, Wienecke T, Hansen JM, et al. Vasoactive intestinal peptide causes marked cephalic vasodilatation but does not induce migraine. Cephalalgia 2007;28:226–36.
241. Tunis MM, Wolff HG. Long term observations of the reactivity of the cranial arteries in subjects with vascular headache of the migraine type. Arch Neurol Psychiatry 1953;70:551–7.
242. Schoonman GG, van der Grond J, Kortmann C, et al. Migraine headache is not associated with cerebral or meningeal vasodilatation—a 3T magnetic resonance angiography study. Brain 2008;131:2192–200.
243. Humphrey PPA, Goadsby PJ. Controversies in headache. The mode of action of sumatriptan is vascular? A debate. Cephalalgia 1994;14:401–10.
244. Humphrey PPA, Feniuk W, Perren MJ, et al. Serotonin and migraine. Ann N Y Acad Sci 1990;600:587–98.
245. Petersen KA, Birk S, Lassen LH, et al. The CGRP-antagonist, BIBN4096BS does not affect cerebral or systemic haemodynamics in healthy volunteers. Cephalalgia 2005;25:139–47.
246. Denuelle M, Fabre N, Payoux P, et al. Brainstem and hypothalamic activation in spontaneous migraine attacks. Cephalalgia 2004;24:775–814.
247. Denuelle M, Fabre N, Payoux P, et al. Hypothalamic activation in spontaneous migraine attacks. Headache 2007;47:1418–26.
248. Matharu MS, Bartsch T, Ward N, et al. Central neuromodulation in chronic migraine patients with suboccipital stimulators: a PET study. Brain 2004;127: 220–30.
249. Afridi S, Matharu MS, Lee L, et al. A PET study exploring the laterality of brainstem activation in migraine using glyceryl trinitrate. Brain 2005;128:932–9.
250. Raskin NH, Hosobuchi Y, Lamb S. Headache may arise from perturbation of brain. Headache 1987;27:416–20.
251. Veloso F, Kumar K, Toth C. Headache secondary to deep brain implantation. Headache 1998;38:507–15.
252. Welch KM, Nagesh V, Aurora S, et al. Periaqueductal grey matter dysfunction in migraine: cause or the burden of illness? Headache 2001;41:629–37.
253. Goadsby PJ. Neurovascular headache and a midbrain vascular malformation—evidence for a role of the brainstem in chronic migraine. Cephalalgia 2002;22: 107–11.
254. Afridi S, Goadsby PJ. New onset migraine with a brainstem cavernous angioma. J Neurol Neurosurg Psychiatr 2003;74:680–2.
255. Goadsby PJ, Lambert GA, Lance JW. Differential effects on the internal and external carotid circulation of the monkey evoked by locus coeruleus stimulation. Brain Res 1982;249:247–54.
256. Goadsby PJ, Lambert GA, Lance JW. The mechanism of cerebrovascular vasoconstriction in response to locus coeruleus stimulation. Brain Res 1985;326: 213–7.

257. Goadsby PJ, Duckworth JW. Low frequency stimulation of the locus coeruleus reduces regional cerebral blood flow in the spinalized cat. Brain Res 1989; 476:71–7.

258. Goadsby PJ, Zagami AS, Lambert GA. Neural processing of craniovascular pain: a synthesis of the central structures involved in migraine. Headache 1991;31:365–71.

259. Kaube H, Giffin NJ. The electrophysiology of migraine. Curr Opin Neurol 2002; 15:303–9.

260. Schoenen J, Ambrosini A, Sandor PS, et al. Evoked potentials and transcranial magnetic stimulation in migraine: published data and viewpoint on their pathophysiologic significance. Clin Neurophysiol 2003;114:955–72.

261. Afra J, Sandor P, Schoenen J. Habituation of visual and intensity dependence of cortical auditory evoked potentials tend to normalise just before and during migraine attacks. Cephalalgia 2000;20:347.

262. Proietti-Cecchini A, Afra J, Schoenen J. Intensity dependence of the cortical auditory evoked potentials as a surrogate marker of central nervous system serotonin transmission in man: demonstration of a central effect for the 5HT1B/1D agonist zolmitriptan (311C90, Zomig). Cephalalgia 1997;17:849–54.

263. Schoenen J, Wang W, Albert A, et al. Potentiation instead of habituation characterizes visual evoked potentials in migraine patients between attacks. Eur J Neurol 1995;2:115–22.

264. Wang W, Schoenen J. Interictal potentiation of passive oddball auditory event-related potentials in migraine. Cephalalgia 1998;18:261–5.

265. Di Clemente L, Coppola G, Magis D, et al. Interictal habituation deficit of the nociceptive blink reflex: an endophenotypic marker for presymptomatic migraine? Brain 2007;130:765–70.

266. Schoenen J, Timsit-Berthier M. Contingent negative variation: methods and potential interest in headache. Cephalalgia 1993;13:28–32.

267. Kropp P, Gerber WD. Prediction of migraine attacks using a slow cortical potential, the contingent negative variation. Neurosci Lett 1998;257:73–6.

268. Maertens de Noordhout A, Timsit-Berthier M, Schoenen J. Contingent negative variation (CNV) in migraineurs before and during prophylactic treatment with beta-blockers. Cephalalgia 1985;5(Suppl 3):34–5.

269. Coppola G, Vandenheede M, Di Clemente L, et al. Somatosensory evoked high-frequency oscillations reflecting thalamo–cortical activity are decreased in migraine patients between attacks. Brain 2005;128:98–103.

270. Gantenbein A, Goadsby PJ, Kaube H. Introduction of a clinical scoring system for migraine research applied to electrophysiological studies. Cephalalgia 2004; 24:1095–6.

271. Kruuse C, Thomsen LL, Birk S, et al. Migraine can be induced by sildenafil without changes in middle cerebral artery diameter. Brain 2003;126:241–7.

272. Limmroth V, May A, Auerbach P, et al. Changes in cerebral blood flow velocity after treatment with sumatriptan or placebo and implications for the pathophysiology of migraine. J Neurol Sci 1996;138:60–5.

273. Niebur E, Hsiao SS, Johnson KO. Synchrony: a neural mechanism for attentional selection? Curr Opin Neurobiol 2002;12:190–4.

274. Angelini L, de Tommaso M, Guido M, et al. Steady-state visual evoked potentials and phase synchronization in migraine patients. Phys Rev Lett 2004;93. 038103-1–038103-4.

275. Goadsby PJ. Migraine pathophysiology. The brainstem governs the cortex. Cephalalgia 2003;23:565–6.

Transient Neurologic Dysfunction in Migraine

Rod Foroozan, MD[a],*, F. Michael Cutrer, MD[b]

KEYWORDS

- Migraine • Aura • Persistent aura • Retinal migraine
- Pathophysiology • Genetics

One of the most striking characteristics of migraine is the occurrence of transient neurologic dysfunction during the course of acute attacks. The symptoms, collectively termed "aura," are the source of significant concern when first experienced by migraineurs. The prominence of these symptoms in medical historical writings that pertain to migraine has obscured the fact that they occur in only about a quarter of migraine sufferers and that they do not occur in every attack experienced by those who have the aura. Although within the general population migraine is likely to be one of the most common if not the most common setting for the combination of neurologic symptoms and headache, it is by no means the only setting in which the combination occurs. Care should be taken that neurologic symptoms identified as "migrainous" are truly consistent with the aura in terms of duration, development, and quality. Misidentification of neurologic symptoms as migrainous may delay correct diagnosis and treatment.

In this article we will discuss the aura as it occurs in the context of a migraine attack and review each of the major types: visual, sensory, and language aura. Because visual aura is the most common and the most well studied, it will be discussed in some detail and a thorough differential diagnosis presented.

GENERAL CLINICAL FEATURES OF MIGRAINE WITH AURA

Until the most recent International Headache Society (IHS) criteria were published in 2004 (International Classification of Headache Disorders 2 [ICHD2], 2004), the aura was classified into four types: (1) visual aura, by far the most common; (2) sensory aura and (3) language aura, which occur less commonly; and (4) motor aura, the least common. At present, the International Headache Society recognizes motor aura as

[a] Department of Ophthalmology, Baylor College of Medicine, Cullen Eye Institute, 6565 Fannin NC-205, Houston, TX 77030, USA
[b] Department of Neurology, Mayo Clinic, 200 First Street SW, Rochester, MN 55902, USA
* Corresponding author.
E-mail address: foroozan@bcm.tmc.edu (R. Foroozan).

Neurol Clin 27 (2009) 361–378
doi:10.1016/j.ncl.2008.11.002
0733-8619/08/$ – see front matter © 2009 Elsevier Inc. All rights reserved.

neurologic.theclinics.com

a key manifestation of a specific type of migraine, hemiplegic migraine (HM). The reclassification is based on increasing genetic data in the familial hemiplegic form of hemiplegic migraine. While a detailed discussion of familial hemiplegic migraine (FHM) is beyond the scope of this review, it should be pointed out that patients with FHM usually report typical auras also.

Migraine with typical aura is a recurrent condition characterized by reversible neurologic symptoms, which typically develop over 5 to 20 minutes and resolve within 60 minutes. Migraine headache usually follows the aura, although, less commonly, pain may not be present. Visual symptoms are the most common manifestations in migraine aura. Typical aura with migraine has been characterized by the following criteria put forward by the IHS,[1] and the sensitivity and specificity of these criteria appear to be high:[2]

A. At least two attacks fulfill criteria B to E
B. Fully reversible visual or sensory or speech symptoms but no motor weakness
C. At least two of the three following:
  1. Homonymous visual symptoms includes positive features (flickering lights, spots, lines) or negative features (loss of vision) or unilateral sensory symptoms
  2. At least one symptom develops gradually within 5 minutes or different symptoms occur in succession
  3. Each symptom lasts between 5 and 60 minutes
D. Headache that meets criteria for B–D for migraine without aura, begins during the aura, or follows the aura within 60 minutes
E. Not attributed to another disorder

There are certain characteristics of visual and sensory auras that may be used to distinguish them from ischemia-related symptoms. Both sensory and visual auras have a slow migratory or spreading quality in which symptoms slowly spread across the affected body part or the visual field, followed by a gradual return to normal function in the areas first affected after 20 to 60 minutes. This spreading quality is not characteristic of an ischemic event in which neurologic deficits tend to appear somewhat suddenly and tend to be equally distributed within the relevant vascular territory.[3] In stroke, the affected area can certainly expand as blood flow drops in additional vessels; however, ischemic change is a more step-wise and less a smoothly spreading process. Although a migratory pattern is also seen in partial seizure disorders, its progression is generally much more rapid. Neither ischemia nor seizure are associated with the return of function in the areas first affected, even as symptoms are simultaneously appearing in newly affected areas.

Another feature which is suggestive of migraine aura is a tendency for different neurologic symptoms to occur sequentially. Almost all patients experiencing more than one type of aura during a single attack first recount the appearance of one aura type (most often visual), which is then followed by another aura type. Some patients experience all three typical auras in sequence during a single attack. In almost twenty years of asking patients to describe their aura, none have reported the appearance of all aura types at the same time.[3] In contrast to migraine aura, the simultaneous manifestation of multiple types of neurologic symptoms is, however, quite common in cerebral ischemia.

In addition, migraine aura often has a biphasic quality inherent in its neurologic symptoms—with positive phenomena (eg, shimmering lights, zigzagging visual disturbances, or tingling paresthesias) appearing first, only to be followed within a few minutes by negative symptoms (eg, scotoma, loss of visual image or numbness, or loss of sensation). Ischemic events do not tend to exhibit a bimodal progression of symptoms and while there may be a biphasic progression in the course of a seizure, progression is likely to occur at a much faster rate. In the language aura, making the same biphasic analogy is more difficult. While patients experiencing the language aura report both paraphasic errors and word retrieval errors (abnormal function), migraineurs seldom become mute (loss of function) during language aura. Assessing basic language function is complex given the importance of context. Obtaining accurate descriptions of language dysfunction during aura is also problematic because of the difficulties in laying down precise memories while language is disturbed.

The unilateral motor symptoms previously considered motor aura before their reassignment to the HM category actually differ in a couple of basic characteristics from the more common forms of aura. There is no apparent spread of symptoms over the course of an hour. In FHM, motor symptoms do not have positive and negative phases. No twitching or migratory spasm before weakness is noted by patients with hemiplegic migraine. However, the most prominent difference is the much greater average duration of motor weakness with HM. Patients with HM often have unilateral weakness for hours to days—which is much longer than the 60 minutes or less reported in the other aura types. As our knowledge of the pathophysiological mechanisms of each aura type improves, so will our understanding of whether or not the motor aura arises from a process analogous to those underlying the more common aura types.

EPIDEMIOLOGY OF MIGRAINE AURA

In a large population-based study, nosographic analysis of migraine aura from the mid 1990's, 163 patients were identified with migraine aura in a random, Danish sampling of 4,000 people.[4] In this sample, visual aura was by far the most common symptom, occurring in 99% of subjects; this was followed by sensory and, then, by language auras. In 64% of patients, only visual aura occurred; whereas the other aura types typically happened in combination with another aura type (usually visual).[5] Among 491 patients with migraine with aura, drawn from 1148 migraine patients entered into the Mayo Clinic Headache Registry, 489 (99%) reported having at least two episodes of visual aura, 225 (45%) language aura, 198 (40%) sensory aura, and 53 (11%) motor aura. Also noted in this population was a higher occurrence of nonvisual aura symptoms in the absence of visual disturbance (Cutrer, unpublished data, 2006).

TRANSIENT NEUROLOGIC DISTURBANCE IN MIGRAINE
Visual System Disturbance

Afferent visual dysfunction associated with migraine
Migraine is one of the most commonly seen disorders which cause transient visual loss. Afferent visual dysfunction is the most common sensory symptom in migraine with aura. Although efferent dysfunction has been reported with migraine (ophthalmoplegic migraine),[6] we will focus solely on the afferent manifestation of visual loss and visual hallucinations.

Migraine visual aura
One classic form of visual aura is the fortification spectra (teichopsia), a jagged figure which builds or spreads outward (more commonly than inward) and leaves variable areas of visual loss behind (**Fig. 1**).[3,7,8] The fortification lines are typically arranged at right angles to one another and begin from a paracentral area or "germ" (**Fig. 2**).[7]

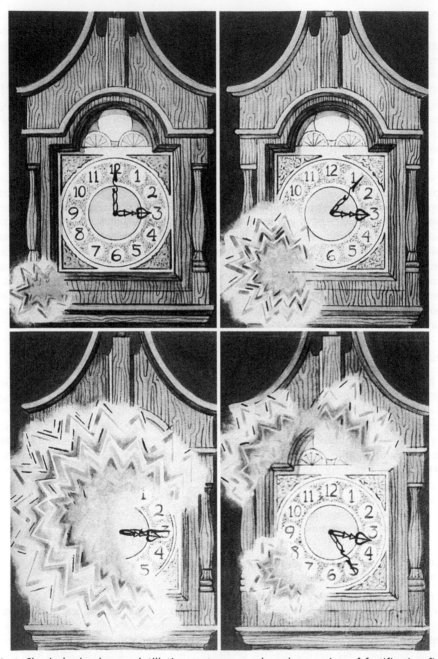

Fig. 1. Classical migrainous scintillating scotoma march and expansion of fortification figures. Initial small paracentral scotoma (*top left*). Enlarging scotoma 7 minutes later (*top right*). Scotoma obscuring much of central vision 15 minutes later (*bottom left*). Break-up of scotoma at 20 minutes (*bottom right*). *From* Hupp SL, Kline LB, Corbett JJ. Visual disturbances of migraine. Surv Ophthalmol 1989;33(4):221–36; with permission.

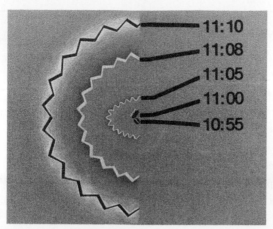

Fig. 2. Expansion of the visual aura of migraine from a "germ" in the paracentral visual field occurring over 15 minutes. *Reproduced from* Hupp SL, Kline LB, Corbett JJ. Visual disturbances of migraine. Surv Ophthalmol 1989;33(4):221–36; with permission.

There are often scintillations (which may be the most common visual symptom in migraine visual aura) that assume a semicircle or C shape, surrounding an area of visual loss (scotoma). The scintillations may be white, gray, or have colors similar to a kaleidoscope. Visual field defects often begin around fixation and spread outward. Scintillating scotomas are typically within one hemifield. Most commonly, these visual symptoms last 20 to 30 minutes in their entirety.

Other characteristic visual phenomena associated with migraine include sparkles, visual distortion (metamorphopsia), the appearance of objects being too large (macropsia) or too small (micropsia), visual perseveration (palinopsia), and the appearance of multiple images (cerebral polyopia). General visual blurring, like looking through a film or water, even without clear visual field loss, may be present. Objects may be seen as shimmering (such as "heat waves" on pavement) or rotating. Distortions of body image have been described in the "Alice in Wonderland" syndrome, thought to be more common in younger patients with migraine aura.[9] Central color vision loss (dyschromatopsia) and loss of facial recognition (prosopagnosia) may occur.[10] Environmental tilt may be present. Patients may complain of excessive brightness or light sensitivity (photophobia).

For diagnostic purposes, it may be helpful to show illustrations of migraine aura to patients with similar visual phenomena. A number of authors have detailed their own experience with migraine visual aura, often with accompanying illustrations.[3] A number of examples of visual hallucinations related to migraine are depicted by Schott.[11] Although each of these symptoms may be characteristic of migraine, other ocular and neurologic disorders may cause visual symptoms and should be distinguished from migraine visual aura (**Box 1**).

Migraine aura may occur in the absence of headache (previously termed acephalgic migraine or migrainous accompaniments). This has been labeled by the IHS as typical aura without headache. The aura fulfills all of the criteria for migraine with aura. Visual dysfunction is the most common feature of migraine aura without headache, occurring 75% of the time.[7]

Persistent migraine visual aura

Persistent migraine visual aura most commonly consists of positive visual phenomena. These most commonly are formed (shapes or figures) or unformed (lights

Box 1
Causes of transient visual disturbance of afferent visual system

Monocular

    Refractive error—myopia

    Vitreoretinal traction

    Inflammation—vitritis/retinitis/optic neuritis

    Amaurosis fugax—retinal microembolism

    Papilledema

    Optic disc drusen

    Congenital dysplasia of the optic disc

    Coagulopathies

    Vasculitis

    Hypotension—arrhythmia/orthostatic

    Anemia

    Ocular migraine

Binocular

    Migraine

    Seizure

    Occipital mass lesion—tumor or arteriovenous malformation

    Occipital ischemia—embolic, vasculitis, hypoperfusion

Reprinted from Hupp SL, Kline LB, Corbett JJ. Visual disturbances of migraine. Surv Ophthalmol 1989;33(4):221–36; with permission.

or sparkles) visual hallucinations.[12] The hallucinations are rarely more complex (metamorphopsia, palinopsia). Other ocular and neurologic conditions may cause these types of visual symptoms so that the diagnosis of persistent migraine visual aura is generally one of exclusion. There are no clear guidelines as to what tests should be performed to exclude other conditions (for example seizures, toxic-metabolic conditions, retinal inflammatory conditions, and psychiatric disease) which may cause persistent visual symptoms.

The IHS lists persistent migraine aura as a diagnosis with the following criteria:[1]
    Previous attacks fulfilling criteria for migraine with aura.
    The present attack is typical of previous attacks, but one or more aura symptoms persist for more than 2 weeks.
    Not attributed to another disorder.

There are no neuroimaging findings suggesting infarction. Most patients have hallucinations which are unformed and cover the entire visual field of both eyes. Although in some patients there is a clear history of migraine before the onset of symptoms,[13] in others the link to migraine is more tenuous. Prior reports have noted that most patients with persistent migraine visual aura have no abnormalities on routine neuroimaging, electroencephalography, and ophthalmic examination. One report has noted hyperhomocysteinaemia in two patients with persistent visual auras which spontaneously resolved, but a cause-and-effect relationship remains unclear.[14]

Two descriptive patterns have been particularly common in patients with persistent visual aura. One is "visual snow" (sometimes referred to as primary persistent visual disturbance); the other is "television static." There have been Web sites created with forums for discussion for patients with these symptoms (eg, www.visualsnow.com). Some patients notice symptoms only under certain lighting conditions or in certain circumstances. Not all patients with these symptoms have a clear history of migraine and, in some, the diagnosis of persistent migraine visual aura has been inferred because no other causes were evident. These visual symptoms may represent a distinct clinical disorder. Some authors have suggested that they be regarded as distinct from those with persistent migraine visual aura.[15]

The cause of persistent migraine visual aura remains unclear, but may be related to abnormal cortical neuronal inhibition. Single photon emission computed tomography and perfusion MRI have been reported to be abnormal during the persistent aura, which lasted 7 months, within one hemifield of a patient.[16] Perfusion MRI performed after the symptoms resolved was normal. Cortical spreading edema, with restricted diffusion which spontaneously resolved, has been noted in a patient with persistent migraine visual aura.[17] However, in patients with persistent visual aura (visual snow) no abnormality was noted on diffusion- or perfusion-weighted MRI.[15]

In some patients persistent aura may resolve spontaneously after a period of weeks to months; however, in others they may persist. Treatment of persistent visual aura has been attempted on a patient-by-patient basis, without clear success for one particular agent. Some success has been reported with antiepileptic agents including lamotrigine and valproate.[18,19]

Persistent visual loss

Although most commonly transient, visual loss associated with migraine may be persistent. The visual loss may include loss of visual acuity or visual field. Fixed visual loss associated with migraine has been reported from involvement of multiple areas of the afferent visual pathway. Although migraine has been associated with pathology in each of these sites in the visual pathway, conclusive evidence is largely still lacking to support a definitive cause-and-effect relationship.

Retinopathy (choroidopathy) Persistent visual loss related to migraine has been described from retinal artery and vein occlusions, and retinal hemorrhages (see section on retinal migraine). Central serous choroidopathy and choroidopathy presumably from ischemia have been attributed to migraine.[20]

Anterior ischemic optic neuropathy Anterior ischemic optic neuropathy (AION) is thought to involve infarction of the optic nerve head. It is the most common acute optic neuropathy which affects patients over the age of 50 years. Painless visual loss occurs over a period of days and is associated with signs of an optic neuropathy including a relative afferent pupillary defect (when unilateral or asymmetric), dyschromatopsia, and nerve fiber bundle or central visual field defects. Optic disc edema is present acutely, presumably because the anterior portion of the optic nerve is affected, and there is subsequent resolution of the disc swelling and the development of optic disc pallor over weeks to months.

Patients in whom migraine has been reported to be a cause of AION have generally been younger (under the age of 50 years).[21–25] Most patients reported with migraine-associated AION developed unilateral optic neuropathy, and were women. The severity of visual loss is variable with visual acuities from 20/15 (with mild nerve fiber bundle visual field defects) to light perception. In some patients reported to have migraine-associated AION, including the youngest reported, an 11 year old with sickle cell trait, the diagnosis is not clear because there was no documentation of optic disc edema.[26] The onset of visual loss has been temporally related to an episode of migraine headache, and in all reported patients there was a history of chronic migraine.

Posterior ischemic optic neuropathy Posterior ischemic optic neuropathy (PION) is an uncommon type of ischemic optic neuropathy, which results from infarction of the intraorbital, intracanalicular, or intracranial optic nerve. The diagnosis of PION is made after other causes of retrobulbar optic neuropathy have been excluded. The clinical findings are similar to AION except that, acutely following the ischemic event in PION, funduscopic examination of the optic discs is normal, in contradistinction to the presence of optic disc edema in AION.

Three patients (in two reports) with migraine-associated PION have been reported.[27,28] All three were women in their 20s who developed unilateral optic neuropathy with little or no loss of visual acuity and nerve fiber bundle type visual field defects. Two of the three patients had no other identifiable vascular risk factors apart from migraine.

Optic neuropathy related to ergotamine derivatives and treatment of migraine Ergot derivatives are known to cause vasoconstriction and may cause unwanted ischemic side effects such as stroke and myocardial infarction. Two reports of ischemic optic neuropathy[29,30] and a third with bilateral "papillitis" and optic disc edema with a macular star[31] have been reported. Ergotamine-induced vasospasm was suggested as the cause.

Migraine and optic disc drusen Optic disc drusen (hyaline bodies) are crystalline structures located within the anterior portion of the optic nerve. They occur in about 1 in 500 people and are bilateral in 75% of patients.[32] The precise pathophysiology of optic disc drusen remains unclear, but continued calcium deposition due to abnormal axonal metabolism is thought to be the underlying cause. Optic disc drusen may be buried (not visible ophthalmoscopically) before they become visible during ophthalmoscopy. In both cases the optic disc may become elevated or swollen and resemble optic disc edema from elevated intracranial pressure. Patients are typically asymptomatic or have mild nerve fiber bundle visual field defects;[33] however, vascular complications, including retinal artery occlusions, retinal parapapillary hemorrhages,[34] and AION, have been reported in patients with optic disc drusen.

An association of migraine and optic disc drusen has been reported.[35] A 25 year old with migraine had sequential central retinal artery occlusions over an 8 year period and was found to have optic disc drusen.[36] The authors suggested that optic disc drusen and migraine may have combined to cause the visual loss. They also suggested that the apparent association of migraine and optic disc drusen may reflect the referral of patients with headache and elevated optic discs. Given how common each of these disorders is, the association between migraine and optic disc drusen may be coincidental.

Migraine and stroke Persistent visual loss may occur as a result from stroke involving the posterior visual pathways.[37,38] The precise relationship between migraine and stroke remains unclear. Some studies have suggested that oral contraceptives may increase the risk of stroke in patients with migraine. Migraine aura has been reported to be risk factor for stroke in young women.[37] The IHS specifies that migrainous infarction occurs when the stroke can be directly attributable to migraine.[1]

Stroke from migraine would be expected to cause a homonymous hemianopia,[39] an exception being the unilateral temporal visual field loss associated with the temporal crescent syndrome.

Retinal migraine

Migraine has long been listed as one cause of monocular transient visual loss (TVL). The assumption has been that transient loss of perfusion of the ocular circulation may occur in a similar fashion that is thought to occur in relation to vasospasm from migraine. The terminology for this potential process has been confusing and has included "ocular migraine" and "retinal migraine." The term retinal migraine has been attributed to Carroll's[40] description in 1970. In addition, the assumption has been that only the retinal circulation may be involved. However, TVL may also occur from impairment of the circulation to the choroid or optic nerve.

Visual symptoms include graying of vision or complete visual loss, sparkles or flashes, and a shade over a portion of the visual field in one eye. In most patients visual symptoms last less than 30 minutes.[7] Some of the ambiguity in the diagnosis of TVL from migraine comes from the difficulty patients have distinguishing monocular visual loss from visual loss within the same hemifield in both eyes.[41] In addition, monocular temporal visual symptoms from disorders of the visual cortex (temporal crescent syndrome) may cause confusion with disorders involving the anterior visual pathways. As alternative theories of the pathogenesis of migraine have evolved, so has the notion that retinal migraine is a common cause of TVL.

The IHS has provided criteria for the diagnosis of retinal migraine.[1] They include:

Description:
   Repeated attacks of monocular visual disturbance, including scintillations, scotomata, or blindness, associated with migraine headache

Diagnostic criteria:
   A. At least two attacks fulfilling criteria B and C
   B. Fully reversible monocular positive or negative visual phenomena (scintillations, scotomata, or blindness) confirmed by examination during an attack or (after proper instruction) by the patient's drawing of a monocular field defect during an attack
   C. Headache, fulfilling criteria B–D for Migraine without aura begins during the visual symptoms or follows them within 60 minutes
   D. Normal ophthalmologic examination between attacks
   E. Not attributed to another disorder

The criteria suggest that retinal migraine is a cause for recurrent, stereotypical episodes of monocular TVL which occurs during a migraine headache.[42] The criteria also imply that before the diagnosis of retinal migraine is made patients should undergo a thorough evaluation to exclude other causes of monocular TVL.

An extension of this definition (this point is controversial; see the next two paragraphs and the section on persistent visual loss) has included patients with persistent monocular visual loss, including those with retinal infarction, and even those who have had visual symptoms and fulfilled the other criteria but lacked the headache.[43] Some reports have included photographic evidence of retinal ischemia, including changes within the retinal vasculature, suggestive of central or branch retinal artery occlusions, which have occurred in the setting of an otherwise typical migraine headache.[44–46]

The incidence of retinal migraine and the existence of the condition itself remain hotly contested topics.[41,47–50] In a review, IHS criteria were used to identify 46 patients (6 new patients and 40 from the literature) with retinal migraine.[43] In some cases patients were included with incomplete evaluations of monocular visual loss when the episodes occurred in the context of migraine headaches. The typical attack was characterized by visual loss lasting less than 1 hour and occurring on the same side as the headache. The authors of this report noted that patients with retinal migraine were more commonly women with aura. Symptoms could be negative (visual loss) or positive (scintillations). The monocular visual loss from retinal migraine may accompany or may precede the headache, whereas in migraine with aura the visual symptoms typically precede the headache. Forty-three percent of patients ultimately experienced permanent monocular visual loss, possibly representing a form of migrainous infarction. They noted that this high rate of permanent visual loss may suggest the benefit of prophylactic therapy. Finally, the authors proposed changing the term "retinal migraine" to "migraine associated with monocular visual symptoms."

These findings differ from those of another report, a literature review, which used a more strict IHS definition and categorized 142 patients with transient (103 patients) or fixed (39 patients) visual symptoms attributed to retinal migraine reported in 60 different manuscripts.[51] Of these, only 16 with monocular TVL had findings suggestive of retinal migraine. Only 5 fulfilled the criteria for definite retinal migraine. Furthermore, none of the patients with persistent visual loss (for example from retinal arterial occlusion and ischemic optic neuropathy) could be categorized as having definite retinal migraine. Instead they suggested that the cause of monocular TVL in the patients presumed to have retinal migraine may be vasospasm or some other cause of anterior visual pathway pathology in the presence of headache or eye pain. Patients with vasospasm involving the ocular circulation have responded favorably to calcium-channel blockers.[52]

It appears that using a strict definition of retinal migraine proposed by the IHS, the majority of patients reported with monocular TVL and reported as having retinal migraine do not strictly fulfill the IHS criteria, and suggest the need for a thorough evaluation to exclude other causes of TVL. Nevertheless, there are some descriptions of monocular visual loss which appear to fit the criteria inarguably.[53]

The underlying cause of retinal migraine remains unclear. The same two broad theories as for cortical migraine have been suggested: vasospasm, which may account for some patients with persistence of visual loss from arterial occlusion, and neuronal spreading depression. Thus far, the evidence for spreading depression within the retina has not been as supported as that for the cerebral cortex.[51]

Visual field loss in migraine

Visual field abnormalities related to migraine and migraine aura are well known[54] and, most commonly, resolve completely. However, there is also a high rate of visual field defects in patients with migraine who are otherwise visually asymptomatic between attacks.[55] Using automated perimetry, 21 (35%) of 60 patients with migraine were found to have some abnormality on visual field testing.[56] Visual field loss was more common in those who were older or had a longer duration of disease. In another study, 3 (20%) of 15 patients were noted to have deficits on automated perimetry.[57] Kinetic perimetry, performed at least 7 days after an episode of migraine, has also revealed defects which have improved over time.[58] Test–retest variability during automated perimetry has been noted to be increased in patients with migraine.[59] Both length of migraine history and frequency of attacks appear to correlate with lower sensitivity on perimetry.[60] Generalized decreased sensitivity and focal deficits can be seen.

Visual field deficits have been noted using short-wavelength automated perimetry;[61] and some authors have suggested a deficit in a specific retinal circuit.[62] Several reports have linked migraine with glaucoma, including low-tension glaucoma.[63] Visual field defects in some studies have suggested precortical (anterior visual pathway) pathology. A study of 16 patients with migraine (15 with aura), used both static and temporally modulated targets with an automated perirmeter. Perimetry was conducted 7 days after the onset of a headache. Visual field losses were noted with temporal modulation perimetry in 11 of 16 migraine patients, even in the presence of normal static visual fields. The authors suggested that this pattern is similar to that seen in the early stages of glaucoma.[57]

Sensory System Dysfunction in Migraine

The migraine sensory aura most often starts as unilateral tingling or "paresthesias" in a hand or distal arm, which slowly migrates proximally, only to jump from the arm to the ipsilateral face before reaching the shoulder. The crawling, tingling sensation moves from the cheek and side of the nose, across the perioral region and lips, then spreads inside the mouth, to involve the ipsilateral buccal mucosa and half of the tongue.[3] Paresthesias or a "feeling of needles and pins" are usually the first sensory symptoms, leaving numbness in their wake,[64] although auras which consist of numbness primarily also occur. Russell and Olesen, in a study of 51 patients with sensory aura, reported that the hand (96% of cases) and face (67%) were the body parts most commonly affected, whereas the leg (24%) and torso (18%) were much less likely to be involved. The sensory symptoms, recorded in Russell and Olesen's series of individuals, progressed for less than 30 minutes (82%). The unilateral symptoms of sensory aura are frequently quite distressing for patients, especially at their first appearance, because of their similarity to those of stroke or transient ischemic attack. Although the presence of migraine aura does, in fact, seem to be an independent risk factor of ischemic stroke in women who have a low level of other cardiovascular risk factors,[65] the overall increase in absolute risk attributable to migraine with aura when compared with other factors is modest. There are clinical features that help to distinguish sensory aura from stroke. The spread of paresthesias across the face and into the mouth to affect half the tongue is a classical feature of migraine sensory aura and is rarely seen in cases of cerebrovascular ischemia.[66]

Language System Aura Dysfunction

Because it is relatively uncommon, language disturbance during migraine aura may be overlooked in the history unless the patient is specifically asked about it. While speech disturbance may result from numbness and tingling in the mouth or tongue, as the sensory aura gradually migrates intraorally, this is distinct from language aura. In language aura, patients have impaired language comprehension, marked word-finding difficulties, and a decreased ability to read or write—implying more than just a pure sensory or proprioceptive disturbance. Interestingly, language aura seems to occur with a higher frequency in patients with hemiplegic migraine than in those with typical aura only (approximately 20% in typical aura versus 47% in hemiplegic migraine).[67] In another series of patients with language aura, 76% had paraphasic errors, 72% had other production problems and 38% had impaired comprehension.[4] Fortunately, the very distressing symptoms of language disturbance tend to persist for less than 30 minutes in most patients.[4] A recent questionnaire based on case series reported other instances of symptomatic cortical dysfunction including proper name anomia, ideational apraxia, and proposagnosia.[10]

PATHOPHYSIOLOGY OF MIGRAINE AURA

The aura has figured prominently in migraine pathophysiological research. Until the 1980s, the vasogenic theory of migraine was used to explain the aura. It postulated that the aura occurred as the consequence of an initial vasoconstrictive phase in the migraine attack. However, as early as the 1940s, proponents of the neurogenic theory of migraine hypothesized that the aura was the clinical manifestation of a spreading abnormality which moved over the visual cortex at a rate of 3 to 5 mm per minute. This spreading abnormality was believed to be atypical for ischemia. Around the same time, Leao,[68] a neurophysiologist, described an electrophysiological phenomenon, characterized by cortical hyperexcitation followed by suppression, which originated and migrated over areas of contiguous cortex in experimental animals at a slow rate of 3 to 4 mm per minute, after chemical or mechanical stimulations. This phenomenon, which Leao called cortical spreading depression (CSD), has been proposed as the cause of migraine aura, based on its slow rate of cortical spread which is similar to that extrapolated for migraine aura across visual cortex.[69] The fact that both CSD and aura move across neurovascular boundaries strengthens this hypothesis. The neurogenic theory proposes that the drops in blood flow observed during migraine aura are the direct consequence of reduced metabolic demand in abnormally functioning neurons, rather than the vasoconstriction. Evidence from functional imaging techniques, applied during the aura phase in humans, has increasingly supported the neurogenic theory.

Functional Neuroimaging and the Migraine Aura

Beginning in the early 1980s, various functional imaging techniques[70–72] employed during aura symptoms have supported a CSD or CSD-like phenomenon as the underlying mechanism of the migraine aura. One of the most recent of these studies applied blood-oxygen-level–dependent (BOLD) imaging, to aura. BOLD imaging is based on known increases in MRI signal intensity that occur in response to decreases in local deoxyhemoglobin concentration.[73] In this study, BOLD imaging was performed before, during and after exercise-induced visual auras.[74] BOLD imaging was also performed during aura symptoms in two spontaneous auras. During visual aura there was a loss of cortical activation to visual stimuli in the occipital lobe contralateral to the visual field in which a scotoma was reported by the patient. As the visual symptoms resolved, cortical activation within the affected occipital lobe returned to normal. In the study of the induced aura, BOLD imaging was initiated after exercise but before the onset of symptoms, was performed continuously during the visual symptoms, and was continued well into the headache phase after complete resolution of the visual symptoms. With the onset of the aura symptoms, loss of cortical activation to visual stimulation was observed first in V3a, an area of visual association cortex, rather than in the primary visual cortex. Over the next 30 to 40 minutes, the portion of visual cortex which was unresponsive to visual stimulation expanded to involve neighboring occipital cortex at a rate of 3.5 mm per minute, eventually encompassing large areas of the ipsilateral primary visual and association cortices. The BOLD functional MRI (fMRI) findings observed during human migraine aura are very similar to those that have been seen in CSD induced in animal experiments,[75] indicating that a human process analogous to CSD might be the source of migraine visual aura. It is important to note that findings from two cases of spontaneous migraine visual aura studied with BOLD imaging were the same as those observed during later time points in the exercise-induced aura.

Findings from fMRI performed on patients experiencing prolonged or persistent aura have been inconsistent.[15,16,76,77]

Altered Cortical Function in Migraine with Aura

There is accumulating evidence that differences in patients who experience migraine aura have altered cortical function. Such differences may account for their susceptibility to recurrent episodes of aura. In the 1980s and 1990s,[31] P magnetic resonance spectroscopic (MRS) studies indicated altered phosphocreatinine/inorganic phosphate ratios (index of brain phosphorylation potential),[78,79] indicating altered neuronal energy metabolism. Other MRS studies have shown low magnesium levels in the occipital cortex of migraine aura sufferers,[80] suggesting lowered thresholds for induction of a CSD or CSD-like phenomenon by way of disinhibition of NMDA receptor activity.[81] Interestingly, a more recent MRS study of migraine aura revealed that patients who experienced purely visual aura had baseline elevated lactate levels which showed no changes despite prolonged visual stimulation between migraine attacks. Conversely, patients who reported experiencing episodes of visual aura symptoms plus an additional aura type (sensory, language, or motor) had levels of brain lactate which were not elevated compared with those in healthy controls, but increased rather sharply with prolonged visual stimulation.[82] The causes of these unexpected findings are not clear.

Electrophysiological studies, which have employed various evoked potential modalities, have consistently demonstrated a decrease in habituation in the cortex of migraineurs with aura after repeated stimulation compared with normal controls. This altered habituation response has led to the hypothesis that a deficiency in habituation related to abnormal functioning in the subcortical aminergic pathways is critical in vulnerability to aura.[83] Other electrophysiological evidence from transcranial magnetic stimulation-based studies also indicates altered cortical excitability in migraineurs who experience aura.[84] Although all of the details of altered cortical processing in patients who experience the aura are not yet available, the body of evidence indicating that such differences exist is growing. There seems to be an increasing likelihood that such differences are important in the generation of the aura.

Genetic Factors

Currently, it is clear that the propensity to experience recurrent episodes of migraine aura are to a large extent genetically determined. Several genetic loci have been linked to typical migraine with aura (**Table 1**). This list excludes the genetic loci linked to FHM.

Table 1
Loci with reported association with migraine aura

Chromosome/Locus	Gene/Protein	Migraine Type	Reference
1 p36	MTHF-R	MA	86
4 q24	?	MA	87
6 p12–21	?	MA MO	88
6 q25.1	Estrogen receptor 1 (ESR1)	MA & MO	89
11 q22–23	Progesterone receptor (PGR)	MA & MO	90
11 q23	Dopamine D2 (DRD2) Ncol	MA	91
11 q23	Dopamine D2 (DRD2) Ncol	MA	92
11 q24	?	MA	93
15 q11–q13	?GABA-A	MA	94
17 q11.1–q12	Human serotonin transporter (SLC6A4)	MA & MO	95

Abbreviations: MA, migraine with aura; MO, migraine without aura; MTHF-R, Methylenetetrahydrofolate reductase.

However, one should remember that patients with FHM may also experience typical auras.

The genetic determinants of migraine aura probably consist of a number of loci which, based on the presence of certain polymorphisms, confer greater or lesser susceptibility to aura. Each of these potential "susceptibility genes" individually have a low-to-moderate effect.[85] It is the vector sum of these effects that determine, for a given individual, his or her overall level of susceptibility to aura and many of the clinical features of their migraine syndrome in general. It is also possible that when susceptibility conferring polymorphisms occur in the same individual, they might act synergistically to produce the migraine phenotype. Such complex genetic interactions will probably be difficult to detect by traditional single-locus linkage analysis and will probably require association studies performed in very large samples.

SUMMARY

Neurologic symptoms that accompany migraine in about one quarter of migraine patients are classically transient and occur as the result of cortical phenomena. Visual symptoms of migraine aura are by far the most common type. The visual aura may include positive and negative symptoms which occur within the homonymous visual field and characteristically last in the range of 30 minutes. Persistent migraine visual aura is uncommon and may be a distinct entity from primary persistent visual disturbance (visual snow). Transient monocular visual symptoms associated with migraine (often referred to as "retinal migraine") may be less frequent than originally suggested. Migraine has rarely been associated with fixed visual loss (most commonly from stroke, ischemic optic neuropathy, or retinal vascular occlusion), but evidence for a cause-and-effect mechanism remains somewhat limited. Other aura symptoms include unilateral sensory symptoms and language disturbance. Until recently, motor symptoms were included as an aura type. However, because of increasing genetic information as to the origin of motor aura, it has been reclassified as an integral part of a distinct migraine subtype known as hemiplegic migraine. Although patients with hemiplegic migraine also generally experience more typical visual, sensory, and language auras, the motor symptoms are of longer duration and it is unclear whether they arise from an analogous phenomenon. Recent data from functional neuroimaging suggest that the more common aura symptoms may arise from a cortical spreading depression-like process. The tendency for aura appears to be influenced by complex genetic factors and the overall susceptibility is likely to be based on polymorphisms at multiple loci and may be modulated by epigenetic factors.

REFERENCES

1. International classification of headache disorders, 2nd edition. Cephalalgia 2004;24:1–160.
2. Eriksen MK, Thomsen LL, Olesen J. Sensitivity and specificity of the new international diagnostic criteria for migraine with aura. J Neurol Neurosurg Psychiatr 2005;76(2):212–7.
3. Cutrer FM, Huerter K. Migraine aura. Neurologist 2007;13(3):118–25.
4. Russell MB, Olesen J. A nosographic analysis of the migraine aura in a general population. Brain 1996;119:335–61.
5. Russell MB, Iversen HK, Olesen J. Improved description of the migraine aura by a diagnostic aura diary. Cephalalgia 1994;14:107–17.
6. Carlow TJ. Oculomotor ophthalmoplegic migraine: is it really migraine? J Neuro-ophthalmol 2002;22(3):215–21.

7. Hupp SL, Kline LB, Corbett JJ. Visual disturbances of migraine. Surv Ophthalmol 1989;33(4):221–36.
8. Spector RH. Migraine. Surv Ophthalmol 1984;29(3):193–207.
9. Evans RW, Rolak LA. The Alice in Wonderland syndrome. Headache 2004;44(6):624–5.
10. Vincent MB, Hadjikhani N. Migraine aura and related phenomena: beyond scotomata and scintillations. Cephalalgia 2007;27(12):1368–77.
11. Schott GD. Exploring the visual hallucinations of migraine aura: the tacit contribution of illustration. Brain 2007;130(Pt 6):1690–703.
12. Liu GT, Schatz NJ, Galetta SL, et al. Persistent positive visual phenomena in migraine. Neurology 1995;45(4):664–8.
13. San-Juan OD, Zermeno PF. Migraine with persistent aura in a Mexican patient: case report and review of the literature. Cephalalgia 2007;27(5):456–60.
14. Cupini LM, Stipa E. Migraine aura status and hyperhomocysteinaemia. Cephalalgia 2007;27(7):847–9.
15. Jager HR, Giffin NJ, Goadsby PJ. Diffusion- and perfusion-weighted MR imaging in persistent migrainous visual disturbances. Cephalalgia 2005;25(5):323–32.
16. Relja G, Granato A, Ukmar M, et al. Persistent aura without infarction: description of the first case studied with both brain SPECT and perfusion MRI. Cephalalgia 2005;25(1):56–9.
17. Bereczki D, Kollar J, Kozak N, et al. Cortical spreading edema in persistent visual migraine aura. Headache 2008;48(8):1226–9.
18. Rothrock JF. Successful treatment of persistent migraine aura with divalproex sodium. Neurology 1997;48(1):261–2.
19. Chen WT, Fuh JL, Lu SR, et al. Persistent migrainous visual phenomena might be responsive to lamotrigine. Headache 2001;41(8):823–5.
20. Narita AS, Elder JE. Ocular migraine in an eight-year-old girl. Aust N Z J Ophthalmol 1994;22(4):275–7.
21. Katz B. Bilateral sequential migrainous ischemic optic neuropathy. Am J Ophthalmol 1985;99(4):489.
22. Katz B, Bamford CR. Migrainous ischemic optic neuropathy. Neurology 1985;35(1):112–4.
23. O'Hara M, O'Connor PS. Migrainous optic neuropathy. J Clin Neuroophthalmol 1984;4(2):85–90.
24. McDonald WI, Sanders MD. Migraine complicated by ischaemic papillopathy. Lancet 1971;2(7723):521–3.
25. Weinstein JM, Feman SS. Ischemic optic neuropathy in migraine. Arch Ophthalmol 1982;100(7):1097–100.
26. Lana-Peixoto MA, Barbosa A. Anterior ischaemic optic neuropathy in a child with AS haemoglobinopathy and migraine. Br J Ophthalmol 1998;82(2):199–200.
27. Lee AG, Brazis PW, Miller NR. Posterior ischemic optic neuropathy associated with migraine. Headache 1996;36(8):506–10.
28. Foroozan R, Marx DP, Evans RW. Posterior ischemic optic neuropathy associated with migraine. Headache 2008;48(7):1135–9.
29. Chiari M, Manzoni GC, Van de Geijn EJ. Ischemic optic neuropathy after sumatriptan in a migraine with aura patient. Headache 1994;34(4):237–8.
30. Sommer S, Delemazure B, Wagner M, et al. [Bilateral ischemic optic neuropathy secondary to acute ergotism]. J Fr Ophtalmol 1998;21(2):123–5.
31. Wollensak J, Grajewski O. [Bilateral vascular papillitis following ergotamin medication]. [author's transl]. Klin Monatsbl Augenheilkd 1978;173(5):731–7.

32. Auw-Haedrich C, Staubach F, Witschel H. Optic disk drusen. Surv Ophthalmol 2002;47(6):515–32.
33. Wilkins JM, Pomeranz HD. Visual manifestations of visible and buried optic disc drusen. J Neuroophthalmol 2004;24(2):125–9.
34. Gaynes PM, Towle PA. Hemorrhage in hyaline bodies (drusen) of the optic disc during an attack of migraine. Am J Ophthalmol 1967;63(6):1693–6.
35. Ramirez H, Blatt ES, Hibri NS. Computed tomographic identification of calcified optic nerve drusen. Radiology 1983;148(1):137–9.
36. Newman NJ, Lessell S, Brandt EM. Bilateral central retinal artery occlusions, disk drusen, and migraine. Am J Ophthalmol 1989;107(3):236–40.
37. Bousser MG, Baron JC, Iba-Zizen MT, et al. Migrainous cerebral infarction: a tomographic study of cerebral blood flow and oxygen extraction fraction with the oxygen-15 inhalation technique. Stroke 1980;11(2):145–53.
38. Robinson BE. Permanent homonymous migraine scotomata. AMA Arch Ophthalmol 1954;53(4):566–7.
39. Wakakura M, Ichibe Y. Permanent homonymous hemianopias following migraine. J Clin Neuroophthalmol 1992;12(3):198–202.
40. Carroll D. Retinal migraine. Headache 1970;10(1):9–13.
41. Lepore FE. Retinal migraine. J Neuroophthalmol 2007;27(3):242–3, author reply 4–5.
42. Evans RW, Grosberg BM. Retinal migraine: migraine associated with monocular visual symptoms. Headache 2008;48(1):142–5.
43. Grosberg BM, Solomon S, Friedman DI, et al. Retinal migraine reappraised. Cephalalgia 2006;26(11):1275–86.
44. Doyle E, Vote BJ, Casswell AG. Retinal migraine: caught in the act. Br J Ophthalmol 2004;88(2):301–2.
45. Glenn AM, Shaw PJ, Howe JW, et al. Complicated migraine resulting in blindness due to bilateral retinal infarction. Br J Ophthalmol 1992;76(3):189–90.
46. Pandit JC, Fritsche P. Permanent monocular blindness and ocular migraine. J R Soc Med 1997;90(12):691–2.
47. Grosberg BM, Solomon S. Retinal migraine: two cases of prolonged but reversible monocular visual defects. Cephalalgia 2006;26(6):754–7.
48. Solomon S, Grosberg BM, Friedman DI, et al. Retinal migraine. J Neuroophthalmol 2007;27(3):243–4, author reply 4–5.
49. Winterkorn JM. "Retinal migraine" is an oxymoron. J Neuroophthalmol 2007;27(1):1–2.
50. Daroff RB. Retinal migraine. J Neuroophthalmol 2007;27(1):83.
51. Hill DL, Daroff RB, Ducros A, et al. Most cases labeled as "retinal migraine" are not migraine. J Neuroophthalmol 2007;27(1):3–8.
52. Winterkorn JM, Kupersmith MJ, Wirtschafter JD, et al. Brief report: treatment of vasospastic amaurosis fugax with calcium-channel blockers. N Engl J Med 1993;329(6):396–8.
53. Robertson DM. I am a retinal migraineur. J Neuroophthalmol 2008;28(1):81–2.
54. Ebner R. Visual field examination during transient migrainous visual loss. J Clin Neuroophthalmol 1991;11(2):114–7.
55. McKendrick AM, Vingrys AJ, Badcock DR, et al. Visual dysfunction between migraine events. Invest Ophthalmol Vis Sci 2001;42(3):626–33.
56. Lewis RA, Vijayan N, Watson C, et al. Visual field loss in migraine. Ophthalmology 1989;96(3):321–6.
57. McKendrick AM, Vingrys AJ, Badcock DR, et al. Visual field losses in subjects with migraine headaches. Invest Ophthalmol Vis Sci 2000;41(5):1239–47.

58. Drummond PD, Anderson M. Visual field loss after attacks of migraine with aura. Cephalalgia 1992;12(6):349–52.

59. McKendrick AM, Badcock DR. Decreased visual field sensitivity measured 1 day, then 1 week, after migraine. Invest Ophthalmol Vis Sci 2004a;45(4):1061–70.

60. McKendrick AM, Badcock DR. An analysis of the factors associated with visual field deficits measured with flickering stimuli in between migraine. Cephalalgia 2004;24(5):389–97.

61. Yenice O, Temel A, Incili B, et al. Short-wavelength automated perimetry in patients with migraine. Graefes Arch Clin Exp Ophthalmol 2006;244(5):589–95.

62. Tibber MS, Shepherd AJ. Transient tritanopia in migraine: evidence for a large-field retinal abnormality in blue-yellow opponent pathways. Invest Ophthalmol Vis Sci 2006;47(11):5125–31.

63. Corbett JJ, Phelps CD, Eslinger P, et al. The neurologic evaluation of patients with low-tension glaucoma. Invest Ophthalmol Vis Sci 1985;26(8):1101–4.

64. Lord GDA. Clinical characteristics of the migrainous aura. In: Amery WK, Wauquier A, editors. The prelude to the migraine attack. London: Baillière Tindall; 1986. p. 87–98.

65. Kurth T, Schürks M, Logroscino G, et al. Migraine, vascular risk, and cardiovascular events in women: prospective cohort study. BMJ 2008;337:a636.

66. Fisher CM. Late-life migraine accompaniments: further experience. Stroke 1986; 17:1033–42.

67. Bradshaw P, Parsons M. Hemiplegic migraine, a clinical study. QJM 1965;34: 3465–85.

68. Leao AAP. Spreading depression of activity in the cerebral cortex. J Neurophysiol 1944;7:359–90.

69. Milner P. Note on a possible correspondence between the scotomas of migraine and spreading depression of Leao. Electroencephalogr Clin Neurophysiol 1958; 10:705.

70. Olesen J, Larsen B, Lauritzen M. Focal hyperemia followed by spreading oligemia and impaired activation of rCBF in classic migraine. Ann Neurol 1981; 9:344–52.

71. Lauritzen M, Skyhoj Olsen T, Lassen NA, et al. Changes of regional cerebral blood flow during the course of classical migraine attacks. Ann Neurol 1983; 13:633–41.

72. Cutrer FM, Sorensen AG, Weisskoff RM, et al. Perfusion-weighted imaging defects during spontaneous migrainous aura. Ann Neurol 1998;43(1):25–31.

73. Sorensen AG, Rosen BR. Functional MRI of the brain. In: Atlas S, editor. Magnetic resonance imaging of the brain and spine. 2nd edition. Philadelphia: Lippcott-Raven Publishers; 1996.

74. Hadjikhani N, Sanchez Del Rio M, Wu O, et al. Mechanisms of migraine aura revealed by functional MRI in human visual cortex. Proc Natl Acad Sci U S A 2001; 98(8):4687–92.

75. James MF, Smith MI, Bockhorst KH, et al. Cortical spreading depression in the gyrencephalic feline brain studied by magnetic resonance imaging. J Physiol 1999;519(Pt 2):415–25.

76. Smith M, Cros D, Sheen V. Hyperperfusion with vasogenic leakage by fMRI in migraine with prolonged aura. Neurology 2002;58(8):1308–10.

77. Gekeler F, Holtmannspotter M, Straube A, et al. Diffusion-weighted magnetic resonance imaging during the aura of pseudomigraine with temporary neurologic symptoms and lymphocytic pleocytosis. Headache 2002;42(4):294–6.

78. Welch KMA, Levine SR, D'Andrea G, et al. Brain pH during migraine studied by in-vivo 31-phosphorus NMR spectroscopy. Cephalalgia 1988;8:273–7.
79. Welch KMA, Levine SR, D'Andrea G, et al. Preliminary observations on brain energy metabolites in migraine studied by in vivo 31-phosphorus NMR spectroscopy. Neurology 1989;39:538–41.
80. Welch KMA, Barkley GL, Ramadan NM, et al. NMR spectroscopic and magnetoencephalographic studies in migraine with aura: support for the spreading depression hypothesis. Pathol Biol 1992;40(4):349–54.
81. van Harreveld A, Fifekova E. Mechanisms involved in spreading depression. J Neurobiol 1973;4:375–87.
82. Sandor PS, Dydak U, Schoenen J, et al. MR-spectroscopic imaging during visual stimulation in subgroups of migraine with aura. Cephalalgia 2005;25(7):507–18.
83. Ambrosini A, de Noordhout AM, Sandor PS, et al. Electrophysiological studies in migraine: a comprehensive review of their interest and limitations. Cephalalgia 2003;23(Suppl 1):13–31.
84. Aurora SK, Welch KM, Al-Sayed F. The threshold for phosphenes is lower in migraine. Cephalalgia 2003;23(4):258–63.
85. Lea RA, Nyholt DR, Curtain RP, et al. A genome-wide scan provides evidence for loci influencing a severe heritable form of common migraine. Neurogenetics 2005;6(2):67–72.
86. Kara I, Sazci A, Ergul E, et al. Association of the C677T and A1298C polymorphisms in the 5,10 Methylenetetrahydrofolate reductase gene in patients with migraine risk. Brain Res Mol Brain Res 2003;111(1–2):84–90.
87. Wessman M, Kallela M, Kaunisto MA, et al. A susceptibility locus for migraine with aura, on chromosome 4q24. Am J Hum Genet 2002;70:652–62.
88. Carlsson A, Forsgren L, Nylander P-O, et al. Identification of a susceptibility locus for migraine with and without aura on 6p12.2-p21.1. Neurology 2002;59:1804–7.
89. Colson N, Lea R, Quinlan S, et al. The estrogen receptor 1G594A polymorphism is associated with migraine susceptibility in two independent case/control groups. Neurogenetics 2004;5:129–33.
90. Colson N, Lea R, Quinlan S, et al. Investigation of hormone receptor genes in migraine. Neurogenetics 2005;6:17–23.
91. Peroutka SJ, Price SC, Wilhoit TL. Comorbid migraine with aura, anxiety, and depression is associated with dopamine D2 receptor (DRD2) Ncol alleles. Mol Med 1998;4(1):14–21.
92. Peroutka SJ, Wilhoit T, Jones K. Clinical susceptibility to migraine with aura is modified by dopamine D2 receptor (DRD2) Ncol alleles. Neurology 1997;49(1):201–6.
93. Cader ZM, Noble-Topham S, Dyment DA, et al. Significant linkage to migraine with aura on chromosome 11q24. Hum Mol Genet 2003;12(19):2511–7.
94. Russo L, Mariotti P, Sangiorgi E, et al. A new susceptibility locus for migraine with aura in the 15q11-q13 genomic region containing three GABA-A receptor genes. Am J Hum Genet 2005;76(2):327–33.
95. Ogilvie AD, Russell MB, Dhall P. Altered allelic distributions of the serotonin transporter gene in migraine without aura and migraine with aura. Cephalalgia 1998;18(1):23–6.

Vestibular Migraine

Hannelore Neuhauser, MD, MPH[a,b,*], Thomas Lempert, MD[b,c]

KEYWORDS

- Migraine • Vestibular • Vertigo • Dizziness
- Vestibular migraine • Migraine-associated dizziness
- Migrainous vertigo

That migraine may manifest with attacks of vertigo has been repeatedly documented from the early days of neurology.[1] Clinical recognition of vertigo linked to migraine could be summarized as "not seeing the forest for the trees" until quite recently, however. Starting with Kayan and Hood's classic article,[2] the clinical features of vestibular migraine (VM) have been well delineated in several large case series.[3–9] Because VM is an evolving entity and knowledge on the pathophysiology and treatment of VM remains scarce, it is not surprising that terminology is confusing and that generally accepted diagnostic criteria are still lacking. Various terms, including *migraine-associated vertigo*, *migraine-associated dizziness*, *migraine-related vestibulopathy*, *migrainous vertigo*, *benign recurrent vertigo*, and *basilar migraine*, have all been applied to roughly the same patient population. *Vestibular migraine* has been convincingly advocated as a term that stresses the particular vestibular manifestation of migraine, and thus best avoids confounding with nonvestibular dizziness or motion sickness associated with migraine.[10] Therefore, the term *migrainous vertigo* used so far by the authors' group is replaced by the term *vestibular migraine* in this article. The term *basilar migraine*, however, should be restricted to patients who fulfill the diagnostic criteria of the International Headache Society (IHS)[11] for basilar migraine.

Interestingly, the awareness of a causal link between vertigo and migraine was promoted by epidemiologic observation indicating a more than chance association of migraine with vertigo and dizziness. Dizziness and vertigo rank among the most common complaints in the general population and are frequently reported by patients who have migraine. The prevalence of migraine has been shown to be elevated among patients with dizziness,[7] however, particularly among patients who have unclassified vertigo.[12] Conversely, significantly more patients who had migraine reported vertigo compared with patients who had tension headache[2] and with headache-free controls.[13,14] In the general population, migraine headaches and vestibular vertigo concur approximately

a Department of Epidemiology, Robert Koch Institut, General Pape Str. 62-64, 12101 Berlin, Germany
b Vestibular Research Group, Charité, Department of Neurology, Augustenburger Pl. 1, 13353, Berlin, Germany
c Department of Neurology, Neurologische Abteilung, Schlosspark-Klinik, Heubnerweg 2, 14059 Berlin, Germany
* Corresponding author.
E-mail address: neuhauserh@rki.de (H. Neuhauser).

Neurol Clin 27 (2009) 379–391
doi:10.1016/j.ncl.2008.11.004
0733-8619/08/$ – see front matter © 2009 Elsevier Inc. All rights reserved.

neurologic.theclinics.com

three times more often than expected by chance. Because migraine has a lifetime prevalence of 14%[15] and vestibular vertigo has a lifetime prevalence of 7%,[16] chance concurrence is expected in 1% of the population but was actually found in 3.2% in a large population-based study.[17] Therefore, clinicians must determine whether an individual patient has VM (ie, vestibular vertigo) that is caused by migraine, dizziness or vertigo of an unrelated cause (which occurs in a migraineur by chance), or one of several vestibular and nonvestibular dizziness syndromes with increased prevalence in migraineurs. These include Ménière's disease (MD), benign paroxysmal positional vertigo (BPPV), motion sickness, and orthostatic hypotension. In the following sections, the authors deal first with the core syndrome of VM and then with other dizziness syndromes that are statistically associated with migraine.

DIAGNOSTIC CRITERIA

In the current IHS classification, vertigo is not included as a migrainous symptom in adults except in the framework of basilar migraine,[11] which involves vertigo in more than 60% of the patients.[18] As an aura symptom of basilar migraine, vertigo should last between 5 and 60 minutes and should be followed by migrainous headache. In addition, a second aura symptom from the posterior circulation should be reported. In fact, less than 10% of patients who have VM in published case series fulfill the criteria for basilar migraine,[4–7] which makes basilar migraine an inappropriate category for these patients. As a consequence, most adult patients who have VM cannot be classified with the current IHS criteria.

To date, there are no internationally approved criteria for the diagnosis of VM. Like migraine itself, VM cannot be diagnosed by specific biologic markers but only on the basis of history. A proposal from the authors' group uses operational clinical criteria modeled on the IHS classification of headaches.[7] Two separate diagnostic categories seem to be useful: definite VM and the more sensitive but less specific category of probable VM (**Table 1**). A diagnostic interview applying this classification has been developed.[19] In accordance with most researchers, the proposed criteria conceptualize VM as an episodic vestibular disorder. Several reports have included patients with nonspecific dizziness[3–5] or with permanent symptoms,[4,20] however. There is little doubt that these patients have dizziness related to migraine, but for the sake of specificity, it is useful to define the core syndrome first and then to consider exceptions.

PREVALENCE OF VESTIBULAR MIGRAINE

The prevalence of definite VM according to these criteria was 7% in a group of 200 consecutive clinic patients with dizziness and 9% in a group of 200 clinic patients who had migraine.[7] In a two-stage population-based study (n = 4869 adults) with screening interviews followed by expert telephone interviews, the lifetime prevalence of VM was estimated at 0.98% (95% confidence interval: 0.7–1.37) using the same criteria.[17] Of note, definite VM accounted for only a third of migraineurs with a history of vestibular vertigo, which indicates the need for a thorough neurotologic workup for exclusion of other diagnoses.[17]

CLINICAL FEATURES
Demographic Aspects

VM may occur at any age.[3,4,6] It has a female preponderance, with a reported female-to-male ratio between 1.5 and 5 to 1.[4–7] Familial occurrence is not uncommon, probably based on an autosomal dominant pattern of inheritance with decreased

Table 1
Diagnostic criteria for definite vestibular migraine

Definite Vestibular Migraine
A   Episodic vestibular symptoms of at least moderate severity
B   Current or previous history of migraine according to the 2004 criteria of the IHS
C   One of the following migrainous symptoms during two or more attacks of vertigo: migrainous headache, photophobia, phonophobia, visual aura, or other aura
D   Other causes ruled out by appropriate investigations Comment: Vestibular symptoms are rotational vertigo or another illusory self- or object motion. They may be spontaneous or positional. Vestibular symptoms are "moderate" if they interfere with but do not prohibit daily activities and "severe" if patients cannot continue daily activities.
Probable vestibular migraine
A   Episodic vestibular symptoms of at least moderate severity
B   One of the following: (1) current or previous history of migraine according to the 2004 criteria of the IHS; (2) migrainous symptoms during vestibular symptoms; (3) migraine precipitants of vertigo in more than 50% of attacks: food triggers, sleep irregularities, or hormonal change; or (4) response to migraine medications in more than 50% of attacks
C   Other causes ruled out by appropriate investigations

penetrance in men.[21] In most patients, migraine begins earlier in life than VM.[6,7] Some patients have been free from migraine attacks for years when VM first manifests itself.[6] Not infrequently, migraine headaches are replaced by vertigo attacks in women around the time of menopause. VM seems to occur more often in patients who have migraine without aura than in patients who have migraine with aura.[2,5,6]

Vestibular Migraine in Children

Benign paroxysmal vertigo of childhood is an early manifestation of VM that is recognized by the IHS classification of headaches. It is characterized by brief attacks of vertigo or disequilibrium, anxiety, and often nystagmus or vomiting recurring for months or years in otherwise healthy young children.[22] Many of these children later develop migraine, often years after vertigo attacks have ceased.[23] A family history of migraine in first-degree relatives is twofold increased compared with controls.[24] In a population-based study, the prevalence of recurrent vertigo probably related to migraine was estimated at 2.8% in children between the ages of 6 and 12 years.[24]

Clinical Presentation in Adults and Distinction from other Diagnoses

Because migraineurs can present with dizziness or vertigo attributable to a variety of causes, a first diagnostic step is the distinction of vertigo (which is a vestibular symptom) and dizziness (which is not). This distinction can usually be made by careful history taking: rotational vertigo or other illusory sensations of motion indicate vertigo (ie, vestibular symptoms), whereas a sensation of lightheadedness, giddiness, drowsiness, or impending fainting implies dizziness of nonvestibular origin. Nonspinning dizziness only during standing or walking usually indicates a neurologic gait problem rather than vestibular vertigo. A residual gray area remains, however, as a semantic problem or because mild vestibular dysfunction may present with dizziness rather than vertigo.

Patients who have VM typically report spontaneous or positional vertigo. Some experience a sequence of spontaneous vertigo transforming into positional vertigo after several hours or days.[25,26] This positional vertigo is distinct from BPPV with regard to duration of individual attacks (often as long as the head position is maintained in VM versus seconds only in BPPV), duration of symptomatic episodes (minutes to days in VM versus weeks to months in BPPV), and nystagmus findings (**Table 2**). Altogether, 40% to 70% of patients experience positional vertigo in the course of the disease but not necessarily with every attack.[2,21,27] Head motion intolerance, quite similar to motion sickness (ie, imbalance, illusory motion or nausea aggravated or provoked by head movements) is a frequent additional symptom.[4,13] Visual vertigo (ie, vertigo provoked by moving visual scenes, such as traffic or cinema) can be another prominent feature of VM.[4,20,28] Nausea and imbalance are frequent but nonspecific accompaniments of acute VM. The duration and frequency of attacks can vary between patients and in individual patients over time. The duration of vertigo ranges from seconds (approximately 10%) and minutes (30%) to hours (30%) and several days (30%).[2,3,5,6,29] For some patients, it may take weeks to recover fully from an attack. The attacks may occur days, months, or even years apart in an irregular fashion. Overall, only 10% to 30% of patients have vertigo with the typical duration of a migraine aura (ie, 5–60 minutes).[6,7]

VM often misses not only the duration criterion for an aura as defined by the IHS but the temporal relation to migraine headaches: vertigo can precede headache, as would be typical for an aura; may begin with headache; or may appear late in the headache phase. Many patients experience attacks with and without headache.[3,5,7] Quite frequently, patients have an attenuated headache with their vertigo as compared with their usual migraine.[5,8] In some patients, vertigo and headache never occur together.[3,5,7] In these cases, diagnosis must be based on migrainous symptoms during the attack other than headache. Along with the vertigo, patients may experience photophobia, phonophobia, osmophobia, and visual or other auras (**Table 3**). These phenomena are of diagnostic importance because they may represent the only apparent connection of vertigo and migraine. Patients need to be specifically asked about these migrainous symptoms because they often do not volunteer them. A dizziness diary can be useful for prospective recording of associated features. Hearing loss and tinnitus are not prominent symptoms of VM but have been reported in individual patients who have VM.[2,4,5,30] Hearing loss is usually mild and transient, without progression in the course of the disorder.[5] Patients with severe fluctuating hearing loss suggestive of MD and migrainous features during the attack implying VM[2,5,31] have been reported, however. Asking for migraine-specific precipitants of vertigo attacks may provide valuable diagnostic information (menstruation; deficient or irregular sleep; excessive stress; specific foods, such as matured cheese, red wine, and glutamate; and, finally, sensory stimuli, such as bright or scintillating lights, intense smells, or noise). Sometimes, migrainous accompaniments and typical precipitants may be missing, but VM is still considered the most likely diagnosis after other potential causes have been investigated and seem unlikely. In this case, a favorable response to antimigraine drugs supports the suspicion of an underlying migraine mechanism. Apparent efficacy of a drug should not be regarded as a definite confirmation of the diagnosis, however, because spontaneous improvement, placebo response, and additional drug effects (eg, anxiolytic, antidepressant) have to be taken into account.

In summary, the clinical presentation of VM is variable in many respects and the connection to migraine can be subtle. The key to the diagnosis is the repeated concurrence of migrainous symptoms and vertigo, migraine-specific precipitants, and sometimes response to antimigraine drugs.

Clinical and Neurotologic Findings in Patients who have Vestibular Migraine

In most patients, the general neurologic and otologic examination is normal in the symptom-free period.[3] Approximately 10% to 20% of patients who have VM have

Table 2
Recurrent vertigo in patients who have migraine: differential diagnosis of vestibular migraine

Disorder	Key Features
BPPV	Vertigo lasting seconds to 1 minute provoked by changes in head position; positive positional test result with typical torsional nystagmus
MD	Vertigo lasting 20 minutes to 3 hours with concurrent hearing loss, tinnitus, and aural fullness; progressive hearing loss over years[46]
Central positional vertigo	History similar to BPPV but latency, duration, and direction of positional nystagmus not typical for BPPV; frequently, additional neurologic or neurotologic signs
Vertebrobasilar transient ischemic attack	Attacks lasting mostly minutes, with brain stem symptoms, including vertigo, ataxia, dysarthria, diplopia, or visual field defects (rarely isolated recurrent vertigo); usually elderly patients with vascular risk factors
Vascular compression of the eighth nerve	Brief attacks of vertigo (seconds) several times per day with or without cochlear symptoms; often response to carbamazepine
Perilymph fistula	Vertigo after head trauma, barotrauma, or stapedectomy or provoked by coughing, sneezing, straining, or loud sounds
Autoimmune inner ear disease	Frequent attacks of variable duration, often bilateral, with rapidly progressing hearing loss
Insufficient compensation of unilateral vestibular loss	Brief and mild spells of vertigo during rapid head movements, oscillopsia with head turns to affected ear; positive result of head thrust test to affected side
Schwannoma of the eighth nerve	Rarely presents with (mild) attacks of vertigo; key symptoms are slowly progressive unilateral hearing loss and tinnitus; abnormal BAER

Abbreviation: BAER, brainstem auditory evoked responses.

unilateral hypoexcitability to caloric stimulation, and approximately 10% have directional preponderance of nystagmus responses.[3,6,32] Such findings, however, are not specific for VM because they can be found in migraine patients who do not have vestibular symptoms[33,34] and in many other vestibular syndromes. Neuro-ophthalmologic evaluation may reveal mild central oculomotor deficits in the absence of other brain stem or cerebellar signs.[6] In one study, patients who had VM became nauseous after caloric testing four times more often than migraineurs who had other vestibular disorders.[35]

A neurotologic study of 20 patients during the acute phase of VM showed imbalance with increased sway on tandem Romberg or tandem walking in all patients but 1. Fourteen patients had pathologic nystagmus: a peripheral type of spontaneous nystagmus was observed in 3 patients, a central type of spontaneous nystagmus was observed in 3 patients, a central positional nystagmus was observed in 5 patients, and a combined central spontaneous and positional nystagmus was observed in 3 patients. Unlike benign paroxysmal positional nystagmus, VM positional nystagmus was always persistent as long as the provoking position was maintained and was usually not beating in the plane of positioning. A unilateral deficit of the horizontal vestibulo-ocular

Table 3 Clinical features of definite vestibular migraine in 33 patients	
Clinical Features	%
Vestibular symptoms[a]	
Rotational vertigo	70
Other illusory self- or object motion	18
Positional vertigo	42
Head motion intolerance[b]	48
Duration of vestibular symptoms	
Seconds to 5 minutes	18
5 to 60 minutes	33
1 hour to 1 day	21
>1 day	2
Migrainous symptoms during vertigo	
Migrainous headache	94
Always	47
Sometimes	48
No headache	6
Photophobia	70
Phonophobia	64
Visual or other auras	36

[a] Several patients had more than one type of vestibular symptoms.
[b] None of the patients had only head motion intolerance.
Data from Neuhauser H, Leopold M, von Brevern M, et al. The interrelations of migraine, vertigo and migrainous vertigo. Neurology 2001;56(4):436–41.

reflex was observed in 3 patients, and 1 of these 3 patients did not recover peripheral function on follow-up. Overall, findings during acute VM pointed to central vestibular dysfunction in 10 patients (50%) and to peripheral vestibular dysfunction in 3 patients (15%) and were inconclusive with regard to the involved structures in 7 patients (35%).[36]

In clinical practice, history usually provides more clues for the diagnosis than vestibular testing, because there are no abnormalities that are specific for VM. Therefore, in patients with a clear-cut history, no additional vestibular tests are required. Nevertheless, vestibular testing in the interval can be useful to reassure the patient and doctor that there is no severe abnormality, such as complete canal paresis, which would suggest another diagnosis. Conversely, testing during or shortly after an attack can reveal more profound peripheral or central abnormalities that should improve or disappear within a few weeks.

PATHOPHYSIOLOGY

The neural mechanisms of VM are still obscure, because systematic investigations based on proper methodology and patient identification are just at their beginning. Several hypotheses have been put forward.[19] Spreading depression, which is the presumed mechanism of the migraine aura, may play a role in patients who have short attacks.[3] Spreading depression is a cortical mechanism that could produce vestibular symptoms when the multisensory cortical areas that process vestibular signals become involved, which are mainly located in the posterior insula and at the temporoparietal junction.[37] Several findings during the acute stage of VM, however, including canal paresis and complex positional nystagmus, cannot be explained by cortical dysfunction.[36]

Several neurotransmitters that are involved in the pathogenesis of migraine (eg, calcitonin gene–related peptide, serotonin, noradrenaline, dopamine) are also known to modulate the activity of central and peripheral vestibular neurons and could contribute to the pathogenesis of VM.[3–5,38] One may speculate that unilateral release of these substances—in analogy to the often unilateral location of headaches—might cause a static vestibular imbalance leading to rotatory vertigo, whereas bilateral release would instead cause a state of altered vestibular excitability leading to a motion sickness type of dizziness.

In the past decade, genetic defects of ion channels have been identified as the cause of various paroxysmal neurologic disorders. The finding of an abnormal voltage-gated calcium-channel gene in familial hemiplegic migraine (FHM) and episodic ataxia type 2 (EA-2),[39] both of which can have vertigo and migraine headache as prominent symptoms, has prompted the search for a susceptibility gene for VM in the same region. So far, however, no such genetic defect has been identified.[40,41]

The only hypothesis that is actually based on an experimental model of VM relates to the known reciprocal connections between the trigeminal and vestibular nuclei. Trigeminal activation by painful electrical stimulation of the forehead produced spontaneous nystagmus in patients who had migraine but not in controls, indicating that migraineurs have a lowered threshold for cross-talk between these neighboring brain stem structures.[42]

TREATMENT

In many patients, VM attacks are severe, long, and frequent enough to warrant acute or prophylactic treatment. Unfortunately, current treatment recommendations are based on expert opinion rather than on solid data from randomized placebo-controlled trials. Indeed, apart from one small and inconclusive study on the use of zolmitriptan for acute VM,[43] no proper study has been undertaken.

A few case reports suggest that medication used for migraine prophylaxis may be effective, including propranolol,[44] metoprolol,[6] tricyclic antidepressants,[9] pizotifen,[9,20] and flunarizine[6] (which is not licensed in the United States). The carboanhydrase inhibitors acetazolamide[45] and dichlorphenamide,[46] which are not normally used for migraine prophylaxis, have also been applied successfully (**Table 4**). All these reports are difficult to interpret in the absence of controls and a well-documented pretreatment period, however, because the frequency and duration of attacks vary considerably in the natural course of the disorder.[3] Expected side effects, such as orthostatic hypotension with beta-blockers or weight gain with pizotifen, can influence the selection of the drug. Patients should monitor the frequency and severity of their attacks in a diary. Treatment response should be evaluated after 3 months. A greater than 50% reduction in attack frequency is a reasonable goal.

Treatment of acute VM with acute migraine medication can be attempted with triptans[16,47] and vestibular suppressants, such as promethazine, dimenhydrinate, and meclizine.[47] A retrospective study found that the effect of triptans on vertigo was correlated to its effect on headache.[48] Nonpharmaceutic approaches in the treatment of VM should not be neglected and may be even more effective than drugs in individual patients. A thorough explanation of the migrainous origin of the attacks can relieve unnecessary fears. Avoidance of identified triggers, regular sleep and

Table 4
Prophylactic treatment of vestibular migraine

Drug	Daily Dose	Side Effects
Propranolol[44]	40–240 mg	Fatigue, hypotension, impotence, depression, nightmares, bronchial constriction
Metoprolol[6]	50–200 mg	Fatigue, hypotension, impotence, depression, nightmares, bronchial constriction
Amitriptylin[9]	50–100 mg	Sedation, orthostatic hypotension, dry mouth, weight gain, constipation, urinary retention, conduction block
Pizotifen[8,20]	1.5–6 mg	Weight gain, sedation
Flunarizine[6]	5–10 mg	Weight gain, sedation, depression, reversible parkinsonism
Acetazolamide[45]	250–750 mg	Paresthesia, nausea, sedation, hypokalemia, hyperglycemia
Dichlorphenamide[46]	17.5–75 mg	Paresthesia, nausea, sedation, hypokalemia, hyperglycemia

meals, and regular exercise have a firm place in migraine prophylaxis. Selected patients may profit from vestibular rehabilitation.[49]

MIGRAINE AND MÉNIÈR'S DISEASE

An increased prevalence of migraine in patients who have MD is well documented,[31,50] although the pathophysiologic nature of this association is not clear yet. The prevalence of migraine according to the IHS criteria was almost twice as high in a group of 78 patients who had idiopathic unilateral or bilateral MD according to the criteria of the American Academy of Otolaryngology[51] than in the age- and gender-matched control group (56% versus 25%; $P<.001$).[31] Migraine may lead to a greater susceptibility of developing MD and influence its course, as suggested by a recent study in which patients who had MD had an earlier onset of symptoms and a greater susceptibility to bilateral hearing loss when they also had migraine.[52] Vestibular function tests provide only modest assistance in differentiation between the two conditions.[53] In most patients, the distinction can be made, considering that hearing loss is an occasional, mild, and nonprogressive feature in VM,[5] whereas it is a regular accompaniment of MD, progressing to severe hearing loss within a few years. Nevertheless, there are patients who have migraine and recurrent vertigo for whom it is not possible to differentiate with certainty whether they have VM or MD.[31] A possible explanation would be that MD and VM are different manifestations of the same underlying susceptibility that leads to a spectrum of migrainous, vertiginous, and cochlear symptoms and may have a genetic basis.[52]

MIGRAINE AND BENIGN PAROXYSMAL POSITIONAL VERTIGO

BPPV is the most common cause of recurrent vestibular symptoms in unselected patients[6,54] and in migraineurs[7] presenting to a dizziness clinic. Although clinically two separate entities, there is evidence for a link between migraine and BPPV. Migraine has been found to be three times more common in patients who have idiopathic BPPV than in patients who have BPPV secondary to trauma or surgical procedures.[55] Moreover, migraine was two times more common in patients who had idiopathic BPPV than in age- and gender-matched controls.[56]

MIGRAINE AND MOTION SICKNESS

Motion sickness occurs more frequently in patients who have migraine (30%–70%) than in controls who have tension headache or in headache-free controls (20%–40%).[2,13,28] The association is more pronounced in children[57] and in migraine with aura.[13] Migraineurs also report more "visual vertigo" induced by optokinetic stimuli.[13,28] In addition, headache, scalp tenderness, and photophobia can be more easily provoked by optokinetic stimulation in patients who have migraine than in controls.[58] In an individual patient, it may be difficult to differentiate between episodic motion sickness and attacks of VM induced by motion stimuli. The distinction can be made regarding the type and duration of symptoms. Nausea and dizziness improving after cessation of the motion stimulus point to a diagnosis of motion sickness, whereas rotational or positional vertigo persisting after the motion stimulus has ended suggests VM. Chronic VM[20] may be explained by a constantly lowered threshold to motion stimuli. Interestingly, motion sickness could be prevented using rizatriptan in migraineurs who had VM but not in patients who had migraine alone.[59]

MIGRAINE AND CEREBELLAR DYSFUNCTION

Cerebellar dysfunction causes imbalance that patients may experience as dizziness. Some families who have FHM, a rare subtype of migraine, develop progressive cerebellar ataxia and nystagmus.[60] Interestingly, mutations in the CACNA1A gene coding for the α_{1A}-subunit of a neuronal Ca^{2+} channel, which is heavily expressed in the cerebellum, have been identified not only in FHM but in EA-2[61] and spinocerebellar ataxia type 6.[62] EA-2 is characterized by short bouts of cerebellar ataxia, often with vertigo, and interictal nystagmus. Approximately half of the patients who have EA-2 have migraine.[63] FHM and EA-2 are associated with typical symptoms of basilar migraine.[63,64] In more common types of migraine, cerebellar symptoms are not usually present, but subclinical hypermetria and other subtle subclinical cerebellar signs in patients who have migraine with or without aura have been reported.[34,65] Researchers suggested dysfunctional Ca^{2+} channels as a possible cause. This hypothesis relies on findings of involvement of the CACNA1A gene region in some families who have non-hemiplegic migraine with and without aura.[66] The mild oculomotor deficits of cerebellar origin observed in patients who have VM represent another possible link between migraine and cerebellar dysfunction.[6]

MIGRAINE AND NONVESTIBULAR DIZZINESS

Patients who have migraine report not only more vertigo but significantly more dizzy spells than controls (32% versus 13%).[13] These can usually be attributed to nonvestibular causes. One should remember, however, that mild vestibular dysfunction may also present with dizziness rather than vertigo.

Migraine, Orthostatic Hypotension, and Syncope

Syncope during migraine attacks has been reported in 5% of 500 unselected migraineurs.[67] A recent large population-based study showed an elevated prevalence of syncope (46% versus 31%) and orthostatic intolerance (32% versus 12%) in migraineurs compared with controls.[68] Interestingly, orthostatic hypotension can be induced by small doses of dopamine agonists and counteracted by dopamine antagonists in migraineurs but not in controls, suggesting hypersensitivity to dopaminergic stimulation as the underlying mechanism.[69]

Migraine and Dizziness Attributable to a Comorbid Psychiatric Disorder

The interrelations between migraine, dizziness, and certain psychiatric disorders are intricate. There are bidirectional associations of migraine with major depression and panic disorder, with migraine being a risk factor for first-onset major depression and panic disorder and vice versa.[70,71] Dizziness is the second most common symptom of panic attacks after palpitations[72] and can be a symptom of major depression as well. To complicate things further, patients with panic and anxiety have an increased rate of vestibular test abnormalities,[73] which may reflect an elevated risk for patients who have vestibular disorders to develop an anxiety disorder.[74] Patients who have VM show the highest rate of concurrent anxiety or depressive disorders as compared with other vertigo syndromes.[75] Because of the frequent association of dizziness, migraine, and anxiety, a new syndrome called migraine-anxiety–related dizziness has been proposed.[76]

Dizziness Attributable to Antimigraine Medication

Dizziness is listed as a side effect of many medications, some of which are used in the treatment of migraine. Therefore, it is useful to elicit a detailed drug history and ascertain the onset of dizziness in relation to changes in medication. Beta-blockers may cause orthostatic hypotension, particularly at the beginning of treatment. Antidepressants, particularly tricyclic antidepressants, which are used in the prophylactic therapy of migraine, can cause sleepiness, blurred vision, lightheadedness, and postural hypotension.

REFERENCES

1. Liveing E. On megrim: sick headache and some allied health disorders: a contribution to the pathology of nerve storms. London:1873:129–48.
2. Kayan A, Hood JD. Neuro-otological manifestations of migraine. Brain 1984; 107(Pt 4):1123–42.
3. Cutrer FM, Baloh RW. Migraine-associated dizziness. Headache 1992;32(6): 300–4.
4. Cass SP, Furman JM, Ankerstjerne K, et al. Migraine-related vestibulopathy. Ann Otol Rhinol Laryngol 1997;106(3):182–9.
5. Johnson GD. Medical management of migraine-related dizziness and vertigo. Laryngoscope 1998;108(Suppl 85):1–28.
6. Dieterich M, Brandt T. Episodic vertigo related to migraine (90 cases): vestibular migraine? J Neurol 1999;246(10):883–92.
7. Neuhauser H, Leopold M, von Brevern M, et al. The interrelations of migraine, vertigo, and migrainous vertigo. Neurology 2001;56(4):436–41.
8. Behan PO, Carlin J. Benign recurrent vertigo. New York: Raven Press; 1982.
9. Reploeg MD, Goebel JA. Migraine-associated dizziness: patient characteristics and management options. Otol Neurotol 2002;23(3):364–71.
10. Brandt T, Strupp M. Migraine and vertigo: classification, clinical features, and special treatment considerations. Headache Currents 2006;3(1):12–9.
11. International Headache Society Classification Subcommittee. International classification of headache disorders. 2nd edition. Cephalalgia 2004;24(Suppl 1): 1–160.

12. Lee H, Sohn SI, Jung DK, et al. Migraine and isolated recurrent vertigo of unknown cause. Neurol Res 2002;24(7):663–5.
13. Kuritzky A, Ziegler DK, Hassanein R. Vertigo, motion sickness and migraine. Headache 1981;21(5):227–31.
14. Vukovic V, Plavec D, Galinovic I, et al. Prevalence of vertigo, dizziness, and migrainous vertigo in patients with migraine. Headache 2007;47(10):1427–35.
15. Jensen R, Stovner LJ. Epidemiology and comorbidity of headache. Lancet Neurol 2008;7(4):354–61.
16. Neuhauser HK, von Brevern M, Radtke A, et al. Epidemiology of vestibular vertigo: a neurotological survey of the general population. Neurology 2005;65(6):898–904.
17. Neuhauser HK, Radtke A, von Brevern M, et al. Migrainous vertigo. Prevalence and impact on quality of life. Neurology 2006;67(6):1028–33.
18. Sturzenegger MH, Meienberg O. Basilar artery migraine: a follow-up study of 82 cases. Headache 1985;25(8):408–15.
19. Furman JM, Marcus DA, Balaban CD. Migrainous vertigo: development of a pathogenetic model and structured diagnostic interview. Curr Opin Neurol 2003; 16(1):5–13.
20. Waterston J. Chronic migrainous vertigo. J Clin Neurosci 2004;11(4):384–8.
21. Oh AK, Lee H, Jen JC, et al. Familial benign recurrent vertigo. Am J Med Genet 2001;100(4):287–91.
22. Basser LS. Benign paroxysmal vertigo of childhood. (A variety of vestibular neuronitis.)Brain 1964;87(3):141–52.
23. Watson P, Steele JC. Paroxysmal dysequilibrium in the migraine syndrome of childhood. Arch Otolaryngol 1974;99:177–9.
24. Abu-Arafeh I, Russell G. Paroxysmal vertigo as a migraine equivalent in children: a population-based study. Cephalalgia 1995;15(1):22–5 [discussion 24].
25. Moretti G, Manzoni GC, Caffarra P, et al. "Benign recurrent vertigo" and its connection with migraine. Headache 1980;20(6):344–6.
26. Slater R. Benign recurrent vertigo. J Neurol Neurosurg Psychiatry 1979;42(4): 363–7.
27. von Brevern M, Radtke A, Clarke AH, et al. Migrainous vertigo presenting as episodic positional vertigo. Neurology 2004;62(3):469–72.
28. Drummond PD. Triggers of motion sickness in migraine sufferers. Headache 2005;45(6):653–6.
29. Versino M, Sances G, Anghileri E, et al. Dizziness and migraine: a causal relationship? Funct Neurol 2003;18(2):97–101.
30. Parker W. Migraine and the vestibular system in adults. Am J Otol 1991;12(1): 25–34.
31. Radtke A, Lempert T, Gresty MA, et al. Migraine and Meniere's disease: is there a link? Neurology 2002;59(11):1700–4.
32. Celebisoy N, Gökçay F, Sirin H, et al. Migrainous vertigo: clinical, oculographic and posturographic findings. Cephalalgia 2008;28(1):72–7.
33. Toglia JU, Thomas D, Kuritzky A. Common migraine and vestibular function. Electronystagmographic study and pathogenesis. Ann Otol Rhinol Laryngol 1981;90(3 Pt 1):267–71.
34. Harno H, Hirvonen T, Kaunisto MA, et al. Subclinical vestibulocerebellar dysfunction in migraine with and without aura. Neurology 2003;61(12):1748–52.
35. Vitkovic J, Paine M, Rance G. Neuro-otological findings in patients with migraine- and nonmigraine-related dizziness. Audiol Neurootol 2008;13(2):113–22.
36. von Brevern M, Zeise D, Neuhauser H, et al. Acute migrainous vertigo: clinical and oculographic findings. Brain 2005;128(Pt 2):365–74.

37. Fasold O, von Brevern M, Kuhberg M, et al. Human vestibular cortex as identified with caloric stimulation in functional magnetic resonance imaging. Neuroimage 2002;17(3):1384–93.

38. Babalian A, Vibert N, Assie G, et al. Central vestibular networks in the guinea-pig: functional characterization in the isolated whole brain in vitro. Neuroscience 1997; 81(2):405–26.

39. Ophoff RA, Terwindt GM, Vergouwe MN, et al. Familial hemiplegic migraine and episodic ataxia type-2 are caused by mutations in the Ca2+ channel gene CACNL1A4. Cell 1996;87:543–52.

40. Kim JS, Yue Q, Jen JC, et al. Familial migraine with vertigo: no mutations found in CACNA1A. Am J Med Genet 1998;79(2):148–51.

41. von Brevern M, Ta N, Shankar A, et al. Migrainous vertigo: mutation analysis of the candidate genes CACNA1A, ATP1A2, SCN1A, and CACNB4. Headache 2006; 46(7):1136–41.

42. Marano E, Marcelli V, Di Stasio E, et al. Trigeminal stimulation elicits a peripheral vestibular imbalance in migraine patients. Headache 2005;45(4):325–31.

43. Neuhauser H, Radtke A, von Brevern M, et al. Zolmitriptan for treatment of migrainous vertigo: a pilot randomized placebo-controlled trial. Neurology 2003;60(5):882–3.

44. Harker LA, Rassekh CH. Episodic vertigo in basilar artery migraine. Otolaryngol Head Neck Surg 1987;96(3):239–50.

45. Baloh RW, Foster CA, Yue Q, et al. Familial migraine with vertigo and essential tremor. Neurology 1996;46(2):458–60.

46. Asprella Libonati G, Gagliardi G. La malattia di Meniere e vertigine emicranica: terapia intercritica, terapia medica. Otoneurologia 2004;18:40–2.

47. Baloh RW. Neurotology of migraine. Headache 1997;37(10):615–21.

48. Bikhazi P, Jackson C, Ruckenstein MJ. Efficacy of antimigrainous therapy in the treatment of migraine-associated dizziness. Am J Otol 1997;18(3):350–4.

49. Whitney SL, Wrisley DM, Brown KE, et al. Physical therapy for migraine-related vestibulopathy and vestibular dysfunction with history of migraine. Laryngoscope 2000;110(9):1528–34.

50. Rassekh CH, Harker LA. The prevalence of migraine in Meniere's disease. Laryngoscope 1992;102(2):135–8.

51. Committee on Hearing and Equilibrium Guidelines for the Diagnosis and Evaluation of Therapy in Menière's Disease. American Academy of Otolaryngology–Head and Neck Foundation, Inc. Otolaryngol Head Neck Surg 1995;113:181–5.

52. Cha YH, Brodsky J, Ishiyama G, et al. The relevance of migraine in patients with Ménière's disease. Acta Otolaryngol 2007;127(12):1241–5.

53. Shepard NT. Differentiation of Ménière's disease and migraine-associated dizziness: a review. J Am Acad Audiol 2006;17(1):69–80.

54. Bath AP, Walsh RM, Ranalli P, et al. Experience from a multidisciplinary "dizzy" clinic. Am J Otol 2000;21(1):92–7.

55. Ishiyama A, Jacobson KM, Baloh RW. Migraine and benign positional vertigo. Ann Otol Rhinol Laryngol 2000;109(4):377–80.

56. Lempert T, Leopold M, von Brevern M, et al. Migraine and benign positional vertigo. Ann Otol Rhinol Laryngol 2000;109(12 Pt 1):1176.

57. Barabas G, Matthews WS, Ferrari M. Childhood migraine and motion sickness. Pediatrics 1983;72(2):188–90.

68. Drummond PD. Motion sickness and migraine: optokinetic stimulation increases scalp tenderness, pain sensitivity in the fingers and photophobia. Cephalalgia 2002;22(2):117–24.

59. Marcus DA, Furman JM. Prevention of motion sickness with rizatriptan: a double-blind, placebo-controlled pilot study. Med Sci Monit 2006;12(1):1–7.
60. Ophoff RA, van Eijk R, Sandkuijl LA, et al. Genetic heterogeneity of familial hemiplegic migraine. Genomics 1994;22(1):21–6.
61. Denier C, Ducros A, Vahedi K, et al. High prevalence of CACNA1A truncations and broader clinical spectrum in episodic ataxia type 2. Neurology 1999;52(9): 1816–21.
62. Zhuchenko O, Bailey J, Bonnen P, et al. Autosomal dominant cerebellar ataxia (SCA6) associated with small polyglutamine expansions in the alpha 1A-voltage-dependent calcium channel. Nat Genet 1997;15(1):62–9.
63. Baloh RW, Yue Q, Furman JM, et al. Familial episodic ataxia: clinical heterogeneity in four families linked to chromosome 19p. Ann Neurol 1997;41(1):8–16.
64. Haan J, Terwindt GM, Ophoff RA, et al. Is familial hemiplegic migraine a hereditary form of basilar migraine? Cephalalgia 1995;15(6):477–81.
65. Sandor PS, Mascia A, Seidel L, et al. Subclinical cerebellar impairment in the common types of migraine: a three-dimensional analysis of reaching movements. Ann Neurol 2001;49(5):668–72.
66. May A, Ophoff RA, Terwindt GM, et al. Familial hemiplegic migraine locus on 19p13 is involved in the common forms of migraine with and without aura. Hum Genet 1995;96(5):604–8.
67. Lance JW, Anthony M. Some clinical aspects of migraine. A prospective survey of 500 patients. Arch Neurol 1966;15(4):356–61.
68. Thijs RD, Kruit MC, van Buchem MA, et al. Syncope in migraine: the population-based CAMERA study. Neurology 2006;66(7):1034–7.
69. Bes A, Dupui P, Guell A, et al. Pharmacological exploration of dopamine hypersensitivity in migraine patients. Int J Clin Pharmacol Res 1986;6(3):189–92.
70. Breslau N, Schultz LR, Stewart WF, et al. Headache and major depression: is the association specific to migraine? Neurology 2000;54(2):308–13.
71. Breslau N, Schultz LR, Stewart WF, et al. Headache types and panic disorder: directionality and specificity. Neurology 2001;56(3):350–4.
72. Margraf J, Taylor B, Ehlers A, et al. Panic attacks in the natural environment. J Nerv Ment Dis 1987;175(9):558–65.
73. Jacob RG, Furman JM, Durrant JD, et al. Panic, agoraphobia, and vestibular dysfunction. Am J Psychiatry 1996;153(4):503–12.
74. Eagger S, Luxon LM, Davies RA, et al. Psychiatric morbidity in patients with peripheral vestibular disorder: a clinical and neuro-otological study. J Neurol Neurosurg Psychiatry 1992;55(5):383–7.
75. Eckhardt-Henn A, Best C, Bense S, et al. Psychiatric comorbidity in different organic vertigo syndromes. J Neurol 2008;255(3):420–8.
76. Furman JM, Balaban CD, Jacob RG, et al. Migraine-anxiety related dizziness (MARD): a new disorder? J Neurol Neurosurg Psychiatry 2005;76(1):1–8.

Diagnostic Testing for Migraine and Other Primary Headaches

Randolph W. Evans, MD

KEYWORDS

- Headache • Diagnostic testing • Magnetic resonance imaging
- Computerized tomography • Migraine
- Trigeminal autonomic cephalalgias • Hemicrania continua
- New daily persistent headache

Most primary headaches can be diagnosed without diagnostic testing using a comprehensive history and neurologic and focused general physical examinations.

In some cases, however, diagnostic testing is necessary to distinguish primary from secondary causes that may share similar features. The differential diagnosis is one of the longest in all of medicine, with more than 300 different types and causes. In this article, the reasons for diagnostic testing and the use of neuroimaging, electrencephalography, lumbar puncture, and blood testing are evaluated. The use of diagnostic testing in adults and children who have a normal neurologic examination, migraine, trigeminal autonomic cephalalgias (TACs), hemicrania continua (HC), and new daily persistent headache (NDPH) are reviewed.

REASONS FOR DIAGNOSTIC TESTING

The indications for diagnostic testing are variable and neurologists must make decisions on a case-by-case basis when presented with a suspected primary headache if secondary headache is a consideration. Clinical situations where neurologists consider diagnostic testing are listed in **Box 1**.

There are many other reasons why neurologists recommend diagnostic testing: "our stubborn quest for diagnostic certainty;"[1] faulty cognitive reasoning; the medical decision rule that it is better to impute disease than to risk overlooking it busy practice conditions where tests are ordered as a shortcut; patient expectations; financial incentives; professional peer pressure, where recommendations for routine and esoteric tests are expected as a demonstration of competence; and medicolegal issues.[2,3] The attitudes and demands of patients and families and the practice of defensive medicine are especially important reasons in the case of headaches. In the era of managed care, equally compelling reasons for not ordering diagnostic studies include

1200 Binz #1370, Houston, TX 77004, USA
E-mail address: rwevans@pol.net

Neurol Clin 27 (2009) 393–415
doi:10.1016/j.ncl.2008.11.009
0733-8619/08/$ – see front matter © 2009 Elsevier Inc. All rights reserved.

neurologic.theclinics.com

Box 1

Reasons to consider neuroimaging for headaches

Temporal and headache features

1. The "first or worst" headache
2. Subacute headaches with increasing frequency or severity
3. A progressive headache or NDPH
4. Chronic daily headache
5. Headaches always on the same side
6. Headaches not responding to treatment

Demographics

7. New-onset headaches in patients who have cancer or who test positive for HIV infection
8. New-onset headaches after age 50
9. Patients who have headaches and seizures

Associated symptoms and signs

10. Headaches associated with symptoms and signs, such as fever, stiff neck, nausea, and vomiting
11. Headaches other than migraine with aura associated with focal neurologic symptoms or signs
12. Headaches associated with papilledema, cognitive impairment, or personality change

From Evans RW. Headaches. In: Evans RW, editor. Diagnostic testing in neurology. Philadelphia: W.B. Saunders; 1999. p. 2; with permission.

---

physician fears of deselection and at-risk capitation. Lack of funds and underinsurance continue to be barriers to appropriate diagnostic testing for many patients.

DIAGNOSTIC TESTING OPTIONS
CT versus MRI

CT detects most abnormalities that may cause headaches. CT generally is preferred to MRI for evaluation of acute subarachnoid hemorrhage, acute head trauma, and bony abnormalties. There are several disorders, however, that may be missed on routine CT of the head, including vascular disease, neoplastic disease, cervicomedullary lesions, and infections (**Box 2**). MRI is more sensitive than CT in the detection of posterior fossa and cervicomedullary lesions, ischemia, white matter abnormalities (WMA), cerebral venous thrombosis (CVT), subdural and epidural hematomas, neoplasms (especially in the posterior fossa), meningeal disease (such as carcinomatosis, diffuse meningeal enhancement in low cerebrospinal fluid [CSF] pressure syndrome, and sarcoid), and cerebritis and brain abscess. Pituitary pathology is more likely to be detected on a routine MRI of the brain than a routine CT.

Another concern with CT is exposure to ionizing radiation. The average radiation dose of a CT scan of the head (with or without contrast—both studies double the dose) is an effective dose of 2.0 millisieverts (mSv), which is equivalent to 100 chest radiographs.[4] The most common malignancies associated with radiation exposure include leukemia and breast, thyroid, lung, and stomach cancers. The latency period for solid tumors usually is long, an average of 10 to 20 years, with a persistent lifelong risk. Leukemia has an earlier latency period with an increased risk 2 to 5 years after

Box 2
Causes of headache that can be missed on routine CT scan of the head
Vascular disease
Saccular aneurysms
AVMs (especially posterior fossa)
Subarachnoid hemorrhage
Carotid or vertebral artery dissections
Infarcts
CVT
Vasculitis
WMA
Subdural and epidural hematomas
Neoplastic disease
Neoplasms (especially in the posterior fossa)
Meningeal carcinomatosis
Pituitary tumor and hemorrhage
Cervicomedullary lesions
Chiari malformations
Foramen magnum meningioma
Infections
Paranasal sinusitis
Meningoencephalitis
Cerebritis and brain abscess
Other
Low CSF pressure syndrome
Idiopathic hypertrophic pachymeningitis
From Evans RW. Headaches. In: Evans RW, editor. Diagnostic testing in neurology. Philadelphia: W.B. Saunders; 1999. p. 3; with permission.

radiation exposure. The pediatric population is at increased risk, as a result of increased radiosensitivity and more years of remaining life, for potentially developing cancer. Consider the radiation exposure of some patients who have multiple trips to an emergency department, have migraine and multiple CT scans, and also have multiple CT scans of the head and sinuses in an outpatient setting. For a single CT scan of the head, the estimated lifetime attributable risk for death from cancer by age is approximately as follows: age 10 years, 0.025%; age 20 years, 0.01%; and age 50 years, 0.003%.[5] Although these are small numbers, are individual studies justified? Up to 2% of all cancer deaths in the United States may be attributable to radiation exposure associated with CT use. The Food and Drug Administration has estimated that exposure to 10 mSv (equivalent to one CT of the abdomen) may be associated with an increased risk for developing fatal cancer in one of every 2000 patients [FDA].[6]

Thus, MRI generally is preferred over CT for evaluation of headaches. The yield of MRI may vary depending on the field strength of the magnet, the use of paramagnetic contrast, the selection of acquisition sequences, and the use of magnetic resonance (MR) angiography and MR venography (MRV). MRI may be contraindicated, however, in the presence of an aneurysm clip or pacemaker. In addition, approximately 8% of patients are claustrophobic, approximately 2% to the point at which they cannot tolerate the study.

Neuroimaging During Pregnancy and Lactation

When there are appropriate indications, neuroimaging should be performed during pregnancy.[7] With the use of lead shielding, a standard CT scan of the head exposes the uterus to less than 1 mrad. The radiation dose for a typical cervical or intracranial arteriogram is less than 1 mrad. The fetus is most susceptible to the teratogenic effects of radiation between the second and 20th weeks of embryonic age[8] with a threshold radiation dose estimated at between 5 and 15 rad.[9] Although there is no known risk associated with iodinated contrast use during pregnancy, contrast should be avoided without indication.[10]

MRI is more sensitive for rare disorders that may occur during pregnancy, such as pituitary apoplexy, CVT (with the addition of MRV), and metastatic choriocarcinoma. There is no known risk associated with MRI during pregnancy[11] but there is some controversy because the magnets induce an electric field and raise the core temperature slightly (less than 1°C). A survey of pregnant MRI workers found no adverse fetal outcome,[12] and no adverse fetal effects from MRI have been documented to date. Children exposed in utero at 1.5 tesla were found to have no exposure-related abnormalities at 9 months of age[13] and up to 9 years of age.[14]

According to the 2007 American College of Radiology Guidance Document for Safe Practices,[10]

> Present data have not conclusively documented any deleterious effects of MR imaging exposure on the developing fetus. Therefore, no special consideration is recommended for the first, versus any other, trimester in pregnancy. Pregnant patients can be accepted to undergo MR scans at any stage of pregnancy if, in the determination of a level 2 MR personnel-designated attending radiologist, the risk-benefit ratio to the patient warrants that the study be performed. The radiologist should confer with the referring physician and document the following in the radiology report or the patient's medical record:
>
> 1. The information requested from the MR study cannot be acquired via nonionizing means (eg, ultrasonography).
> 2. The data are needed to potentially affect the care of the patient or fetus during the pregnancy.
> 3. The referring physician does not feel it is prudent to wait until the patient is no longer pregnant to obtain these data.
>
> ...MR contrast agents should not be routinely provided to pregnant patients. The decision to administer a gadolinium-based MR contrast agent to pregnant patients should be accompanied by a well-documented and thoughtful risk–benefit analysis.[15]

There is no known risk of gadolinium to the fetus.[10]

Lactating women may be advised to discard breast milk for 24 hours after receiving intravenous iodinated contrast or gadolinium. Only a tiny fraction of iodinated contrast or gadolinium entering the infant gut is actually absorbed, however. "The very small potential risk associated with absorption of contrast medium may be insufficient to warrant stopping breast-feeding for 24 hours after either iodinated or gadolinium contrast agents."[11]

Electroencephalography

The electroencephalogram (EEG) was a standard test for evaluation of headaches in the pre-CT scan era. Gronseth and Greenberg[16] reviewed the literature from 1941 to 1994 on the usefulness of EEG in the evaluation of patients who had headache. Most of the articles had serious methodologic flaws. The only significant abnormality reported in studies with a relatively nonflawed design was prominent driving in response to photic stimulation (the H-response) in migraineurs who had a sensitivity ranging from 26%[17] to 100%[18] and a specificity from 80%[19] to 91%.[18] This finding, although interesting, is not necessary for the clinical diagnosis of migraine. If the purpose of the EEG is to exclude an underlying structural lesion, such as a neoplasm, CT or MRI imaging is far superior.

A report of the Quality Standards Subcommittee of the American Academy of Neurology (AAN) suggests the following practice parameter: "The electroencephalogram (EEG) is not useful in the routine evaluation of patients with headache. This does not exclude the use of EEG to evaluate headache patients with associated symptoms suggesting a seizure disorder such as atypical migrainous aura or episodic loss of consciousness. Assuming head imaging capabilities are readily available, EEG is not recommended to exclude a structural cause for headache."[20]

A report of the Quality Standards Subcommittee of the AAN and the Practice Committee of the Child Neurology Society[21] makes the following pediatric recommendations: "EEG is not recommended in the routine evaluation of a child with recurrent headaches, as it is unlikely to provide an etiology, improve diagnostic yield, or distinguish migraine from other types of headaches (Level C; class II and class III evidence)."

Lumbar Puncture

MRI or CT scan always is performed before a lumbar puncture for evaluation of headaches except in some cases where acute meningitis is suspected. Lumbar puncture can be diagnostic for meningitis or encephalitis, meningeal carcinomatosis or lymphomatosis, subarachnoid hemorrhage, and high (eg, pseudotumor cerebri) or low CSF pressure. In cases of blood dyscrasias, the platelet count should be 50,000 or greater before safely performing a lumbar puncture. The CSF opening pressure always should be measured when investigating headaches. When measuring the opening pressure, it is important for patients to relax and at least partially extend the head and legs to avoid recording a falsely elevated pressure.

After neuroimaging is performed, lumbar puncture often is indicated in the following circumstances: the first or worst headache, headache with fever or other symptoms or signs suggesting an infectious cause, a subacute or progressive headache (eg, in an HIV-positive patient or a person who has carcinoma), and an atypical chronic headache (eg, to rule out pseudotumor cerebri in an obese woman who does not have papilledema).

There are many potential complications of lumbar puncture, the most common of which is low CSF pressure headache, which occurs approximately 30% of the time using the conventional bevel-tip or Quincke needle.[22] The risk for headache can be reduced dramatically to approximately 5% to 10% by using an atraumatic needle, such as the Sprotte or Whitacre, and replacing the stylet before withdrawing the needle.[23]

Blood Tests

Blood tests generally are not helpful for diagnosis of headaches. There are many indications, however, such as the following: erythrocyte sedimentation rate or C-reactive protein to consider the possibility of temporal arteritis in a person 50 years or older who has new-onset migraine, as only 2% of migraineurs have an onset at age 50 years or older; erthyrocyte sedimentation rate, rheumatoid arthritis factor, and antinuclear antibody test in patients who have headache and arthralgia to evaluate for possible collagen vascular disease, such as lupus;[24] monospot in teenagers who have headaches, sore throat, and cervical adenopathy; complete blood cell count (CBC), liver function tests, HIV test, or Lyme antibody test in some patients who have a suspected infectious basis; an anticardiolipin antibody and lupus anticoagulant in migraineurs who have extensive WMA on MRI; thyroid-stimulating hormone because headache may be a symptom in 14% of cases of hypothyroidism; CBC because headache may be a symptom when the hemoglobin concentration is reduced by one half or more; serum urea nitrogren and creatinine to exclude renal failure, which can cause headache; serum calcium because hypercalcemia can be associated with headaches; CBC and platelets because thrombotic thrombocytopenic purpura can cause headaches; and endocrine studies in patients who have headaches and a pituitary tumor.

Additionally, blood tests may be indicated as a baseline and for monitoring for certain medications, such as valproic acid for migraine prophylaxis, carbamazepine for trigeminal neuralgia, and lithium for chronic cluster headaches.

HEADACHES AND A NORMAL NEUROLOGIC EXAMINATION
Neuroimaging Studies in Adults

The yield of abnormal neuroimaging studies in studies of patients who have headaches as the only neurologic symptom and normal neurologic examinations depends on several factors, including the duration of the headache, study design (prospective versus retrospective), who orders the scan, and the type of scan performed.[25] The percentage of abnormal scans is higher when ordered by neurologists[26] or a tertiary care center[27] compared with primary care physicians and represents case selection bias. In reported CT scan series, the yield may vary depending on the generation of scanner and whether or not iodinated contrast was used. The yield of MRI may vary depending on the field strength of the magnet, the use of paramagnetic contrast, the selection of acquisition sequences, and the use of MR angiography.

Frishberg[25] reviewed eight CT scan studies of 1825 patients who had unspecified headache types and varying durations of headache.[26-33] The summarized findings from these studies is combined with four additional studies of 1566 CT scans in patients who had headache and normal neurologic examinations[34-37] for a total of 3389 scans. The overall percentages of various pathologies is as follows: brain tumors, 1%; arteriovenous malformations (AVMs), 0.2%; hydrocephalus, 0.3%; aneurysm, 0.1%; subdural hematoma, 0.2%; and strokes (including chronic ischemic process), 1.1%.

There are four studies of patients who had chronic headaches and a normal neurologic examination. Combining three of these studies with 1282 patients, the only clinically significant pathology was one low-grade glioma and one saccular aneurysm.[33,34,36] A fourth study of 363 consecutive CT scans, however, found significant pathology in 11 (3%), including two of intraventricular cysts, four meningiomas, and five malignant neoplasms.[35]

Weingarten and colleagues[33] extrapolated various types of data from 100,800 adult patients who belonged to a health maintenance organization. The estimated prevalence (in patients who had chronic headache and a normal neurologic examination) of a CT scan demonstrating an abnormality requiring neurosurgical intervention may have been as low as 0.01%. It is not certain whether or not detection of additional pathology on MRI scan would change this percentage. For example, complaints of headache with a normal neurologic examination may be seen in patients who have Chiari type I malformation, which is easily detected on MRI but not CT scans.[38] Pituitary hemorrhage can produce a migraine-like acute headache with a normal neurologic examination.[39] Pituitary infarction, with severe headache, photophobia, and CSF pleocytosis, initially can be similar to aseptic meningitis or meningoencephalitis.[40] Pituitary pathology is more likely to be detected on a routine MRI than CT scan.

Wang and coworkers[41] retrospectively reviewed the medical records and MRI images of 402 adult patients (286 women and 116 men) who had been evaluated by the neurology service and who had a primary complaint of chronic headache (a duration of 3 months or more) and no other neurologic symptoms or findings. Major abnormalities (a mass, caused mass effect, or was believed the likely cause of patient's headache) were found in 15 patients (3.7%) and included glioma, meningioma, metastases, subdural hematoma, AVM, hydrocephalus (three patients), and Chiari I malformations (two patients). They were found in 0.6% of patients who had migraine, 1.4% of those who had tension headaches, 14.1% of those who had atypical headaches, and 3.8% of those who had other types of headaches.

Tsushima and Endo[42] retrospectively reviewed the clinical data and MR studies of 306 adult patients (136 men and 170 woman) all of whom were referred for MRI evaluation of chronic or recurrent headache with a duration of 1 month or month, had no other neurologic symptoms or focal findings at physical examination, and had no prior head surgery, head trauma, or seizure: 55.2% had no abnormalities, 44.1% had minor abnormalities, and 0.7% (two) had clinically significant abnormalities (pituitary macroadenoma and subdural hematoma). Neither contrast material enhancement (n = 195) nor repeated MRI (n = 23) contributed to the diagnosis.

Sempere and colleagues[43] reported a study of 1876 consecutive patients (1243 women and 633 men), ages 15 or older, mean age 38 years, who had headaches that had an onset at least 4 weeks previously and who were referred to two neurology clinics in Spain. One third of the headaches were new onset, and two thirds had been present for more than 1 year. Subjects had the following types: migraine (49%), tension (35.4%), cluster (1.1%), posttraumatic (3.7%), and indeterminate (10.8%). Normal neurologic examinations were found in 99.2% of the patients. CT scan was performed in 1432 patients and MRI in 580; 136 patients underwent both studies.

Neuroimaging studies detected significant lesions in 22 patients (1.2%), of whom 17 had a normal neurologic examination. The only variable or red flag associated with a higher probability of intracranial abnormalities was an abnormal neurologic examination with a likelihood ratio of 42. The diagnoses in these 17 patients were pituitary adenoma (n = 3), large arachnoid cyst (n = 2), meningioma (n = 2), hydrocephalus (n = 2), and Arnold-Chiari type I malformation, ischemic stroke, cavernous angioma, AVM, low-grade astrocytoma, brainstem glioma, colloid cyst, and posterior fossa papilloma (one of each). Of these 17 patients, eight were treated surgically for hydrocephalus (n = 2), and pituitary adenoma, large arachnoid cyst, meningioma, AVM, colloid cyst, and papilloma (one of each).

The rate of significant intracranial abnormalities in patients who had headache and normal neurologic examination was 0.9%. Neuroimaging studies discovered incidental findings in 14 patients (75%): three pineal cysts, three intracranial lipomas, and eight arachnoid cysts. The yield of neuroimaging studies was higher in the group with indeterminate headache (3.7%) than in the migraine (0.4%) or tension-type headache (0.8%) groups. The study does not provide information on WMA in migraineurs. MRI performed in patients who had normal CT revealed significant lesions in two cases: a small meningioma and an acoustic neurinoma. No saccular aneurysms were detected; MR angiography was not obtained.

The studies do not give information about the detection of paranasal sinus disease, however, which may be the cause of some headaches. For example, sphenoid sinusitis may cause a severe, intractable, new-onset headache that interferes with sleep and is not relieved by simple analgesics. The headache may increase in severity with no specific location. There may be associated pain or paraesthesias in the facial distribution of the fifth nerve and photophobia or eye tearing with or without fever or nasal drainage. The headache may mimic other causes, such as migraine or meningitis.[44]

Neuroimaging in Children

Several studies have investigated the findings of neuroimaging in children who had headaches. Dooley and colleagues reported the retrospective findings of CT scans of 41 children who had headaches and normal neurologic examinations referred to a secondary or tertiary care facility.[45] Only one scan was abnormal demonstrating a choroid plexus papilloma. Chu and Shinnar[46] obtained brain imaging studies in 30 children, ages 7 or younger, who had headaches and were referred to pediatric neurologists. The studies were normal except for five that had incidental findings.

Maytal and coworkers[47] obtained MRI or CT scans or both in 78 children, ages 3 to 18, who had headaches. With the exception of six patients, the neurologic examinations were normal. The studies were normal except for incidental cerebral abnormalities in four and mucoperiosteal thickening of the paranasal sinuses in seven. Wöber-Bingöl and colleagues[48] prospectively obtained MRI scans in 96 children, ages 5 to 18, who had headaches and normal neurologic examinations and who were referred to an outpatient headache clinic. The studies were normal except for 17 (17.7%) that had incidental findings.

Medina and colleagues[49] retrospectively reported MRI findings in 315 children, ages 3 to 20 (mean 11 years), who had headaches. The neurologic examinations were abnormal in 89 patients. Thirteen (4%) had surgical space-occupying lesions. After analyzing risk factors for these lesions and the prior literature, Medina and colleagues suggested guidelines for neuroimaging in children who have headache (**Box 3**).

Lewis and Dorbad[50] retrospectively reviewed records of children, ages 6 to 18, who had migraine and chronic daily headache with normal examinations. Of 54 patients who had migraine who underwent CT (42) or MRI (12) scans, the yield of abnormalities was 3.7%, none clinically relevant. Of 25 patients who had chronic daily headache who underwent CT (17) or MRI (8) scans, the yield of abnormalities was 16%, none clinically relevant.

Carlos and colleagues,[51] in a retrospective chart review, identified all pediatric migraine patients who had a CT or MRI to investigate their headaches. Ages ranged from 3 to 18. Of the 93 patients, 35 had CT, 14 had MRI, and 9 had both. Twenty-two had abnormalities but none was believed related to the patients' headaches. Alehan[52] prospectively obtained neuroimaging (49 MRI scans and 11 CT scans) in 60 of 72 consecutive children diagnosed with migraine or tension-type headaches. Ten percent had findings related to their headache with no neoplasms, and no patients required surgery.

Mazzotta and colleagues[53] performed a prospective study at several pediatric headache centers of 6535 first-time referrals; patients up to age 18 were studied. Based on the indications of the diagnostic flow-chart, 1485 underwent neuroimaging testing. Incidental findings were observed in 138 (9.3%) subjects. Abnormal results were observed in 273 (18.5%) subjects. Findings that led to diagnosis of secondary

---

Box 3
Reasons to consider neuroimaging for children who have headaches

1. Persistent headaches of less than 6-months' duration that do not respond to medical treatment

2. Headache associated with abnormal neurologic findings, especially if accompanied by papilledema, nystagmus, or gait or motor abnormalities

3. Persistent headaches associated with an absent family history of migraine

4. Persistent headache associated with substantial episodes of confusion, disorientation, or emesis

5. Headaches that awaken a child repeatedly from sleep or occur immediately on awakening

6. Family history or medical history of disorders that may predispose one to central nervous system lesions and clinical or laboratory findings suggestive of central nervous system involvement

Data from Medina S, Pinter JD, Zurakowski D, et al. Children with headache: clinical predictors of surgical space-occupying lesions and the role of neuroimaging. Radiology 1997;202:819–24.

---

headache were observed in 135 (9.1%), including sinusitis in 57% and intracranial space-occupying lesions in 17.4%.

A report of the Quality Standards Subcommittee of the AAN and the Practice Committee of the Child Neurology Society[21] makes the following recommendations:

1. Obtaining a neuroimaging study on a routine basis is not indicated in children who have recurrent headaches and a normal neurologic examination (level B; class II and class III evidence).
2. Neuroimaging should be considered in children who have an abnormal neurologic examination (eg, focal findings, signs of increased intracranial pressure, significant alteration of consciousness), the coexistence of seizures, or both (level B; class II and class III evidence).
3. Neuroimaging should be considered in children in whom there are historical features to suggest the recent onset of severe headache or change in the type of headache or if there are associated features that suggest neurologic dysfunction (level B; class II and class III evidence).

American Academy of Neurology Practice Parameter

A report of the Quality Standards Subcommittee of the AAN[54] makes the following recommendations for nonacute headache:

The following symptoms significantly increased the odds of finding a significant abnormality on neuroimaging in patients with nonacute headache: rapidly increasing headache frequency; history of lack of coordination; history of localized neurologic signs or a history such as subjective numbness or tingling; and history of headache causing awakening from sleep (although this can occur with migraine and cluster headache). The absence of these symptoms did not significantly lower the odds of finding a significant abnormality on neuroimaging.

Consider Neuroimaging in Patients with an unexplained abnormal finding on the neurologic examination (Grade B).

Consider neuroimaging in patients with atypical headache features or headaches that do not fulfill the strict definition of migraine or other primary headache disorder (or have some additional risk factor, such as immune deficiency), when a lower threshold for neuroimaging may be applied (Grade C).

No evidence-based recommendations are established for the following: presence or absence of neurologic symptoms (Grade C); tension-type headache (Grade C); and relative sensitivity of MRI as compared with CT in the evaluation of migraine or other nonacute headache (Grade C).

Risk/Benefit and Cost/Benefit of Neuroimaging

Table 1 summarizes the estimated risks and benefits of neuroimaging in patients who have headaches and normal neurologic examinations. (Radiation exposure and the increased long-term risk for are cancer discussed previously.) Although for many patients the scan helps to relieve anxiety, for others the scan may produce anxiety when nonspecific abnormalities are found, such as incidental anatomic variants or white matter lesions. I suspect that many neurologists have seen patients who have isolated headaches referred by primary care physicians with a request to rule out multiple sclerosis when white matter lesions are detected.

Although the cost of finding significant pathology is high, the cost of neuroimaging is decreasing significantly under some managed care contracts. Cost/benefit estimates should include the cost to physicians of malpractice suits filed when patients who have significant pathology do not have neuroimaging and the cost to patients and society of premature death and disability of undetected treatable lesions.

Table 1
Balance sheet. CT or MRI in patients with headaches and normal neurologic examinations. Technology: CT with intravenous contrast or MRI without contrast. Indications: (1) migraine and (2) any headache

	CT	MRI	No Test
Health outcomes			
Benefits			
Discovery of potentially treatable lesions			
1. Migraine	0.3%	0.4%	0
2. Any headache	2.4%	2.4%	0
Relief of anxiety	30%	30%	0
Harms			
Iodine reaction			
Mild	10%		
Moderate	1%		
Severe	0.01%		
Death	0.002%		
Claustrophobia			
Mild	5%	15%	0
Moderate (needs sedation)	1%	5%–10%	
Severe (unable to comply)	1%–2%		
False-positive studies	No data	No data	
Cost (charges)	Varies widely depending on payor		

Data from Frishberg BM. The utility of neuroimaging in the evaluation of headache in patients with normal neurologic examinations. Neurology 1994;44:1196.

NEUROIMAGING IN MIGRAINE
Incidence of Pathology

Frishberg[25] reviewed four CT scan studies,[55–58] four MRI scan studies,[59–62] and one combined MRI and CT scan study[63] of 897 scans of patients who had migraine. These findings are combined with more recent reports of one CT scan study of 284 patients[36] and six studies of MRI scans of 444 patients[64–69] for a total of 1625 scans of patients who had various types of migraine. Other than WMA, the studies showed no significant pathology except for four brain tumors (three of which were incidental findings) and one AVM (in a patient who had migraine and a seizure disorder). Sempere[43] found a similarly low yield of 0.4%.

White Matter Abnormalities and Subclinical Infarcts

Fourteen MRI studies have investigated WMA on scans of patients who had migraine. WMA are foci of hyperintensity on proton density and T2-weighted images in the deep and periventricular white matter resulting from interstitial edema or perivascular demyelination. WMA are easily detected on MRI but are not seen on CT scan.[63]

The percentages of WMA for all types of migraine range from 12%[61] to 46%.[62] WMA have been reported as more frequent in the frontal region of the centrum semiovale[59,65] and no more frequent[67] than in the white matter of the parietal, temporal, and occipital lobes. Six of the eight studies using controls found a higher incidence of WMA in migraineurs. The incidence of WMA in controls ranged from 0%[70] to 14%.[66] One small study reported a similar incidence of WMA in patients who had tension-type headaches, 34.3%, as in those who had migraine, 32.1%, and greater than the 7.4% in controls.[65]

Four studies found similar percentages of WMA comparing migraine with aura to migraine without,[64,65,67,71] whereas two reported a higher percentage in migraine with aura.[59,66] Three small studies of basilar migraine found WMA in 17%[60,64] and 38%.[66] WMA are variably reported as present more often in adult migraineurs more than 40 years old and less than 60[64,71] and equally present[66] compared with those 40 or younger. Cooney and coworkers[64] found an increased frequency of WMA associated with age over 50 and with medical risk factors (hypertension, atherosclerotic heart disease, diabetic mellitus, autoimmune disorder, or demyelinating disease) but not with gender, migraine subtype, or duration of migraine symptoms.

Migraine with aura is associated with an increased frequency of right-to-left shunts, mostly resulting from patent foramen ovale, which hypothetically could cause WMA as a result of paradoxic microembolism of platelets or the shunting of vasoactive amines, which have escaped the pulmonary circulation. A study of 185 consecutive subjects who had migraine with aura, 66% with right-to-left shunts, however, found no increase in white matter lesion load as compared with those who did not have shunts.[72] Periventricular WMA were present in 19% and deep WMA in 46%, and 11% showed coexistence of periventricular and deep lesions. Similarly, there was no increase in white matter lesions in another consecutive series of 87 migraineurs, 45% of whom had right-to-left shunts.[73] WMA were present in 61% of patients. In both studies, the only risk factor associated with WMA was older age but not gender, frequency of migraines, smoking, hyperlipidemia, or oral contraceptive use.

In a series of 16 consecutive migraineurs (14 who did not have aura and 2 who had aura), Rovaris and colleagues[70] found white matter lesions in five (31%). The pattern of MRI lesions fulfilled diagnostic criteria suggestive of MS in four—none of the patients had any other neurologic symptoms or signs. Cervical spine MRI studies were obtained in all subjects and in 17 age- and gender-matched controls with the detection of no cord lesions.

Kruit and coworkers[74] obtained MRI scans in a population-based sample of Dutch adults, ages 30 to 60, who had migraine with aura (n = 161) or migraine without aura (n = 134) and in well-matched controls (n = 140). No participants reported a history of stroke or transient ischemic attack or had relevant abnormalities at standard neurologic examination. There was no significant difference between patients who had migraine and controls in overall infarct prevalence (8.1% versus 5%). In the cerebellar region of the posterior circulation territory, however, patients who had migraine had a higher prevalence of infarct than controls (5.4% versus 0.7%). The adjusted odds ratio (OR) for posterior infarct varied by migraine subtype and attack frequency. The adjusted OR was 13.7 for patients who had migraine with aura compared with controls. In patients who had migraine with a frequency of attacks of one or more per month, the adjusted OR was 9.3. The highest risk was in patients who had migraine with aura with one attack or more per month (OR 15.8). Kruit and colleagues[75] hypothesize that focal (possibly migraine-related) hypoperfusion rather than microembolic occlusion is responsible for most of the cerebellar infarcts.

Thirty eight percent of the subjects in the migraine and control groups had at least one medium-sized deep white matter lesion (DWML). Among women, the risk for high DWML load was increased in patients who had migraine compared with controls (OR 2.1); this risk increased with attack frequency (highest in those who had one attack per month; OR 2.6) but was similar in patients who had migraine with or without aura. In men, control patients and patients who had migraine did not differ in the prevalence of DWMLs. There was no association between severity of periventricular white matter lesions (PVWMLs) and migraine, irrespective of gender or migraine frequency or subtype. There were no differences in the distributions and the mean values of grades of severity of PVWMLs between patients who had migraine and controls. These results did not vary by gender, migraine subtype, or migraine attack frequency.

Kruit and colleagues[76] further reported the brainstem and cerebellar hyperintense lesions found in their same migraine population. Infratentorial hyperintensities were identified in 13 of 295 (4.4%) migraineurs and in 1 of 140 (0.7%) controls. Twelve patients had hyperintensities, mostly bilateral, in the dorsal basis pontis (described for the first time in migraine). Those who had infratentorial hyperintensities also had supratentorial white matter lesions more often. The cause may be small-vessel disease (arteriosclerosis), repetitive perfusion deficits, or both.

Although the cause of WMA in migraine is not certain, various hypotheses have been advanced, including increased platelet aggregability with microemboli, abnormal cerebrovascular regulation, and repeated attacks of hypoperfusion during the aura.[59,65,67,74] The presence of antiphospholipid antibodies might be another risk factor for WMA in migraine.[77] The reported incidence of antiphospholipid antibodies in migraine ranges from 0%[78] to 24%.[68] In one MRI study, however, the presence of WMA showed no correlation with the presence of anticardiolipin antibodies.[59] The presence of anticardiolipin antibodies is not an additional risk factor for stroke in migraineurs.[79] Tietjen and colleagues[80] found that, compared with control subjects, there was no increase in frequency of anticardiolipin positivity in adults under age 60 who had transient focal neurologic events or in those who had migraine with or without aura.

A subgroup of migraineurs may have a genetic predisposition for white matter lesions on MRI scans. Cerebral autosomal dominant arteriopathy with subcortical infarcts and leukoencephalopathy (CADASIL) is a familial genetic disease with migraine as a common symptom and severe WMA on MRI as a consistent neuroimaging finding. Chabriat and colleagues[81] described several members of a family who had an autosomal dominant illness manifested by migraine attacks and a significant leukoencephalopathy on MRI but without other specific manifestations of CADASIL. Mourad and colleagues[82] also describe four patients over age 60 who had typical Notch3 mutations leading to CADASIL and who did not have dementia or disability but had extensive WMA on MRI. It is possible that there is a specific gene locus for migraine with white matter changes. Variable gene penetrance could result in CADASIL at one extreme and individuals who have tiny T2 hyperintense white matter foci and migraine alone at the other extreme.

Cerebral Atrophy

Diffuse cerebral atrophy with widening of the lateral ventricles and cerebral sulci is detected equally well by MRI and CT scans.[63] The incidence of cerebral atrophy in migraineurs on CT and MRI scans has been variably reported as 4%,[55] 26%,[57] 28%,[71] 35%,[63] and 58%.[83] Studies describe most cases of atrophy as mild to moderate. The cause of the atrophy, which can be a nonspecific finding based on often subjective criteria, is not certain.[69,71,84] Three more recent studies have found the incidence of atrophy in migraineurs no greater than in controls.[65,69,84] The high incidence of CT changes seen in migraineurs in early studies probably reflects artifact and a failure to recognize the range of normality of this new imaging technique.

Arteriovenous Malformations, Brainstem Vascular Malformations, and Migraine

The prevalence of AVMs is approximately 0.5% in postmortem studies.[85] In contrast to saccular aneurysms, up to 50% of patients present with symptoms or signs other than hemorrhage. Headache without distinctive features (such as frequency, duration, or severity) is the presenting symptom in up to 48% of cases.[86]

Migraine-like headaches with and without visual symptoms can be associated with AVMs especially those in the occipital lobe, the predominant location of approximately 20% of parenchymal AVMs.[87,88] Although headaches always occurring on the same side (side-locked) are present in 95% of patients who have AVMs,[89] 17% of those who have migraine without aura and 15% of patients who have migraine with aura have side-locked headaches.[90]

Migraine resulting from an AVM usually is atypical and rarely meets International Headache Society (IHS) criteria for migraine. In a series of 109 patients who had headache and AVMs, Ghossoub and colleagues[91] reported the following features: nonpulsating, 95%; nausea, vomiting, light, or noise sensitivity, 4.1%; unilateral and homolateral to the AVM, 70%; duration less than 3 hours, 77%; 1 to 2 per month, 82.5%; and usually mild, responding to simple analgesics. Bruyn[89] reported the following features in patients who had migraine-like symptoms and AVM: unusual associated signs (papilledema, field cut, and bruit), 65%; short duration of headache attacks, 20%; brief scintillating scotoma, 10%; absent family history, 15%; atypical sequence of aura, headache, and vomiting, 10%; and seizures, 25%.

The following brainstem vascular malformations are associated with migraine meeting IHS criteria: a hemorrhagic midbrain cavernoma resulting in a contralateral headache,[92] a pontine bleed from a cavernous angioma with initially ipsilateral headache then bilateral with aura,[93] pontine capillary telangiectasia with signs of residual hemorrhage with bilateral headaches initially with aura,[94] and a midbrain/upper pons hemorrhagic AVM/cavernous malformation resulting in a contralateral headache with aura.[95] These malformations provide evidence for the involvement of the brainstem in the initiation of migraine.

Chronic Migraine

American Academy of Neurology practice parameter

A report of the Quality Standards Subcommittee of the AAN[54] makes the following recommendation: "Neuroimaging is not usually warranted in patients with migraine and a normal neurologic examination (Grade B)."

Although the yield is low, **Box 4** lists some reasons to consider neuroimaging in migraineurs.

Trigeminal autonomic cephalalgias

TACs are primary headache syndromes characterized by severe short-lasting headaches typically associated with paroxysmal facial autonomic symptoms. TACs include cluster headache, paroxysmal hemicrania, and short-lasting unilateral neuralgiform headache with conjunctival injection and tearing (SUNCT), with cluster headache the most common.[96,97]

There are 35 case reports of patients who had TACs and TAC-like syndromes (including 20 diagnosed as cluster headaches) showing significant improvement or even disappearance of the headache after therapeutic intervention aimed at the structural lesion (eg, surgery, embolization, radiotherapy, or medical therapy).[98–101] Only 10 of the patients had atypical symptoms, including abnormal attack duration, absence of autonomic symptoms, bilateral autonomic symptoms, or a continuous headache. Patients could have a large cerebral tumor and still meet IHS criteria for a TAC. Secondary causes were as follows: vascular abnormalities, including AVMs, fistula, aneurysms, and arterial dissections (11 patients); tumors (19 patients, including 12 who had pituitary tumor); abnormalities in paranasal sinuses (aspergilloma, foreign object, and mucocele) (three patients); and cervical syrinx (one patient).

Levy and colleagues[102] reported a series of 84 consecutive patients who had pituitary tumors (65% macroadenomas). Using IHS classification, four met criteria for SUNCT, three for cluster, and one for HC. Cavernous sinus invasion was present in two of the three cluster cases. Of the four SUNCT cases, two were prolactinomas

---

Box 4
Reasons to consider neuroimaging in migraineurs

Unusual, prolonged, or persistent aura

Increasing frequency, severity, or change in clinical features

First or worst migraine

Basilar

Confusional

Hemiplegic

Late-life migraine accompaniments

Aura without headache

Headaches always on the same side?

Posttraumatic

Patient or family and friend request

From Evans RW. Diagnosis of headaches and medico-legal aspects. In: Evans RW, Mathew NT, editors. Handbook of headache. 2nd edition. Philadelphia: Lippincott-Williams & Wilkins; 2005. p. 21; with permission.

and two were growth hormone–secreting tumors. Although information is provided on response of all headaches to treatment, response to treatment of the TACs is not provided.

Hemicrania continua According to the IHS second edition,[103] to meet the criteria for HC, another TAC, the headache should be present for more than 3 months with all of the following characteristics: unilateral without side-shift; daily and continuous, without pain-free periods; moderate intensity, but with exacerbations of severe pain; and with a complete response to indomethacin. During exacerbations, the headache must have one of the following ipsilateral features: conjunctival injection or lacrimation; nasal congestion or rhinorrhea; and ptosis or miosis. The headaches usually are unremitting but rare cases of remission are reported. HC can be easily confused with chronic migraine, as approximately 75% who have HC have exacerbations of severe throbbing or stabbing pain, which can be associated with photophobia (59%), phonophobia (59%), nausea (53%), and vomiting (24%).[104] The exacerbations can last from 20 minutes to several days with pain awakening one third of patients. Autonomic features are present in up to 75% with tearing and then conjunctival injection the most common. Thus, a trial of medication effective for HC, such as indomethacin, should be considered for any patient who has chronic unilateral headache that might be HC but can be easily misdiagnosed as migraine.

Rarely, HC many have a secondary cause, which includes the following:[105] mesenchymal tumor of the sphenoid, lung malignancy, HIV (causal association unclear), C7 root irritation reported to aggravate, left lateral medullary infarction with left vertebral artery occlusion on MRI and MR angiography (head pain contralateral to infarction), internal carotid artery dissection, unruptured cavernous internal carotid artery aneurysm,[106] prolactinoma (headache exacerbation with dopamine agonists), venous malformation of the right masseter; sphenoid sinusitis,[107] and cerebellopontine angle epidermoid.[108] Although the yield is probably low, MRI scan of the brain is reasonable when initially evaluating patients presenting with symptoms consistent with HC.

Patients meeting IHS criteria for a TAC rarely have a secondary cause for their headache detected on neuroimaging. Appropriate testing is indicated, however, if atypical symptoms and signs are present.

New daily persistent headache Box 5 lists some primary and secondary causes of NDPHs present for more than 3 months. NDPH is a diagnosis of exclusion. Some of these secondary disorders may have a thunderclap or sudden onset of severe headache whereas others may develop gradually over 1 to 3 days and meet the onset period criteria for NDPH. New-onset daily headaches with a normal neurologic examination also could be the result of various other causes, particularly when seen within the first 2 months after onset, including postmeningitis headache, chronic meningitis, brain tumors, leptomeningeal metastasis, temporal arteritis, chronic subdural hematomas, posttraumatic headaches, sphenoid sinusitis, and hypertension. When the headaches have been present for more than 3 months with a normal neurologic examination, the yield of testing is low. A few additional examples are discussed.

Spontaneous intracranial hypotension (SIH) syndrome often presents as a headache that is present when patients are upright but is relieved by lying down or as an orthostatic headache. As SIH syndrome persists, however, a chronic daily headache may be present without orthostatic features. SIH syndrome also may present as other types of headache, including exertional without any orthostatic features, acute thunderclap onset, paradoxic orthostatic headache (present in recumbency and relieved

---

Box 5
Differential diagnosis of new daily headaches present for more than 3 months

Primary headaches

NDPH

Chronic migraine

Chronic tension-type

Combined features

HC

Secondary headaches (NDPH mimics)

Postmeningitis headache

Chronic meningits

Primary with medication rebound

Neoplasms

Chronic subdural hematoma

Posttraumatic headaches

Sphenoid sinusitis

Hypertension

Low CSF pressure syndrome

Cervical artery dissections

Pseudotumor cerebri (idiopathic and secondary intracranial hypertension)

CVT

AVM

Chiari malformation

Temporal arteritis

Cervicogenic

Temporomandibular joint dysfunction

---

when upright), and intermittent headache resulting from intermittent leaks, or as the acephalgic form with no headache at all.[109] Neck or interscapular pain may precede the onset of headache in some cases by days or weeks. MRI abnormalities of the brain and spine are variably present in approximately 90% of cases. An MRI scan of the brain may reveal diffuse pachymeningeal (dural) enhancement with gadolinium without leptomeningeal (arachnoid and pial) involvement and, in some cases, subdural fluid collections, which return to normal with resolution of the headache.[109,110]

Cervical artery dissections, which can present with headache or neck pain alone,[111] can be a rare cause of new daily headaches.[112] Occasionally, the headaches can persist intermittently for months and even years and can lead to a pattern of chronic daily headaches especially after cervical carotid artery dissection.

Headache is present in up to 90% of cases of CVT and often is the initial symptom and occasionally the only symptom.[113] The headache can be unilateral or bilateral in any location, mild to severe, and intermittent or constant. The onset usually is subacute but can be sudden or thunderclap. The headache almost always is associated with other neurologic signs, such as papilledema, focal deficits, seizures, disorders of consciousness, or cranial nerve palsies. CVT can be a mimic of idiopathic intracranial hypertension.

Neuroimaging studies have variable sensitivities in diagnosing CVT. CT will diagnose only approximately 20% of cases of CVT when demonstrating the hyperdensity of the thrombosed sinus on plain images and the delta sign seen with superior sagittal sinus thrombosis after contrast administration. Helical CT venography is a sensitive diagnostic method. CVT may be missed on routine MRI imaging of the brain although echo-planar T2*-weighted MRI may increase the sensitivity.[114] MRV increases the sensitivity of MR especially within the first 5 days of onset or after 6 weeks. CVT also can be demonstrated on digital subtraction venography.

Chiari I malformation typically is a congenital malformation of cerebellar tonsillar herniation at least 5 cm below the foramen magnum. The headache attributed to Chiari I malformation is occipital or nuchal-occipital with occasional radiation unilaterally to frontotemporal or shoulder regions and sometimes generalized.[38] The pain may be dull, aching, or throbbing and may last less than 5 minutes to several hours to days. Pain may be precipitated by neck flexion or palpation or coughing.

In an imaging study of children, ages 2 to 18, who had headaches,[115] Chiari type I malformation was identified in 14 of 241 (5.8%) patients. Five of 14 (35.7%) patients who had Chiari I malformation had headaches secondary to their malformation. Three patients had surgical decompression with significant headache relief in two. The other nine patients were diagnosed with migraine (35.7%) and tension-type (28.6%) headaches. In adults, one study found an association of chronic migraine with Chiari I.[116] Although headache is the most common presenting complaint of Chiari I malformation, the malformation typically is an incidental finding on MRI studies done for primary headaches.

Secondary pathology should be considered especially when NDPH occurs over age 50. In a study of those over age 65 age who had new-onset headaches, the prevalence of secondary headaches resulting from serious pathology was 15%.[117] Temporal arteritis always should be considered but the diagnosis often is delayed, especially in those under age 70.[118] Temporal arteritis rarely occurs under age 50, with most biopsy-proved large series having no patients under age of 50.[119] A Canadian study reveals the rare exception: of 141 consecutive patients presenting to a neuro-opthalmology practice, there was one patient under age 50 (age 47).[120]

REFERENCES

1. Kassirer JP. Our stubborn quest for diagnostic certainty. A cause of excessive testing. N Engl J Med 1989;320:1489–91.
2. Beresford HR. Medicolegal aspects. In: Evans RW, editor. Diagnostic testing in neurology. Philadelphia: W.B. Saunders; 1999. p. 479–88.
3. Woolf SH, Kamerow DB. Testing for uncommon conditions. The heroic search for positive test results. Arch Intern Med 1990;15:2451–8.
4. Semelka RC, Armao DM, Elias J Jr, et al. Imaging strategies to reduce the risk of radiation in CT studies, including selective substitution with MRI. J Magn Reson Imaging 2007;25:900–9.
5. Brenner DJ, Hall EJ. Computed tomography—an increasing source of radiation exposure. N Engl J Med 2007;357:2277–84.
6. U.S. Food and Drug Administration. What are the radiation risks from CT? Available at: http://www.fda.gov/cdrh/ct/risks.html. 2005. Accessed January 3, 2009.
7. Silberstein SD, Lipton RB, Goadsby PJ. Headache in clinical practice. London: Martin Dunitz; 2002.

8. De Santis M, Di Gianantonio E, Straface G, et al. Ionizing radiations in pregnancy and teratogenesis: a review of literature. Reprod Toxicol 2005;20:323–9.
9. Berlin L. Radiation exposure and the pregnant patient. AJR Am J Roentgenol 1996;167:1377–9.
10. American College of Radiology. Manual on contrast media. Administration of contrast medium to pregnant or potentially pregnant patients 2008:61. Available at: http://www.acr.org/SecondaryMainMenuCategories/quality_safety/contrast_manual.asx. Accessed December 10, 2008.
11. Chen MM, Coakley FV, Kaimal A, et al. Guidelines for computed tomography and magnetic resonance imaging use during pregnancy and lactation. Obstet Gynecol 2008;112(2 Pt 1):333–40.
12. Kanal E, Gillen J, Evans JA, et al. Survey of reproductive health among female MR workers. Radiology 1993;187:395–9.
13. Clements H, Duncan KR, Fielding K, et al. Infants exposed to MRI in utero have a normal paediatric assessment at 9 months of age. Br J Radiol 2000;73:190–4.
14. Kok RD, de Vries MM, Heerschap A, et al. Absence of harmful effects of magnetic resonance exposure at 1.5 T in utero during the third trimester of pregnancy: a follow-up study. Magn Reson Imaging 2004;22:851–4.
15. Kanal E, Barkovich AJ, Bell C, et al. ACR guidance document for safe practices. Am J Roentgenol 2007;2007(188):1447–74.
16. Gronseth GS, Greenberg MK. The utility of electroencephalogram in the evaluation of patients presenting with headache: a review of the literature. Neurology 1995;45:1263–7.
17. Rowan AJ. The electroencephalographic characteristics of migraine. Arch Neurol 1974;37:95–9.
18. Simon RH, Zimmerman AW, Tasman A, et al. Spectral analysis of photic stimulation in migraine. Electroencephalogr Clin Neurophysiol 1982;53:270–6.
19. Smyth VOG, Winter AL. The EEG in migraine. Electroencephalogr Clin Neurophysiol 1964;16:194.
20. American Academy of Neurology. Practice parameter: the electroencephalogram in the evaluation of headache. Neurology 1995;45:1411–3.
21. Lewis DW, Ashwal S, Dahl G, et al. Practice parameter: evaluation of children and adolescents with recurrent headaches: report of the Quality Standards Subcommittee of the American Academy of Neurology and the Practice Committee of the Child Neurology Society. Neurology 2002;59:490–8.
22. Evans RW. Complications of lumbar puncture. In: Evans RW, editor. Neurology and trauma. 2nd edition. New York: Oxford University Press; 2006.
23. Armon C, Evans RW. Addendum to assessment: prevention of post-lumbar puncture headaches: report of the therapeutics and technology assessment subcommittee of the american academy of neurology. Neurology 2005;65:510–2.
24. Amit M, Molad Y, Levy O, et al. Headache and systemic lupus erythematosis and its relation to other disease manifestations. Clin Exp Rheumatol 1999;17:467–70.
25. Frishberg BM. The utility of neuroimaging in the evaluation of headache in patients with normal neurologic examination. Neurology 1994;44:1191–7.
26. Baker H. Cranial CT in the investigation of headache: cost effectiveness for brain tumors. J Neuroradiol 1983;10:112–6.
27. Laffey P, Oaks W, Sawmi R, et al. Computerized tomography in clinical medicine: data supplement. Philadelphia: Medical Directions; 1978.
28. Carrera G, Gorson D, Schnur J, et al. Computerized tomography of the brain in patients with headache or temporal lobe epilepsy: findings and cost effectiveness. J Comput Assist Tomogr 1977;1:200–3.

29. Larson E, Omenn G, Lewis H, et al. Diagnostic evaluation of headache: impact of computerized tomography and cost effectiveness. JAMA 1980;243:359–62.
30. Mitchell C, Osborn R, Grosskreutz S. Computerized tomography in the headache patient: is routine evaluation really necessary? Headache 1993;33:82–6.
31. Russell D, Nakstad P, Sjaastad O. Cluster headache: pneumoencephalographic and cerebral computerized axial tomographic findings. Headache 1978;18:272–3.
32. Sargent J, Lawson C, Solbach P, et al. Use of CT scans in an outpatient headache population: an evaluation. Headache 1979;19:388–90.
33. Weingarten S, Kleinman M, Elperin L, et al. The effectiveness of cerebral imaging in the diagnosis of chronic headache: a reappraisal. Arch Intern Med 1992;152:2457–62.
34. Akpek S, Arac M, Atilla S, et al. Cost effectiveness of computed tomography in the evaluation of patients with headache. Headache 1995;35:228–30.
35. Demaerel P, Boelaert I, Wilms G, et al. The role of cranial computed tomography in the diagnostic work-up of headache. Headache 1996;36:347–8.
36. Dumas MD, Pexman W, Kreeft JH. Computed tomography evaluation of patients with chronic headache. Can Med Assoc J 1994;151:1447–52.
37. Sotaniemi KA, Rantala M, Pyhtinen J, et al. Clinical and CT correlates in the diagnosis of intracranial tumours. J Neurol Neurosurg Psychiatry 1991;54:645–7.
38. Arnett BC. Tonsillar ectopia and headaches. Neurol Clin 2004;22:229–36.
39. Evans RW. Migrainelike headaches in pituitary apoplexy. Headache 1997;37:455–6.
40. Embil JM, Kramer M, Kinnear S, et al. A blinding headache. Lancet 1997;349:182.
41. Wang HZ, Simonson TM, Greco WR, et al. Brain MR imaging in the evaluation of chronic headache in patients without other neurologic symptoms. Acad Radiol 2001;8:405–8.
42. Tsushima Y, Endo K. MR imaging in the evaluation of chronic or recurrent headache. Radiology 2005;235:575–9.
43. Sempere AP, Porta-Etessam J, Medrano V, et al. Neuroimaging in the evaluation of patients with non-acute headache. Cephalalgia 2005;25:30–5.
44. Silberstein SD. Headaches due to nasal and paranasal sinus disease. Neurol Clin 2004;22:1–19.
45. Dooley JM, Camfield O'Neill M, et al. The value of CT scans for children with headaches. Can J Neurol Sci 1990;17:309–10.
46. Chu ML, Shinnar S. Headaches in children younger than 7 years of age. Arch Neurol 1992;49:79–82.
47. Maytal J, Bienkowski RS, Patel M, et al. The value of brain imaging in children with headaches. Pediatrics 1996;96:413–6.
48. Wöber-Bingöl C, Wöber C, Prayer D, et al. Magnetic resonance imaging for recurrent headache in childhood and adolescence. Headache 1996;36:83–90.
49. Medina S, Pinter JD, Zurakowski D, et al. Children with headache: clinical predictors of surgical space-occupying lesions and the role of neuroimaging. Radiology 1997;202:819–24.
50. Lewis DW, Dorbad D. The utility of neuroimaging in the evaluation of children with migraine or chronic daily headache who have normal neurological examinations. Headache 2000;40:629–32.
51. Carlos RA, Santos CS, Kumar S, et al. Neuroimaging studies in pediatric migraine headaches. Headache 2000;40:404.
52. Alehan FK. Value of neuroimaging in the evaluation of neurologically normal children with recurrent headache. J Child Neurol 2002;17:807–9.

53. Mazzotta G, Floridi F, Mattioni A, et al. The role of neuroimaging in the diagnosis of headache in childhood and adolescence: a multicentre study. Neurol Sci 2004;(Suppl 3):S265–6.

54. Silberstein SD. Practice parameter: evidence-based guidelines for migraine headache (an evidence-based review): report of the Quality Standards Subcommittee of the American Academy of Neurology. Neurology 2000;26(55):754–62.

55. Cala L, Mastaglia F. Computerized axial tomography findings in a group of patients with migrainous headaches. Proc Aust Assoc Neurol 1976;13:35–41.

56. Cuetter A, Aita J. CT scanning in classic migraine [letter]. Headache 1983;23: 195.

57. Hungerford G, duBoulay G, Zilkha K. Computerized axial tomography in patients with severe migraine: a preliminary report. J Neurol Neurosurg Psychiatry 1976; 39:990–4.

58. Masland W, Friedman A, Buchsbaum H. Computerized axial tomography of migraine. Res Clin Stud Headache 1978;6:136–40.

59. Igarashi H, Sakai F, Kan S, et al. Magnetic resonance imaging of the brain in patients with migraine. Cephalalgia 1991;11:69–74.

60. Jacome DE, Leborgne J. MRI studies in basilar artery migraine. Headache 1990; 30:88–90.

61. Osborn RE, Alder DC, Mitchell CS. MR imaging of the brain in patients with migraine headaches. AJNR Am J Neuroradiol 1991;12:521–4.

62. Soges LJ, Cacayorin ED, Petro GR, et al. Migraine: evaluation by MR. AJNR Am J Neuroradiol 1988;9:425–9.

63. Kuhn MJ, Shekar PC. A comparative study of magnetic resonance imaging and computed tomography in the evaluation of migraine. Comput Med Imaging Graph 1990;14:149–52.

64. Cooney BS, Grossman RI, Farber RE, et al. Frequency of magnetic resonance imaging abnormalities in patients with migraine. Headache 1996;36:616–21.

65. De Benedittis G, Lorenzetti A, Sina C, et al. Magnetic resonance imaging in migraine and tension-type headache. Headache 1995;35:264–8.

66. Fazekas F, Koch M, Schmidt R, et al. The prevalence of cerebral damage varies with migraine type: a MRI study. Headache 1992;32:287–91.

67. Pavese N, Canapicchi R, Nuti A, et al. White matter MRI hyperintensities in a hundred and twenty-nine consecutive migraine patients. Cephalalgia 1994; 14:342–5.

68. Robbins L. Migraine and anticardiolipin antibodies-case reports of 13 patients and the prevalence of antiphospholipid antibodies in migraineurs. Headache 1991;31:537–9.

69. Ziegler DK, Batnitzky S, Barter R, et al. Magnetic resonance image abnormality in migraine with aura. Cephalalgia 1991;11:147–50.

70. Rovaris M, Bozzali M, Rocca MA, et al. An MR study of tissue damage in the cervical cord of patients with migraine. J Neurol Sci 2001;183:43–6.

71. Prager JM, Rosenblum J, Mikulis DJ, et al. Evaluation of headache patients by MRI. Headache Q 1991;2:192–6.

72. Adami A, Rossato G, Cerini R, et al. Right-to-left shunt does not increase white matter lesion load in migraine with aura patients. Neurology 2008;71:101–7.

73. Del Sette M, Dinia L, Bonzano L, et al. White matter lesions in migraine and right-toleft shunt: a conventional and diffusion MRI study. Cephalalgia 2008;28: 376–82.

74. Kruit MC, van Buchem MA, Hofman PA, et al. Migraine as a risk factor for subclinical brain lesions. J Am Med Assoc 2004;291:427–34.

75. Kruit MC, Launer LJ, Ferrari MD, et al. Infarcts in the posterior circulation territory in migraine. The population-based MRI CAMERA study. Brain 2005;128(Pt 9): 2068–77.
76. Kruit MC, Launer LJ, Ferrari MD, et al. Brain stem and cerebellar hyperintense lesions in migraine. Stroke 2006;37(4):1109–12.
77. Tietjen GE. Migraine and antiphospholipid antibodies. Cephalalgia 1992;12: 69–74.
78. Hering R, Couturier EGM, Steiner TJ, et al. Anticardiolipin antibodies in migraine. Cephalalgia 1991;11:19–21.
79. Daras M, Koppel B, Leyfermann M, et al. Anticardiolipin antibodies in migraine patients: an additional risk factor for stroke? Neurology 1995;45(suppl 4):A367–8.
80. Tietjen GE, Day M, Norris L, et al. Role of anticardiolipin antibodies in young persons with migraine and transient focal neurologic events. A prospective study. Neurology 1998;50:1433–40.
81. Chabriat H, Vahedi K, Iba-Zizen MT, et al. Clinical spectrum of CADASIL: a study of 7 families. Cerebral autosomal dominant arteriopathy with subcortical infarcts and leukoencephalopathy. Lancet 1995;346:934–9.
82. Mourad A, Levasseur M, Bousser MG, et al. (CADASIL with minimal symptoms after 60 years). Rev Neurol (Paris) 2006;162(8–9):827–31 [In French].
83. du Boulay GH, Ruiz JS. CT changes associated with migraine. AJNR Am J Neuroradiol 1983;4:472–3.
84. Rocca MA, Ceccarelli A, Falini A, et al. Diffusion tensor magnetic resonance imaging at 3.0 tesla shows subtle cerebral grey matter abnormalities in patients with migraine. J Neurol Neurosurg Psychiatry 2006;77:686–9.
85. Brown RD, Wiebers DO, Forbes G, et al. The natural history of unruptured intracranial arteriovenous malformations. J Neurosurg 1988;68:352–7.
86. The Arteriovenous Malformation Study Group. Arteriovenous malformations of the brain in adults. N Engl J Med 1999;340:1812–8.
87. Frishberg BM. Neuroimaging in presumed primary headache disorders. Semin Neurol 1997;17:373–82.
88. Kupersmith MJ, Vargas ME, Yashar A, et al. Occipital arteriovenous malformations: visual disturbances and presentation. Neurology 1996;46:953–7.
89. Bruyn GW. Intracranial arteriovenous malformation and migraine. Cephalalgia 1984;4:191–207.
90. Leone M, D'Amico D, Frediani F, et al. Clinical considerations on side-locked unilaterality in long lasting primary headaches. Headache 1993;33:381–4.
91. GhossoubM Nataf F, Merienne L, et al. Characteristics of headache associated with cerebral arteriovenous malformations. Neurochirurgie 2001;47(2–3 Pt 2): 177–83 [In French].
92. Goadsby PJ. Neurovascular headache and a midbrain vascular malformation: evidence for a role of the brainstem in chronic migraine. Cephalalgia 2002;22: 107–11.
93. Afridi S, Goadsby PJ. New onset migraine with a brain stem cavernous angioma. J Neurol Neurosurg Psychiatry 2003;74:680–2.
94. Obermann M, Gizewski ER, Limmroth V, et al. Symptomatic migraine and pontine vascular malformation: evidence for a key role of the brainstem in the pathophysiology of chronic migraine. Cephalalgia 2006;26:763–6.
95. Malik SN, Young WB. Midbrain cavernous malformation causing migraine-like headache. Cephalalgia 2006;26:1016–9.
96. Evans RW. New daily persistent headache. Curr Pain Headache Rep 2003;7: 303–7.

97. Goadsby PJ. Cluster headache. In: Gilman S, editor. MedLink neurology. San Diego (CA): Arbor; 2007. Available at: www.medlink.com. 2007. Accessed January 3, 2009.

98. Favier I, van Vliet JA, Roon KI, et al. Trigeminal autonomic cephalgias due to structural lesions: a review of 31 cases. Arch Neurol 2007;64:25–31.

99. Favier I, Haan J, van Duinen SG, et al. Typical cluster headache caused by granulomatous pituitary involvement. Cephalalgia 2007;27:173–6.

100. Seijo-Martínez M, Castro del Río M, Cervigon E, et al. Symptomatic cluster headache: report of two cases. Neurologia 2000;15:406–10.

101. Seijo-Martínez M, Castro del Río M, Conde C, et al. Cluster-like headache: association with cervical syringomyelia and Arnold-Chiari malformation. Cephalalgia 2004;24:140–2.

102. Levy MJ, Matharu MS, Meeran K, et al. The clinical characteristics of headache in patients with pituitary tumours. Brain 2005;128:1921–30.

103. Headache Classification Committee of the International Headache Society. Classification and diagnostic criteria for headache disorders, cranial neuralgia and facial pain. Second edition. Cephalalgia 2004;24(suppl 1):1–160.

104. Peres MFP. Sleep disorders associated with headaches. Available at. In: Gilman S, editor. MedLink neurology. San Diego (CA): MedLink Corp; 2008. Available at: www.medlink.com. 2008.

105. Boes CJ, Swanson JW. Paroxysmal hemicrania,SUNCT, and hemicrania continua. Semin Neurol 2006;26:260–70.

106. Vikelis M, Xifaras M, Magoufis G, et al. Headache attributed to unruptured saccular aneurysm, mimicking hemicrania continua. J Headache Pain 2005;6:156–8.

107. Meckling SK, Becker WJ. Sphenoid sinusitis presenting as indomethacin responsive "hemicrania continua": a case report. Cephalalgia 1997;17:303.

108. Prakash S, Tandon N, Padmanabhan D, et al. A case of CP angle epidermoid mimicking hemicrania continua: is it different from primary HC? Headache 2008;48:1530–4.

109. Mokri B. Low cerebrospinal fluid pressure syndromes. Neurol Clin 2004;22:55–74.

110. Schievink WI. Spontaneous spinal cerebrospinal fluid leaks and intracranial hypotension. JAMA 2006;295:2286–96.

111. Arnold M, Cumurciuc R, Stapf C, et al. Pain as the only symptom of cervical artery dissection. J Neurol Neurosurg Psychiatry 2006;77(9):1021–4.

112. Mokri B. Headache in cervical artery dissections. Curr Pain Headache Rep 2002;6:209–16.

113. Cumurciuc R, Crassard I, Sarov M, et al. Headache as the only neurological sign of cerebral venous thrombosis: a series of 17 cases. J Neurol Neurosurg Psychiatry 2005;76:1084–7.

114. Selim M, Fink J, Linfante I, et al. Diagnosis of cerebral venous thrombosis with echo-planar T2*-weighted magnetic resonance imaging. Arch Neurol 2002;59(6):1021–6.

115. Schwedt TJ, Guo Y, Rothner AD. "Benign" imaging abnormalities in children and adolescents with headache. Headache 2006;46(3):387–98.

116. Kaplan Y, Oksuz E. Chronic migraine associated with the Chiari type 1 malformation. Clin Neurol Neurosurg 2008;110:818–22.

117. Pascual-Leone A, Pascual APL. Occipital neuralgia: another benign cause of "thunderclap headache". J Neurol Neurosurg Psychiatry 1992;55:411.

118. Gonzalez-Gay MA, Barros S, Lopez-Diaz MJ, et al. Giant cell arteritis: disease patterns of clinical presentation in a series of 240 patients. Medicine (Baltimore) 2005;84:269–76.
119. Lee JL, Naguwa SM, Cheema GS, et al. The geo-epidemiology of temporal (giant cell) arteritis. Clin Rev Allergy Immunol 2008;35:88–95.
120. Ramstead CL, Patel AD. Giant cell arteritis in a neuro-ophthalmology clinic in Saskatoon, 1998–2003. Can J Ophthalmol 2007;42:295–8.

Acute Treatment of Migraine

Stewart J. Tepper, MD*, Roderick C. Spears, MD

KEYWORDS

- Migraine • Acute treatment • Triptans • Ergots
- Rebound • Rescue

Migraine produces moderate to severe pain associated with photophonophobia, nausea, and vomiting, and routine activity typically worsens the symptoms, often resulting in profound impact. Because of the severity, duration, and associated disability, acute treatment of migraine attacks becomes crucial. The goals of acute treatment are rapid treatment in a cost-effective manner, consistent reduction of disability without recurrence of the headache, and reduced use of backup or rescue medications. A key to acute treatment is matching medication to disability as a surrogate marker for disease severity with a stratified care approach.

PATHOPHYSIOLOGY

Migraine is generated centrally, either cortically by cortical spreading depression or in brainstem. These central processes generate meningeal neurogenic inflammation and vasodilation, which are peripheral pain mechanisms, in turn activating nociceptive afferents that carry the pain signals through the trigeminal ganglion to trigeminal nucleus caudalis in the trigeminocervical complex. From there, the pain signals ascend through thalamus to cortex. Meningeal neurogenic inflammatory changes include the release of calcitonin gene-related peptide (CGRP), a profound endogenous vasodilator, and initiation of the arachadonic acid cascade. At this time, there are no acute treatments that reverse the activation of the central processes; acute treatments target the peripheral pain mechanisms, the central integration of the pain, or both.

OUTCOME MEASURES FOR ACUTE TREATMENT

It is essential before writing a prescription for acute treatment of migraine to set up clinical goals and expectations. Unhappily, patients often are given acute medications without clear instructions on how to take them and without establishing desired outcomes.

Center for Headache and Pain, T33, Cleveland Clinic, 9500 Euclid Avenue, Cleveland, OH 44195, USA
* Corresponding author.
E-mail address: teppers@ccf.org (S. J. Tepper).

Neurol Clin 27 (2009) 417–427
doi:10.1016/j.ncl.2008.11.008
0733-8619/08/$ – see front matter © 2009 Elsevier Inc. All rights reserved.

The International Headache Society set the primary measure of efficacy in evaluating acute treatment in migraine acute medication studies as pain-free response at 2 hours.[1] Lipton and Stewart asked patients for their preference for outcomes in acute treatment and received these responses: (1) complete pain relief (pain-free) (2) no recurrence of headache, and (3) rapid onset of pain relief, suggesting that a sustained pain-free response is optimal.[2]

The United States Headache Consortium declared the following goals for acute treatment:

1. Treat attacks rapidly and consistently without recurrence.
2. Restore the patient's ability to function.
3. Minimize the use of back-up and rescue medications.
4. Optimize self-care and reduce subsequent use of resources.
5. Be cost-effective for overall management.
6. Have minimal or no adverse events.[3,4]

An outcomes tool, the Migraine Assessment of Current Therapy (Migraine-ACT), based on previous assessment scales matched to patient-declared needs, has been validated and published:[5]

- Consistency of response: Does your migraine medication work consistently, in the majority of your attacks?
- Global assessment of relief: Does the headache pain disappear within 2 hours?
- Impact: Are you able to function normally within 2 hours?
- Emotional response: Are you comfortable enough with your medication to be able to plan your daily activities?

A Migraine-ACT score of less than or equal to 2 suggests a need to consider changing a patient's acute medication.[6] Thus, a clinician can state to a patient that the clinical goal is 2 hours pain-free or sustained pain-free or show the four questions from Migraine-ACT, explaining that the questionnaire will be used on return visit to evaluate effectiveness of treatment. The important step is to set goals for treatment.

STRATEGIES FOR SELECTING ACUTE TREATMENT

Optimal treatment of migraine necessitates matching disease or patient characteristics to treatment choice—stratified care. Astonishingly, many care providers, and not so astonishingly, many insurance providers, believe that acute treatment should proceed by cost in a one-size-fits-all approach. That is, they select a nonspecific, inexpensive acute medication to prescribe first for patients who have migraine, without regard to patient or attack characteristics, and step up to migraine-specific treatment only if lower-level medications fail. Lipton and Stewart labeled this approach step care across attacks.

A second approach often suggested is having patients start treating an attack with a low-level medication, and, if it fails at 2 hours, instructing the patients to rescue with a migraine-specific medication. This is called step care within attacks.

Lipton and colleagues studied these strategies for treatment, comparing them to stratified care in which patients who had migraine were first evaluated for severity of disability from their migraines and then migraine-specific treatment was given to the more disabled patients. In this approach, disability was a surrogate marker for disease severity.

The Disabilities in Strategies of Care (DISC) study showed unequivocally that matching specificity of treatment to level of disability is a superior way to select treatment, resulting in better patient outcomes and reduced time loss.[7] A subsequent analysis of the DISC study also showed lower costs with stratified care,[8] so step care, despite its popularity, has no evidence for effectiveness compared with stratified care.

The DISC study used zolmitriptan as migraine-specific treatment. An approach to selecting the right treatment first time involves (1) establishing a diagnosis of migraine, (2) establishing level of disability, and (3) establishing suitability of patients for a triptan or ergot as a migraine-specific treatment if disability is at least moderate to severe.

The Migraine Disability Assessment (MIDAS) was used as the measure of disability in the DISC study. This is a five-item questionnaire that can be summarized in a single question: How many days in the last 3 months were you at least 50% disabled from your migraines at work, home, school, or recreational activities?[9] An answer of more than 10 suggests at least moderate to severe disability and the need for migraine-specific treatment. Another validated disability tool is the Headache Impact Test (HIT-6), for which a score of greater than 60 suggests severe impact from migraine.[10]

Thus, the quickest way to decide on an acute treatment class (that is, specific versus nonspecific) for a patient who has episodic migraine is to ask about the severity of disability or impact, preferably using MIDAS or HIT-6. If disability is high and a patient has no vascular contraindications, a triptan or dihydroergotamine (DHE) should be used as first-line treatment from the beginning, avoiding step care.

NONSPECIFIC ACUTE MIGRAINE TREATMENT

There is a large group of disparate nonspecific acute medications for migraine, and evidence for effectiveness is as varied as the classes of drugs studied. Some of the medications are nonsteroidal anti-inflammatory drugs (NSAIDs), aspirin (ASA), acetaminophen (APAP), analgesic combinations with or without caffeine, opioids, butalbital, isometheptene, also often in combinations, and medication classes including antihistamines, antinauseants, antiepilepsy drugs, and muscle relaxants.

Aspirin-acetaminophen-caffeine (AAC) mixtures are Food and Drug Administration approved for migraine based on a randomized controlled trial (RCT) in which preselected patients who were usually incapacitated (ie, required bed rest for their attacks) or who experienced vomiting 20% or more of the time were excluded. AAC was superior to placebo for pain relief and associated symptoms up to 6 hours post dose for this less disabled group of patients.[11,12]

NSAIDs, such as naproxen, diclofenac,[13,14] and solubilized ibuprofen, also are superior to placebo in RCTs, with the latter tested using a methodology similar to that in the AAC regulatory trial.[15] The United States Headache Consortium states that NSAIDs and AAC can be effective for moderate migraine,[3,4] but the real level of evidence for these nonspecific medications is lower than that for triptans, which were tested on all comers rather than a preselected group who had lower migraine severity.

Evidence for opioid use in acute migraine generally is negative or riddled with methodologic mistakes.[16–21] The United States Headache Consortium states, "Oral opioid combinations may be considered when sedation will not put the patient at risk and/or the risk for abuse has been addressed."[3,20] Jakubowski and colleagues found that even intermittent use of opioids interfered with successful therapeutic reversal of central sensitization and pain-free response when patients who had status migrainosus were given parenteral sumatriptan and ketorolac, and their recommendation states, "We believe it is imperative that migraine patients ... be treated with parenteral COX1/COX2 inhibitors, not with opioids."[22]

There is no positive evidence from RCTs for butalbital mixtures in the acute treatment of migraine. The entire European Union, Asia, and all of Latin America removed butalbital from availability because of lack of evidence for efficacy and excessive risk for habituation and dependence. Butalbital mixtures were the number one medication associated with the development of medication overuse headache in a study of 456 patients in a tertiary headache center, accounting for close to half of the cases of rebound.[23] Bigal and colleagues[24] reported data from the American Migraine Prevalence and Prevention population-based study suggesting that episodic use of butalbital as infrequently as 5 days per month was linked to transformation into chronic daily headache and medication overuse headache. It is wise to never prescribe butalbital for migraine.

SPECIFIC ACUTE MIGRAINE TREATMENT
Triptans

Triptans are serotonin-1B/D ($5HT_{1B/D}$) agonists that work via the serotonin-1D receptors to inhibit CGRP and inflammatory peptide release in the meninges and prevent the pain signal from returning from the periphery to the trigeminal nucleus caudalis. They work via the $5HT_{1B}$ receptor to constrict vessels dilated by CGRP. Because there are some $5HT_{1B}$ receptors in coronary and other arteries, triptans are contraindicated in patients who have vascular disease. Patients who have more than one Framingham risk factor should receive a functional cardiac evaluation before triptan use.[25]

Dr. Robert Kaniecki's mnemonic for selection of triptans is worth remembering: triptans can be chosen via the 3 F's: Fast versus slow, Formulation, and Formulary tier and availability. All triptans come as oral tablets; zolmitriptan also is formulated as a nasal spray; sumatriptan also is available as a nasal spray and a subcutaneous (SC) injection. The doses, formulations, and important pharmacokinetic data on triptans are detailed in **Tables 1** and **2**.[26,27]

Oral triptans can be divided into two groups: fast onset with higher efficacy at 2 hours, and slower onset with lower response rates at 2 hours (**Tables 3** and **4**). Generally speaking, efficacy rates for the group II triptans at 4 hours are similar to response rates for group I triptans at 2 hours. Sumatriptan is available in a rapid release form (brand names Imitrex RT in the United States, Imitrex DF in Canada, and Imigran Radis in the United Kingdom), which may result in higher efficacy than its conventional form, which is still available in Canada and the United Kingdom but not the United States. Zolmitriptan and rizatriptan are available in orally dissolvable tablets, which do not have sublingual absorption or greater or faster efficacy than conventional tablets, but may be more convenient because they do not require water.

Selecting the triptan necessitates determining how fast a migraine worsens. If onset is quick, a group I triptan is necessary. If emesis is common, a nonoral formulation for at least some of the prescriptions is required (nasal or SC). Finally, once the group and formulation are selected, the triptan can be chosen by formulary tier status.

Sumatriptan also is available in the United States in combination with naproxen sodium, a bilayer tablet of 85 mg of rapid release sumatriptan on the top and 500 mg of naproxen sodium on the bottom (brand name Treximet). The Food and Drug Administration mandated regulatory modified factorial studies on this combination medication, and the whole seems more effective than the individual components.[28] Presumably, the NSAID inhibition of the arachadonic acid cascade adds a second mechanism to the acute treatment mechanisms provided by the triptan. Some evidence suggests a triptan-NSAID combination can reduce headache recurrence

Table 1
Triptans

Generic	Brand	Formulations	Doses[a]	Maximum Daily Dose
Sumatriptan	Imitrex	Tablets	25 mg, 50 mg, **100 mg**	200 mg (United States)
		Nasal spray	5 mg, **20 mg**	40 mg
		Subcutaneous injection	4 mg, **6 mg**	12 mg
		Suppositories (European Union)	25 mg	50 mg
Zolmitriptan	Zomig	Tablets	2.5 mg, 5.0 mg	10 mg (United States)
	Zomig-ZMT	Orally disintegrating	2.5 mg, 5.0 mg	10 mg
	Zomig	Nasal spray	5.0 mg	10 mg
Rizatriptan	Maxalt	Tablets	5 mg, **10 mg**	30 mg[b]
	Maxalt-MLT	Orally disintegrating tablet	5 mg, **10 mg**	30 mg[b]
Naratriptan	Amerge	Tablets	1.0 mg, 2.5 mg	5 mg
Almotriptan	Axert	Tablets	6.25 mg, **12.5 mg**	25 mg
Frovatriptan	Frova	Tablets	12.5 mg	25 mg
Eletriptan	Relpax	Tablets	20 mg, **40 mg**	80 mg

[a] Optimal dose, when known, is bolded.
[b] 15 mg if on concomitant propranolol.
From Tepper SJ. Acute treatment of migraine. Continuum 2006;12:87–105.

Table 2
Pharmacokinetics of the triptans

Drug	Time to Peak Plasma Concentration (h)	Half-Life (h)	Bioavailability (%)	Elimination Route/Metabolism
Sumatriptan				Hepatic; MAO-A; 60% renal
50-mg tablet	2	2	14	
20-mg spray	2.5		17	
6-mg SC	1		97	
	0.2			
Zolmitriptan		2.5–3.0	40–48	Hepatic (1 active and 2) inactive metabolites; CYP/MAO-A
2.5-mg tablet	2	2.5–3.0	40–48	
2.5-mg ZMT	3.3			
2.5-mg nasal				
Rizatriptan	1.2 (tablet)	2.0–3.0	45	Hepatic MAO-A; 30%excreted renallyunchanged
	1.6–2.5 (MLT)	2.0–3.0		
Naratriptan	2.0–3.0	5.0–6.3	63 (men) 74 (women)	70% excreted renally unchanged; CYP; not MAO-A
Almotriptan	1.4–3.8	3.2–3.7	80	Hepatic; CYP/MAO-A; 15% active N-desmethyl metabolite 26%–35% excreted renally unchanged
Eletriptan	1.0–2.0	3.6–5.5	50	Hepatic CyP3A4; 15%active N-desmethyl metabolite; not MAO-A
Frovatriptan	2.0–4.0	25	24–30	Hepatic; CYP/MAO-A; 26%–35% excreted renally unchanged

Abbreviations: CYP, cytochrome P450; MAO-A, monoamine oxidase type A.
From Tepper SJ. Acute treatment of migraine. Continuum 2006;12:87–105; with permission; and *modified from* Tepper SJ, Rapoport AM. The triptans: a summary. CNS Drugs 1999;12:403–17; with permission.

Table 3 Group I triptans: fast onset	
Generic Name	**Brand Name**
Sumatriptan	Imitrex, Imigran
Zolmitriptan	Zomig, AscoTop, Zomigon
Rizatriptan	Maxalt, Rizalt
Almotriptan	Axert, Almogran
Eletriptan	Relpax, Rizalt

From Tepper SJ. Acute treatment of migraine. Continuum 2006;12:87–105; with permission.

and that it is a class effect.[29–32] The sumatriptan-naproxen combination could be used in patients who have prolonged migraines with frequent recurrence or in patients who have inadequate response to triptans alone where synergy from the two components might be useful.

Patients who have episodic migraine and fewer than 15 days of headache per month should be instructed to take triptans at the earliest onset of mild pain, before central integration of the migraine with its attendant central sensitization and allodynia develop, that is, nonpainful stimuli perceived as painful. There is evidence that allodynia is a marker for less optimal response to triptans and that a pain-free response is linked to decreased recurrence.[33–35] Thus, it is important to stress early intervention with triptans to increase the likelihood of a one-and-done response, pain-free, with no recurrence and no need for rescue medication.

In summary, the decision to use triptan versus nonspecific treatment requires stratifying disability. If an episodic migraineur has had more than 10 days of greater than or equal to 50% disability in the past 3 months, initial acute treatment should be a triptan in the absence of vascular disease. After selecting the triptan based on speed of action, need for nonoral formulation, and formulary tier, patients should be instructed to treat at the earliest onset of mild pain to increase likelihood of sustained pain-free response. If a triptan alone fails to provide fast, consistent, and prolonged relief, a triptan-NSAID combination should be used, in the absence of gastrointestinal or renal contraindications.

All patients should be followed using a diary and, if possible, using Migraine-ACT. The reason for a diary is not only to evaluate outcomes but also to count the number of acute treatment days per month. Acute treatment days should be kept to fewer than 10 days per month to avoid transformation into medication overuse headache and chronic daily headache. When acute treatment days climb above 10 days per month, preventive medication should be added to reduce frequency of attacks.

Table 4 Group II triptans: slower onset	
Generic Name	**Brand Name**
Naratriptan	Amerge, Naramig
Frovatriptan	Frova

From Tepper SJ. Acute treatment of migraine. Continuum 2006;12:87–105; with permission.

Ergots

Use of ergots has declined in the triptan era because of inconvenience of use. Ergotamine comes only in suppositories, which many patients dislike, and in coated tablets that cannot be cut to smaller doses, and often causes nausea at available doses. DHE is available in a nasal spray (brand name Migranal) and as an injection without an autoinjector. Both have at least the same risk for vasoconstriction as triptans, and both activate many other receptors besides $5HT_{1B/D}$, including α- and β-adrenergic, $5HT_{1A}$, $5HT_{1F}$, $5HT_{2A}$, $5HT_{2C}$, and $5HT_3$, and dopamine$_1$- and dopamine$_2$-receptor subtypes.[36]

Ergotamine is fiercely habituating and must be limited to no more than 1 to 2 days of use per week; this is crucial to avoiding medication overuse headache. DHE is tolerated far better, is useful as an acute treatment of long migraines because of low recurrence, and can be used repetitively for status migrainosus and in detoxification from rebound.

Patients can be taught to self-inject DHE, and common practice is to mix DHE with 0.25 mL to 0.50 mL of 1% to 2% lidocaine in the same syringe (they are miscible) to reduce injection-site burning. Titration to a subnauseating dose is important, as nausea suggests too high a dose and activation of $5HT_2$ and $5HT_3$ receptors. According to AAN guidelines, maximum dosing for DHE is 3 mg per day, up to 21 mg per week.[37]

Intranasal DHE dosing requires one spray (0.5 mg) into each nostril (without sniffing) at the first sign of migraine, followed 15 minutes later by an additional spray into each

Table 5
Parenteral acute treatments of migraine for use in clinic or emergency department

Medication	Dose	Route	Other Facts
Dihydroergotamine	Maximal subnauseating dose up to 1 mg	SC, IM, IV	May be mixed with lidocaine in SC or IM dosing; recurrence is low; nonsedating; contraindicated with vascular disease
Sumatriptan	4 mg, 6 mg	SC	Nonsedating; contraindicated with vascular disease
Metoclopramide	10 mg	IV	Risk for extrapyramidal effects and mild sedation
Promethazine	25 mg to 50 mg	IM, IV	Risk for extrapyramidal effects and sedation
Prochlorperazine	10 mg	IV	Risk for extrapyramidal effects and sedation
Droperidol	2.5 mg to 5.0 mg	IV	Risk for QT prolongation, extrapyramidal effects, hypotension, and sedation
Ondansetron	4–8 mg	IV	Nonsedating antinauseant
Ketorolac	30 mg IV, 60 mg IM	IM, IV	Nonsedating, risk for GI bleeding
Dexamethasone	4 mg to 10 mg	IM, IV	Nonsedating
Valproate	500 mg to 1000 mg	IV	Nonsedating
Magnesium	1 g	IV	Nonsedating; works best for patients who have migraine with aura

From Tepper SJ. Acute treatment of migraine. Continuum 2006;12:87–105; with permission.

nostril, for a total of 2 mg in four sprays. Prolonged nasal stuffiness is the one problematic side effect.

RESCUE AND EMERGENCY ACUTE TREATMENT

As discussed previously and recommended by Jakubowski and colleagues,[22] opioids should not be used for acute treatment of migraine, for rescue in outpatients, or in emergency departments for treatment. Patients often report that they go into status migrainosus because of late or nonspecific treatment; for outpatient rescue, three excellent alternatives are SC sumatriptan, repetitive DHE nasal spray, or a brief several-day course of steroids, such as dexamethasone, until patients are headache-free for 24 hours. Some specialists also use repetitive triptans or repetitive methylergonovine (Methergine), a long-acting ergot, in this manner.

In clinics or emergency departments, a variety of intramuscular (IM) or intravenous (IV) treatments can be used together or separately, with several admonitions: (1) make sure patients are not pregnant before using IV DHE or IV valproate, (2) mixing triptans and ergots in the same day or two triptans in the same day is contraindicated in the prescribing information, and (3) triptans and ergots are prohibited in patients who have vascular disease (see **Table 5**).

SUMMARY

Major points for acute treatment of migraine are

- Establish a clear diagnosis and evaluate the presence and level of disability or impact of migraine.
- Evaluate vascular risk factors.
- Establish outcome goals of 2 hours pain-free or 2 to 24 hours sustained pain-free or use Migraine-ACT.
- Use triptans as first-line acute medications in patients who have disabling migraine in the absence of vascular contraindications.
- Advise patients who have episodic migraine to take the triptan early in the attack, when pain is mild, less than 1 hour from onset.
- Add an NSAID (in the absence of contraindications) to the triptan if recurrence or inadequate pain-free response occurs.
- Do not use opioids or butalbital in patients who have migraine.
- Avoid nonspecific medications in patients who have disabling migraine to avoid transformation into daily headache.
- Follow with a diary and keep acute treatment days to fewer than 10 days per month. Add prevention if acute days exceed 10 days per month.

REFERENCES

1. Tfelt-Hansen P, Block G, Dahlöf C, et al. Guidelines for controlled trials of drugs in migraine: second edition. Cephalalgia 2000;20(9):765–86.
2. Lipton RB, Stewart WF. Acute migraine therapy: do doctors understand what patients with migraine want from therapy? Headache 1999;39:S20–6.
3. Silberstein SD. Practice parameter: evidence-based guidelines for migraine headache (an evidence-based review): report of the Quality Standards Subcommittee of the American Academy of Neurology. Neurology 2000;55(6):754–62.
4. Matchar D, Young WB, Rosenberg JH, et al. Evidence-based guidelines for migraine headache in the primary care setting: pharmacological management

of acute attacks. Available at: http://www.aan.com/practice/guideline/index.cfm? fuseaction=home.welcome&Topics=16&keywords=&Submit=Search+Guidelines; 2000. Accessed July 16, 2008.

5. Dowson AJ, Tepper SJ, Baos V, et al. Identifying patients who require a change in their current acute migraine treatment: the Migraine Assessment of Current Therapy (Migraine-ACT) questionnaire. Curr Med Res Opin 2004;20(7):1125–35.

6. Kilminster SG, Dowson AJ, Tepper SJ, et al. Reliability, validity, and clinical utility of the Migraine-ACT questionnaire. Headache 2006;46(4):553–62.

7. Lipton RB, Stewart WF, Stone AM, et al. Stratified care vs. step care strategies for migraine. The Disability in Strategies of Care (DISC) Study: a randomized trial. JAMA 2000;284(20):2599–605.

8. Sculpher M, Millson D, Meddis D, et al. Cost-effectiveness analysis of stratified versus stepped care strategies for acute treatment of migraine: the Disability in Strategies for Care (DISC) Study. Pharmacoeconomics 2002;20(2):91–100.

9. Lipton RB, Goadsby PJ, Sawyer JPC. Migraine: diagnosis and assessment of disability. Rev Contemp Pharmacother 2000;11:63–73.

10. Kosinski M, Bayliss MS, Bjorner JB, et al. A six-item short-form survey for measuring headache impact: the HIT-6. Qual Life Res 2003;12(8):963–74.

11. Lipton RB, Stewart WF, Ryan RE Jr, et al. Efficacy and safety of acetaminophen, aspirin and caffeine in alleviating migraine headache pain: three double-blind, randomized, placebo-controlled trials. Arch Neurol 1998;55(2):210–7.

12. Goldstein J, Hoffman HD, Armellino JJ, et al. Treatment of severe, disabling migraine attacks in an over-the-counter population of migraine sufferers: results from three randomized, placebo-controlled studies of the combination of acetaminophen, aspirin, and caffeine. Cephalalgia 1999;19(7):684–91.

13. Limmroth V, Przywara S. Analgesics. In: Diener HC, editor. Drug treatment of migraine and other headaches. New York: Karger; 2000. p. 30–43.

14. Krymchantowski A, Tepper SJ. Nonspecific migraine acute treatment. In: Lipton RB, Bigal ME, editors. Migraine and other headache disorders. New York: Informa Healthcare; 2005. p. 273–88.

15. Kellstein DE, Lipton RB, Geetha R, et al. Evaluation of a novel solubilized formulation of ibuprofen in the treatment of migraine headache: a randomized, double-blind, placebo-controlled, dose-ranging study. Cephalalgia 2000;20(4):233–43.

16. Boureau F, Joubert JM, Lasserre V, et al. Double-blind comparison of an acetaminophen 400 mg-codeine 25 mg combination versus aspirin 1000 mg and placebo in acute migraine attack. Cephalalgia 1994;14(2):156–61.

17. Carasso RL, Yehuda S. The prevention and treatment of migraine with an analgesic combination. Br J Clin Pract 1984;38(1):25–7.

18. Gawel MJ, Szalai JF, Stiglick A, et al. Evaluation of analgesic agents in recurring headache compared with other clinical pain models. Clin Pharmacol Ther 1990;47(4):504–8.

19. Silberstein SD, McCrory DC. Opioids. In: Diener HC, editor. Drug treatment of migraine and other headaches. New York: Karger; 2000. p. 222–36.

20. Snow V, Weiss K, Wall EM, et al. Pharmacologic management of acute attacks of migraine and prevention of migraine headache. Ann Intern Med 2002;137(10):840–9.

21. Uzogara E, Sheehan DV, Manschreck TC, et al. A combination drug treatment for acute common migraine. Headache 1986;26(5):231–6.

22. Jakubowski M, Levy D, Goor-Aryeh I, et al. Terminating migraine with allodynia and ongoing central sensitization using parenteral administration of COX1/COX2 inhibitors. Headache 2005;45(7):850–61.

23. Bigal ME, Rapoport AM, Sheftell FD, et al. Transformed migraine and medication overuse in a tertiary headache center - clinical characteristics and treatment outcomes. Cephalalgia 2004;24(6):483–90.

24. Bigal ME, Serrano D, Buse D, et al. Acute migraine medications and evolution from episodic to chronic migraine: a longitudinal population-based study. Headache 2008;48(8):1157–68.

25. Dodick DW, Rosamond W, MaasenVanDenBrink M, et al. Cardiovascular safety and triptans in the acute treatment of migraine. Headache 2004;44(Suppl 1): S1–39.

26. Tepper SJ. Acute treatment of migraine. Continuum 2006;12(6):87–105.

27. Tepper SJ, Rapoport AM. The triptans: a summary. CNS Drugs 1999;12(5): 403–17.

28. Brandes JL, Kudrow D, Stark SR, et al. Sumatriptan-naproxen for acute treatment of migraine: a randomized trial. JAMA 2007;297(13):1443–54.

29. Krymchantowski AV, Adriano M, Fernandes D. Tolfenamic acid decreased migraine recurrence when used with sumatriptan. Cephalalgia 1999;19(3):186–7.

30. Krymchantowski AV. Naproxen sodium decreases migraine recurrence when administered with sumatriptan. Arq Neuropsichiatr 2000;58(2-B):428–30.

31. Krymchantowski AV, Barbosa JS. Rizatriptan combined with rofecoxib vs. rizatriptan for the acute treatment of migraine: an open label pilot study. Cephalalgia 2002;22(4):309–12.

32. Krymchantowski VS, Bigal ME. Rizatriptan versus rizatriptan plus rofecoxib versus rizatriptan plus tolfenamic acid in the treatment of migraine. BMC Neurol 2004;4:10.

33. Burstein R, Collins B, Jakubowski M. Defeating migraine pain with triptans: a race against the development of cutaneous allodynia. Ann Neurol 2004;55(1):19–26.

34. Burstein R, Jakubowski M. Analgesic triptan action in an animal model of intracranial pain: a race against the development of central sensitization. Ann Neurol 2004;55(1):27–36.

35. Sheftell F, O'Quinn S, Watson C, et al. Low migraine headache recurrence with naratriptan: clinical parameters related to recurrence. Headache 2000;40(2): 103–10.

36. Bigal ME, Tepper SJ. Ergotamine and dihydroergotamine: a review. Curr Pain Headache Rep 2003;7(1):55–62.

37. Silberstein SD, Young WB. Safety and efficacy of ergotamine tartrate and dihydroergotamine in the treatment of migraine and status migrainosus. Working Panel of the Headache and Facial Pain Section of the American Academy of Neurology. Neurology 1995;45(3 Pt 1):577–84.

Preventive Migraine Treatment

Stephen D. Silberstein, MD

KEYWORDS

• Migraine • Prevention • Treatment

Migraine is a central nervous system disorder that is characterized by moderate or severe headaches that last 4 to 72 hours. The attacks are often aggravated by routine physical activity and may be associated with a variety of other symptoms, including photophobia, phonophobia, osmophobia, nausea, or vomiting. Approximately 15% of patients experience attacks of migraine with aura. The typical aura consists of visual, sensory, or language symptoms. Aura usually develops over a period of at least 5 minutes and lasts less than 1 hour. Attacks vary widely from patient to patient in regard to frequency, severity, duration, and impact on quality of life. The pharmacologic treatment of migraine may be acute (abortive) or preventive (prophylactic), and patients with frequent or severe headaches often require both approaches.

Preventive therapy is used to try to reduce the frequency, duration, or severity of attacks. Additional benefits include enhancing the response to acute treatments, improving a patient's ability to function, and reducing disability.[1] Preventive treatment may also result in health care cost reductions.[2] Recent US and European guidelines[3,4] have established the circumstances that might warrant preventive treatment. These include (1) recurring migraine that significantly interferes with a patient's quality of life and daily routine despite acute treatment; (2) four or more attacks per month; (3) failure of, contraindication to, or troublesome side effects from acute medications; and (4) frequent, extremely long, or uncomfortable auras.[3,4] A migraine preventive drug is considered successful if it reduces migraine attack frequency by at least 50% within 3 months. A migraine diary is highly recommended for treatment evaluation.[3,4]

US evidence-based guidelines for preventive treatment of migraine include the following:

1. Recurring migraine that significantly interferes with the patient's daily routine despite acute treatment (eg, two or more attacks a month that produce disability that lasts 3 or more days, headache attacks that are infrequent but produce profound disability)

Department of Neurology, Jefferson Headache Center, Thomas Jefferson University Hospital, 111 South Eleventh Street, Gibbon Building, Suite 8130, Philadelphia, PA 19107, USA
E-mail address: stephen.silberstein@jefferson.edu

Neurol Clin 27 (2009) 429–443
doi:10.1016/j.ncl.2008.11.007
0733-8619/08/$ – see front matter © 2009 Elsevier Inc. All rights reserved.

2. Failure of, contraindication to, or troublesome side effects from acute medications
3. Overuse of acute medications
4. Special circumstances, such as hemiplegic migraine or attacks with a risk for permanent neurologic injury
5. Frequent headaches (more than two a week) or a pattern of increasing attacks over time, with the risk for developing medication overuse headache
6. Patient preference, that is, the desire to have as few acute attacks as possible

Prevention is not being used to the extent that it should be; only 13% of all migraineurs currently use preventive therapy to control their attacks.[4] According to the American Migraine Prevalence and Prevention (AMPP) study, 38.8% of patients who have migraine should be considered for (13.1%) or offered (25.7%) migraine preventive therapy.[5]

The major medication groups for preventive migraine treatment include anticonvulsants, antidepressants, β-adrenergic blockers, calcium channel antagonists, serotonin antagonists, botulinum neurotoxins, nonsteroidal anti-inflammatory drugs, and others (including riboflavin, magnesium, and petasites). If preventive medication is indicated, the agent should be chosen from one of the first-line categories based on the drug's relative efficacy in double-blind placebo-controlled trials, its side effect profile, and the patient's preference, in addition to coexistent and comorbid conditions.[6] The following are general principles of preventive therapy, based on the author's experience.

PRINCIPLES OF PREVENTIVE THERAPY

- Start the chosen drug at a low dose, and increase it slowly until therapeutic effects develop, the ceiling dose for the chosen drug is reached, or adverse events (AEs) become intolerable.
- Give each treatment an adequate trial. The full benefit of the drug may not be realized until 6 months have elapsed.
- Set realistic goals. Success is defined as a 50% reduction in attack frequency, a significant decrease in attack duration, or an improved response to acute medication.
- Set realistic expectations regarding AEs. The risk and extent of AEs vary greatly from patient to patient, and we presently have no way of predicting the presence or severity of AEs for an individual patient. Most AEs are self-limited and dose-dependent, and patients should be encouraged to tolerate the early AEs that may develop when a new medication is started.
- Avoid acute headache medication overuse and drugs that are contraindicated because of coexistent or comorbid illnesses.
- Re-evaluate therapy, and, if possible, taper or discontinue the drug after a sustained period of remission (6–9 months).
- Be sure that a woman of childbearing potential is aware of any potential risks, and choose the medication that has the least potential for AE on a fetus.[7]
- To maximize compliance, involve patients in their own care. Take patient preferences into account when deciding between drugs of relatively equivalent efficacy and tolerability.
- Consider comorbidity, which is the presence of two or more disorders whose association is more likely than chance. Conditions that are comorbid with migraine are shown in **Box 1**.[8–11]

Box 1
Migraine comorbid disease
Cardiovascular
Hypertension or hypotension
Raynaud's disease
Mitral valve prolapse (migraine with aura)
Angina or myocardial infarction
Stroke
Psychiatric
Depression
Mania
Panic disorder
Anxiety disorder
Neurologic
Epilepsy
Essential tremor
Positional vertigo
Restless legs syndrome
Gastrointestinal
Irritable bowel syndrome
Other
Asthma
Allergies

Preventive treatment is often recommended for only 6 to 9 months; however, to date, no randomized placebo-controlled trials have been performed to investigate migraine frequency after the preventive treatment has been discontinued. Diener and colleagues[12] assessed 818 patients who had migraine and were treated with topiramate for 6 months to see the effects of topiramate discontinuation. Patients received topiramate in a 26-week open-label phase. They were then randomly assigned to continue this dose or to switch to placebo for a 26-week double-blind phase. Of the 559 patients who completed the open-label phase, 514 entered the double-blind phase and were assigned to topiramate (n = 255) or placebo (n = 259). The mean increase in number of migraine days was greater in the placebo group (1.19 days in 4 weeks, 95% confidence interval [CI]: 0.71–1.66; $P<.0001$) than in the topiramate group (0.10 days in 4 weeks, 95% CI: −0.36–0.56; P = .5756). Patients in the placebo group had a greater number of days on acute medication than did those in the topiramate group (mean difference between groups = 0.95, 95% CI: −1.49 to −0.41; P = .0007). Sustained benefit was reported after topiramate was discontinued, although the number of migraine days did increase. These findings suggest that patients should be treated for 6 months, with the option to continue to 12 months.

SPECIFIC MIGRAINE PREVENTIVE AGENTS
β-Adrenergic Blockers

Beta—blockers, the most widely used class of drugs in prophylactic migraine treatment, are approximately 50% effective in producing a greater than 50% reduction in attack frequency (**Table 1**). Evidence has consistently demonstrated the efficacy[13,14] of the nonselective beta-blocker propranolol[9–11,13–18] and the selective β1-blocker metoprolol.[9,10,15,19–21] Atenolol,[22] bisoprolol,[21,23] nadolol,[24,25] and timolol[13,26] are also likely to be effective. Beta-blockers with intrinsic sympathomimetic activity (eg, acebutolol, alprenolol, oxprenolol, pindolol) are not effective for migraine prevention. Propranolol is effective for migraine prevention at a daily dose of 120 to 240 mg, but no correlation has been found between its dose and its clinical efficacy.

The action of beta—blockers is probably central and could be mediated by (1) inhibiting central β-receptors that interfere with the vigilance-enhancing adrenergic pathways, (2) interaction with 5—HT receptors (but not all effective beta—blockers bind to the 5—HT receptors), and (3) cross-modulation of the serotonin system.[16] Propranolol inhibits nitric oxide (NO) production by blocking inducible NO synthase. Propranolol also inhibits kainate-induced currents and is synergistic with N-methyl-D-aspartate blockers, which reduce neuronal activity and have membrane-stabilizing properties.[17]

Contraindications to the use of beta-blockers include asthma and chronic obstructive lung disease, congestive heart failure, atrioventricular conduction defects, Raynaud's disease, peripheral vascular disease, and brittle diabetes. All beta—

Table 1
Beta-blockers and antidepressants in the preventive treatment of migraine

Agent	Daily Dose	Comment
Beta-blockers		
Atenolol	50–200 mg	Use qd Fewer side effects than propranolol
Metoprolol	100–200 mg	Use the short-acting form bid Use the long-acting form qd
Nadolol	20–160 mg	Use qid Fewer side effects than propranolol
Propranolol	40–400 mg	Use the short-acting form bid or tid Use the long-acting form qd or bid 1–2 mg/kg in children
Timolol	20–60 mg	Divide the dose Short half-life
Antidepressants		
Tertiary amines		
Amitriptyline	10–400 mg	Start at 10 mg at bedtime
Doxepin	10–300 mg	Start at 10 mg at bedtime
Secondary amines		
Nortriptyline	10–150 mg	Start at 10–25 mg at bedtime If insomnia, give early in the morning
Protriptyline	5–60 mg	Start at 10–25 mg at bedtime
Selective serotonin and norepinephrine reuptake inhibitors		
Venlafaxine	75–225 mg	Start at 37.5 mg in morning

Abbreviations: bid, twice daily; qd, every day; tid, three times daily.

blockers can produce behavioral AEs, such as drowsiness, fatigue, lethargy, sleep disorders, nightmares, depression, memory disturbance, and hallucinations.[13] Other potential AEs include gastrointestinal complaints, decreased exercise tolerance, orthostatic hypotension, bradycardia, and impotence. Although stroke has been reported to occur after patients who had migraine with aura were started on beta—blockers, there is neither an absolute nor a relative contraindication to their use by patients who have migraine, with or without aura.

Antidepressants

Antidepressants consist of several different drug classes with different mechanisms of action (see **Table 1**). Only one member of the class of tricyclic antidepressants (TCAs) (amitriptyline) has proved efficacy in migraine.[14] Although the mechanism by which antidepressants work to prevent migraine headache is uncertain, it does not result from treating masked depression. Antidepressants are useful in treating many chronic pain states, including headache, independent of the presence of depression, and the response occurs sooner than the expected antidepressant effect.[21,22] In animal pain models, antidepressants potentiate the effects of coadministered opioids.[23] The antidepressants that are clinically effective in headache prevention inhibit noradrenaline and 5—HT reuptake or are antagonists at the 5—HT$_2$ receptors.[24]

The TCA dose range is wide and must be individualized. Most TCAs are sedating. Start with a low dose of the chosen TCA at bedtime, except when using protriptyline, which should be administered in the morning. If the TCA is too sedating, switch from a tertiary TCA (eg, amitriptyline, doxepin) to a secondary TCA (eg, nortriptyline, protriptyline). AEs are common with TCA use. Antimuscarinic AEs include dry mouth, a metallic taste, epigastric distress, constipation, dizziness, mental confusion, tachycardia, palpitations, blurred vision, and urinary retention. Other AEs include weight gain (rarely seen with protriptyline), orthostatic hypotension, reflex tachycardia, and palpitations. Antidepressant treatment may change depression to hypomania or frank mania (particularly in bipolar patients). Older patients may develop confusion or delirium.[25] The muscarinic and adrenergic effects of these agents may pose increased risks for cardiac conduction abnormalities, especially in the elderly, and these patients should be carefully monitored or other agents should be considered.

Amitriptyline and doxepin are sedating TCAs. Patients with coexistent depression may require higher doses of these drugs to treat underlying depression. Start at a dose of 10 to 25 mg at bedtime. The usual effective dose for migraine ranges from 25 to 200 mg. Nortriptyline, a major metabolite of amitriptyline, is a secondary amine that is less sedating than amitriptyline. Start at a dose of 10 to 25 mg at bedtime. The dosage ranges from 10 to 150 mg/d. Protriptyline is a secondary amine that is similar to nortriptyline. Start at a dose of 5 mg in the morning. The dosage ranges from 5 to 60 mg/d as a single or split dose.

Evidence for the use of selective serotonin reuptake inhibitors (SSRIs) or other antidepressants for migraine prevention is poor. Fluoxetine at doses between 10 and 40 mg was effective in three placebo-controlled trials and not effective in one.[27–29] Other antidepressants not effective in placebo-controlled trials were clomipramine and sertraline; for other antidepressants, only open or non–placebo-controlled trials are available. Because their tolerability profile is superior to that of tricyclics, SSRIs may be helpful for patients with comorbid depression.[30] The most common AEs include sexual dysfunction, anxiety, nervousness, insomnia, drowsiness, fatigue, tremor, sweating, anorexia, nausea, vomiting, and dizziness or lightheadedness. The combination of an SSRI and a TCA can be beneficial in treating refractory depression[31] and, in the author's experience, resistant cases of migraine. The combination may require the TCA dose to be adjusted, because TCA plasma levels may significantly increase.

Recently, venlafaxine, an SSRI and selective norepinephrine reuptake inhibitor (SNRI), has been shown to be effective in a double-blind placebo-controlled trial[32] and in a separate placebo and amitriptyline controlled trial.[33] The usual effective dosage is 150 mg/d. Start with the 37.5-mg extended-release tablet for 1 week, then the 75-mg tablet for 1 week, and then the 150-mg extended-release tablet in the morning. AEs include insomnia, nervousness, mydriasis, and seizures.

Calcium Channel Antagonists

Two types of calcium channels exist: calcium entry channels, which allow extracellular calcium to enter the cell, and calcium release channels, which allow intracellular calcium (in storage sites in organelles) to enter the cytoplasm (**Table 2**).[34] Calcium entry channel subtypes include voltage-gated, opened by depolarization; ligand-gated, opened by chemical messengers, such as glutamate; and capacitative, activated by depletion of intracellular calcium stores. The mechanism of action of the calcium channel antagonists in migraine prevention is uncertain, but possibilities include inhibition of 5−HT release, neurovascular inflammation, or the initiation and propagation of cortical spreading depression.[35] Flunarizine, a nonselective calcium channel antagonist with antidopaminergic properties, was superior to placebo in six of seven randomized clinical trials.[18,20,32–40] The dose is 5 to 10 mg given at night (women seem to need lower doses than men). The most prominent AEs include weight gain, somnolence, dry mouth, dizziness, hypotension, occasional extrapyramidal reactions, and exacerbation of depression. Because of its side effect profile, flunarizine should be considered as a second-line drug for migraine prevention, after beta-blockers. Flunarizine is widely used in Europe but is not available in the United

Table 2
Selected calcium channel blockers and selected anticonvulsants in the preventive treatment of migraine

Agent	Daily Dose	Comment
Selected calcium channel blockers		
Verapamil	120–640 mg	Start at 80 mg bid or tid Sustained-release form can be given qd or bid
Flunarizine	5–10 mg	qd at bedtime Weight gain is the most common side effect
Selected anticonvulsants		
Carbamazepine	600–1200 mg	tid
Gabapentin	600–1200 mg	Dose can be increased to 3000 mg
Topiramate	100 mg	Start at 15–25 mg at bedtime Increase 15–25 mg/wk Attempt to reach 50–100 mg Increase further if necessary Associated with weight loss rather than weight gain
Valproate/divalproex	500–1500 mg	Start at 250–500 mg/d Monitor levels if compliance is an issue Maximum dosage is 60 mg/kg/d

Abbreviations: bid, twice daily; qd, every day; tid, three times daily.

States, where verapamil is the recommended calcium channel antagonist. Verapamil was more effective than placebo in two of three trials, but both positive trials were small and dropout rates were high, rendering the findings uncertain.[41–43] Rigorous randomized controlled trial evidence does not exist to support the use of verapamil for migraine. Nimodipine, nicardipine, diltiazem, and cyclandelate, other nonselective calcium channel antagonists, have not shown superiority over placebo in well-designed clinical trials and cannot be recommended for migraine prophylaxis.

ANTICONVULSANTS

Anticonvulsants are increasingly recommended for migraine prevention because of well-conducted placebo-controlled trials. With the exception of valproic acid, topiramate, and zonisamide, anticonvulsants may substantially interfere with the efficacy of oral contraceptives.[41,44]

Carbamazepine

The only placebo-controlled trial of carbamazepine that suggested a significant benefit had several methodologic issues (see **Table 2**).[42] Carbamazepine, 600 to 1200 mg/d, may be effective in preventive migraine treatment but it is rarely used in clinical practice for this purpose.

Gabapentin

Gabapentin (1800–2400 mg) showed efficacy in a placebo-controlled double-blind trial only when a modified intent-to-treat analysis was used (see **Table 2**). Migraine attack frequency was reduced by 50% in approximately one third of patients.[43] The most common AEs were dizziness or giddiness and drowsiness.

Valproic Acid

Valproic acid is a simple 8-carbon, 2-chain fatty acid. Divalproex sodium (approved by the US Food and Drug Administration [FDA]) is a combination of valproic acid and sodium valproate. Both are effective,[45,46] as is an extended-release form of divalproex sodium.[47] In 1992, Hering and Kuritzky[48] evaluated the efficacy of sodium valproate in migraine treatment in a double-blind, randomized, crossover study. Sodium valproate was effective in preventing migraine or reducing the frequency, severity, and duration of attacks in 86.2% of 29 patients, whose attacks were reduced from 15.6 to 8.8 a month. In 1994, Jensen and colleagues[49] studied 43 patients who had migraine without aura in a triple-blind, placebo- and dose-controlled, crossover study of slow-release sodium valproate. In the valproate group, 50% of the patients had a reduction in migraine frequency to 50% or less, compared with 18% for placebo.

Several subsequent randomized placebo-controlled studies have confirmed these results, with significant responder rates ranging between 43% and 48%[39,49] and dosages ranging from 500–1500 mg/d. Extended-release divalproex sodium has also been shown to be effective for migraine prevention, and compliance and the side effect profile may be more favorable with this formulation.[29]

Nausea, vomiting, and gastrointestinal distress are the AEs that occur most commonly; their incidence decreases, however, particularly after 6 months. Later, tremor and alopecia can occur. Valproate has little effect on cognitive functions and rarely causes sedation. Rare severe AEs include hepatitis and pancreatitis. The frequency varies with the number of concomitant medications used, the patient's age, the presence of genetic and metabolic disorders, and the patient's general state of health. These idiosyncratic reactions are unpredictable.[50] Valproate is teratogenic.[51]

Hyperandrogenism, ovarian cysts, and obesity are of concern in young women who have epilepsy and use valproate.[52] Absolute contraindications are pregnancy and a history of pancreatitis or a hepatic disorder. Other contraindications are thrombocytopenia, pancytopenia, and bleeding disorders.

Valproic acid is available as 250-mg capsules and as syrup (250 mg per 5 mL) (**Table 3**). Divalproex sodium is available as 125-, 250-, and 500-mg capsules and as a sprinkle formulation. Start with 250 to 500 mg/d in divided doses, and slowly increase the dosage. Monitor serum levels if there is a question of toxicity or compliance. The maximum recommended dosage is 60 mg/kg/d.

Topiramate

Topiramate was originally synthesized as part of a research project to discover structural analogs of fructose-1, 6-diphosphate capable of inhibiting the enzyme fructose 1, 6-bisphosphatase, thereby blocking gluconeogenesis, but it has no hypoglycemic activity. Topiramate and divalproex sodium are the only two anticonvulsants that have FDA approval for migraine prevention. Topiramate is not associated with significant reductions in estrogen exposure at dosages less than 200 mg/d. At dosages greater than 200 mg/d, there may be a dose-related reduction in exposure to the estrogen component of oral contraceptives.

Two large, pivotal, multicenter, randomized, double-blind, placebo-controlled clinical trials assessed the efficacy and safety of topiramate (50, 100, and 200 mg/d) in migraine prevention. In the first trial, the responder rate (patients with $\geq$50% reduction in monthly migraine frequency) was 52% with topiramate, 200 mg/d ($P<.001$); 54% with topiramate, 100 mg/d ($P<.001$); and 36% with topiramate, 50 mg/d ($P = .039$), compared with 23% with placebo.[53] The 200-mg dose was not significantly more effective than the 100-mg dose. The second pivotal trial[54] had significantly more patients who exhibited at least a 50% reduction in mean monthly migraines in the groups treated with topiramate at a dosage of 50 mg/d (39%; $P = .009$), 100 mg/d (49%; $P = .001$), and 200 mg/d (47%; $P = .001$).

A third randomized, double-blind, parallel-group, multicenter trial[55] compared two dosages of topiramate (100 mg/d or 200 mg/d) with placebo or propranolol (160 mg/d). Topiramate at a dosage of 100 mg/d was superior to placebo, as measured by average monthly migraine period rate, average monthly migraine days, rate of rescue medication use, and percentage of patients with a 50% or greater decrease in average monthly migraine period rate (37% responder rate). The topiramate

Table 3
Miscellaneous medication in the preventive treatment of migraine

Angiotensin-Converting Enzyme and Angiotensin Receptor Antagonists		
Agent	Daily Dose	Comment
Lisinopril	10–40 mg	Positive small controlled trial
Candesartan	16 mg	Positive small controlled trial
Others		
Feverfew	50–82 mg	Controversial evidence
Petasites	150 mg	75 bid better than placebo in one study
Riboflavin	400 mg	Positive small controlled trial
Coenzyme Q	100–300 mg	Two positive controlled trials
Magnesium	400–600 mg	Controversial evidence

Abbreviation: bid, twice daily.

(100 mg/d) and propranolol groups were similar in change from baseline to the core double-blind phase in average monthly migraine period rate and other secondary efficacy variables.

The most common AE of topiramate is paresthesia; other common AEs are fatigue, decreased appetite, nausea, diarrhea, weight decrease, taste perversion, hypoesthesia, and abdominal pain. In the migraine trials, body weight was reduced an average of 2.3% in the 50-mg group, 3.2% in the 100-mg group, and 3.8% in the 200-mg group. Patients on propranolol gained 2.3% of their baseline body weight. The most common central nervous system AEs were somnolence, insomnia, mood problems, anxiety, difficulty with memory, language problems, and difficulty with concentration. Renal calculi can occur with topiramate use. The reported incidence is approximately 1.5%, representing a two- to fourfold increase over the estimated occurrence in the general population.[56]

A rare AE is acute myopia associated with secondary angle closure glaucoma. No cases of this condition were reported in the clinical studies.[57] Oligohidrosis has been reported in association with an elevation in body temperature. Most reports have involved children.

Start at a dosage of 15 to 25 mg/d given at bedtime (see **Table 3**). Increase dosage by 15 to 25 mg/wk. Do not increase the dose if bothersome AEs develop; wait until they resolve (they usually do). If they do not resolve, decrease the drug to the last tolerable dose and then increase to a lower dose more slowly. Attempt to reach a dosage of 50 to 100 mg given twice a day. It is the author's experience that patients who tolerate the lower doses with only partial improvement often have increased benefit with higher doses. The dosage can be increased to 600 mg/d or higher.

Lamotrigine

Lamotrigine blocks voltage-sensitive sodium channels, leading to inhibition of neuronal glutamate release of glutamate. Chen and colleagues[58] reported on two patients who had migraine with persistent aura-like visual phenomena for months to years. After 2 weeks of lamotrigine treatment, both had resolution of the visual symptoms.

Although open-label studies have suggested that lamotrigine may have a select role in the treatment of patients with frequent or prolonged aura, results from a placebo-controlled study in migraine were negative. Steiner and colleagues[59] compared the safety and efficacy of lamotrigine (200 mg/d) and placebo in migraine prophylaxis in a double-blind, randomized, parallel-group trial. Improvements were greater on placebo, and these changes, which were not statistically significant, indicate that lamotrigine was ineffective for migraine prophylaxis. There were more AEs on lamotrigine than on placebo, most commonly rash. With slow dose escalation, their frequency was reduced, and the rate of withdrawal attributable to AEs was similar in both treatment groups.

Open-label studies have suggested that lamotrigine may have a select role in the treatment of migraine with aura, but no placebo-controlled studies have yet been conducted in this patient population. Lamotrigine and topiramate[60] may have a special role in the treatment of migraine with aura.

OTHER DRUGS
Angiotensin-Converting Enzyme Inhibitors and Angiotensin II Receptor Antagonists

Schrader and colleagues[61] conducted a double-blind, placebo-controlled, crossover study of lisinopril, an angiotensin-converting enzyme inhibitor, in migraine prophylaxis (see **Table 3**). Days with migraine were reduced by at least 50% in 14 participants for active treatment versus placebo and in 17 patients for active treatment versus run-in period. Days with migraine were fewer by at least 50% in 14 participants for active treatment versus placebo. Tronvik and colleagues[62] performed a randomized, double-blind, placebo-controlled, crossover study of candesartan (16 mg), an angiotensin II receptor blocker, in migraine prevention. In a period of 12 weeks, the mean number of days with headache was 18.5 with placebo versus 13.6 with candesartan ($P = .001$) in the intention-to-treat analysis (n = 57). The number of candesartan responders (reduction of ≥50% compared with placebo) was 18 (31.6%) of 57 for days with headache and 23 (40.4%) of 57 for days with migraine. AEs were similar in the two periods. In this study, the angiotensin II receptor blocker candesartan was effective, with a tolerability profile comparable to that of placebo.

Botulinum Toxin Type A

The mechanism by which botulinum toxin may prevent migraine remains poorly understood, but it is unlikely to be related to relief of muscle spasticity. Developing evidence suggests that it may modulate release of neuropeptides, such as calcitonin gene-related peptide, and influence the process of central sensitization that is associated with migraine.

Botulinum toxin type A (Botox; 0, 25, or 75 U) has not been convincingly shown to be effective for the prevention of episodic migraine with or without aura. Although the results of an early placebo-controlled study were positive using a dose of 25 U, the results were confounded by no efficacy at the higher dose (75 U) used in this study.[63] Three recent placebo-controlled trials[64–66] showed no difference between different doses of botulinum toxin (105–260 U) and placebo, however. Based on a significant response to botulinum toxin type A in a subgroup of patients who had chronic migraine and were not on other preventive medications,[67] two large, pivotal, placebo-controlled studies evaluating the efficacy of botulinum toxin type A for chronic migraine are currently underway.

Medicinal Herbs and Vitamins

Feverfew (*Tanacetum parthenium*) is a medicinal herb whose effectiveness has not been totally established.[68] Riboflavin (400 mg) was effective in one placebo-controlled double-blind trial. More than half of the patients responded.[69] *petasites hybridus* (butterbur) root is a perennial shrub, a standardized extract of which (75 mg administered twice daily) was effective in a double-blind placebo-controlled study.[30] The most common AE was belching.

Setting Treatment Priorities

The goals of preventive treatment are to reduce the frequency, duration, or severity of attacks; improve responsiveness to acute attack treatment; improve function; and reduce disability (**Box 2**). The preventive medications with the best-documented efficacy are the beta-blockers and amitriptyline, divalproex, and topiramate. Choice is made based on a drug's proved efficacy, the physician's informed belief about medications not yet evaluated in controlled trials, the drug's AEs, the patient's preferences and headache profile, and the presence or absence of coexisting disorders (see **Table 1**).[27] Coexistent diseases have important implications for treatment. In some instances, two or more conditions may be treated with a single drug. If individuals have more than one disease, certain categories of treatment may be relatively contraindicated.

Box 2
Preventive drugs

High efficacy: low to moderate AEs

    Propranolol, timolol, amitriptyline, valproate, topiramate, and flunarizine

Low efficacy: low to moderate AEs

    Nonsteroidal anti-inflammatory drugs: aspirin, flurbiprofen, ketoprofen, and naproxen sodium

    Beta-blockers: atenolol, metoprolol, and nadolol

    Calcium channel blockers: verapamil

    Anticonvulsants: gabapentin

    Other: fenoprofen, feverfew, vitamin B_2

    Pizotifen

Unproved efficacy: low to moderate AEs

    Antidepressants: doxepin, nortriptyline, imipramine, protriptyline, venlafaxine, fluvoxamine, mirtazapine, paroxetine, protriptyline, sertraline, and trazodone

Proved not effective or low efficacy

    Acebutolol, carbamazepine, clomipramine, clonazepam, indomethacin, lamotrigine, nabumetone, nicardipine, nifedipine, and pindolol

---

The presence of a second illness provides therapeutic opportunities but also imposes certain therapeutic limitations. In some instances, two or more conditions may be treated with a single drug. There are limitations to using a single medication to treat two illnesses, however. Giving a single medication may not treat two different conditions optimally; although one of the two conditions may be adequately treated, the second illness may require a higher or lower dose, and the patient is thus at risk for the second illness not being adequately treated. Therapeutic independence may be needed should monotherapy fail. Avoiding drug interactions or increased AEs is a primary concern when using polypharmacy.

For some patients, a single medication may adequately manage comorbid conditions. This is likely to be the exception rather than the rule, however. Polytherapy may enable therapeutic adjustments based on the status of each illness. TCAs are often recommended for patients who have migraine and depression.[28] Appropriate management of depression often requires higher doses of TCAs, however, which may be associated with more AEs. A better approach might be to treat the depression with an SSRI or SNRI and treat the migraine with an anticonvulsant. For the patient who has migraine and epilepsy,[29] one may achieve control of both conditions with an antiepileptic drug, such as topiramate or divalproex sodium. Divalproex and topiramate are the drugs of choice for the patient who has migraine and bipolar illness.[31,51] When individuals have more than one disease, certain categories of treatment may be relatively contraindicated. For example, beta-blockers should be used with caution for the depressed migraineur, whereas TCAs or neuroleptics may lower the seizure threshold and should be used with caution for the epileptic migraineur.

Although monotherapy is preferred, it is often not the best choice, and it may be necessary to combine preventive medications. Antidepressants are often used with beta-blockers or calcium channel blockers, and topiramate or divalproex sodium may be used in combination with any of these medications.

SUMMARY

Preventive therapy plays an important role in migraine management. With the addition of a preventive medication, patients may experience reduced attack frequency and improved response to acute treatment, which can result in reduced health care resource use and improved quality of life. Despite research suggesting that a large percentage of patients who have migraine are candidates for prevention, only a fraction of these patients are receiving or have ever received preventive migraine medication.

Many preventive medications are available, and guidelines for their selection and use have been established. Because comorbid medical and psychologic illnesses are prevalent in patients who have migraine, one must consider comorbidity when choosing preventive drugs. Drug therapy may be beneficial for both disorders; however, it is also a potential confounder of optimal treatment of either.

No clinical trial data exist to predict among the various therapeutic options and biologic or clinical parameters. The impact of prevention on the natural history of migraine remains to be fully investigated.

REFERENCES

1. Lipton RB, Silberstein SD. Why study the comorbidity of migraine? Neurology 1994;44:4–5.
2. Silberstein SD, Winner PK, Chmiel JJ. Migraine preventive medication reduces resource utilization. Headache: The Journal of Head and Face Pain 2003;43: 171–8.
3. Silberstein SD. Headaches in pregnancy. Neurol Clin 2004;22:727–56.
4. Lipton RB, Diamond M, Freitag F, et al. Migraine prevention patterns in a community sample: results from the American Migraine Prevalence and Prevention (AMPP) study. Headache 2005;45:792–3 [abstract].
5. Silberstein S, Diamond S, Loder E, et al. Prevalence of migraine sufferers who are candidates for preventive therapy: results from the American Migraine Prevalence and Prevention (AMPP) study. Headache 2005;45:770–1 [abstract].
6. Tfelt-Hansen P. Prioritizing acute pharmacotherapy of migraine. In: Olesen J, Tfelt-Hansen P, Welch KMA, editors. The headaches. 2nd edition. New York: Lippincott Williams & Wilkins; 2000. p. 453–6.
7. Silberstein SD. Migraine and pregnancy. Neurol Clin 1997;15:209–31.
8. Olerud B, Gustavsson CL, Furberg B. Nadolol and propranolol in migraine management. Headache 1986;26:490–3.
9. Ryan RE, Sudilovsky A. Nadolol: its use in the prophylactic treatment of migraine. Headache 1983;23:26–31.
10. Ryan RE. Comparative study of nadolol and propranolol in prophylactic treatment of migraine. Am Heart J 1984;108:1156–9.
11. Sudilovsky A, Stern MA, Meyer JH. Nadolol: the benefits of an adequate trial duration in the prophylaxis of migraine. Headache 1986;26:325.
12. Diener HC, Agosti R, Allais G, et al. Cessation versus continuation of 6-month migraine preventive therapy with topiramate (PROMPT): a randomised, double-blind, placebo-controlled trial. Lancet Neurol 2007;6:1054–62.
13. Gray RN, Goslin RE, McCrory DC, et al. Drug treatments for the prevention of migraine headache. Prepared for the Agency for Health Care Policy and

Research, contact no. 290-94-2025. Available from the National Technical Information Service 1999; Accession No. 127953.

14. Silberstein SD. Practice parameter—evidence-based guidelines for migraine headache (an evidence-based review): report of the Quality Standards Subcommittee of the American Academy of Neurology for the United States Headache Consortium. Neurology 2000;55:754-62.
15. Andersson K, Vinge E. Beta-adrenoceptor blockers and calcium antagonists in the prophylaxis and treatment of migraine. Drugs 1990;39:355-73.
16. Koella WP. CNS-related (side-)effects of beta-blockers with special reference to mechanisms of action. Eur J Clin Pharmacol 1985;28:55-63.
17. Ramadan NM. Prophylactic migraine therapy: mechanisms and evidence. Curr Pain Headache Rep 2004;8:91-5.
18. Cortelli P, Sacquegna T, Albani F, et al. Propranolol plasma levels and relief of migraine. Arch Neurol 1985;42:46-8.
19. Sudilovsky A, Elkind AH, Ryan RE, et al. Comparative efficacy of nadolol and propranolol in the management of migraine. Headache 1987;27:421-6.
20. Tfelt-Hansen P, Standnes B, Kangasniemi P, et al. Timolol vs propranolol vs placebo in common migraine prophylaxis: a double-blind multicenter trial. Acta Neurol Scand 1984;69:1-8.
21. Panerai AE, Monza G, Movilia P, et al. A randomized, within-patient, cross-over, placebo-controlled trial on the efficacy and tolerability of the tricyclic antidepressants chlorimipramine and nortriptyline in central pain. Acta Neurol Scand 1990; 82:34-8.
22. Kishore-Kumar R, Max MB, Schafer SC, et al. Desipramine relieves post-herpetic neuralgia. Clin Pharmacol Ther 1990;47:305-12.
23. Feinmann C. Pain relief by antidepressants: possible modes of action. Pain 1985;23:1-8.
24. Richelson E. Antidepressants and brain neurochemistry. Mayo Clin Proc 1990;65: 1227-36.
25. Baldessarini RJ. Drugs and the treatment of psychiatric disorders. In: Gilman AG, Rall TW, Nies AS, et al, editors. The pharmacological basis of therapeutics. 8th edition. New York: Pergamon; 1990. p. 383-435.
26. Abramowicz M. Fluoxetine (Prozac) revisited. Med Lett Drugs Ther 1990;32:83-5.
27. Silberstein SD, Saper JR, Freitag F. Migraine: diagnosis and treatment. In: Silberstein SD, Lipton RB, Dalessio DJ, editors. Wolff's headache and other head pain. 7th edition. New York: Oxford University Press; 2001. p. 121-237.
28. Silberstein SD, Lipton RB, Breslau N. Migraine: association with personality characteristics and psychopathology. Cephalalgia 1995;15:337-69.
29. Mathew NT, Saper JR, Silberstein SD, et al. Migraine prophylaxis with divalproex. Arch Neurol 1995;52:281-6.
30. Lipton RB, Gobel H, Wilks K, et al. Efficacy of petasites (an extract from Petasites rhizone) 50 and 75 mg for prophylaxis of migraine: results of a randomized, double-blind, placebo-controlled study. Neurology 2002;58:A472 [abstract].
31. Bowden CL, Brugger AM, Swann AC. Efficacy of divalproex vs lithium and placebo in the treatment of mania. JAMA 1994;271:918-24.
32. Ozyalcin SN, Talu GK, Kiziltan E, et al. The efficacy and safety of venlafaxine in the prophylaxis of migraine. Headache 2005;45:144-52.
33. Bulut S, Berilgen MS, Baran A, et al. Venlafaxine versus amitriptyline in the prophylactic treatment of migraine: randomized, double-blind, crossover study. Clin Neurol Neurosurg 2004;107:44-8.
34. Greenberg DA. Calcium channels in neurological disease. Ann Neurol 1997;42: 275-82.

35. Wauquier A, Ashton D, Marranes R. The effects of flunarizine in experimental models related to the pathogenesis of migraine. Cephalalgia 1985;5:119–20.
36. Solomon GD. Verapamil and propranolol in migraine prophylaxis: a double-blind crossover study. Headache 1986;26:325.
37. Markley HG, Cleronis JCD, Piepko RW. Verapamil prophylactic therapy of migraine. Neurology 1984;34:973–6.
38. Riopelle R, McCans JL. A pilot study of the calcium channel antagonist diltiazem in migraine syndrome prophylaxis. Can J Neurol Sci 1982;9:269.
39. Smith R, Schwartz A. Diltiazem prophylaxis in refractory migraine. N Engl J Med 1984;310:1327–8.
40. Reveiz-Herault L, Cardona AF, Ospina EG, et al. [Effectiveness of flunarizine in the prophylaxis of migraine: a meta-analytical review of the literature]. Rev Neurol 2003;36:907–12, in Spanish.
41. Hanston PP, Horn JR. Drug interaction. Newsletter 1985;5:7–10.
42. Rompel H, Bauermeister PW. Aetiology of migraine and prevention with carbamazepine (Tegretol). S Afr Med J 1970;44:75–80.
43. Mathew NT, Rapoport A, Saper J, et al. Efficacy of gabapentin in migraine prophylaxis. Headache 2001;41:119–28.
44. Coulam CB, Annagers JR. New anticonvulsants reduce the efficacy of oral contraception. Epilepsia 1979;20:519–25.
45. Klapper JA. Divalproex sodium in migraine prophylaxis: a dose-controlled study. Cephalalgia 1997;17:103–8.
46. Klapper JA. An open label crossover comparison of divalproex sodium and propranolol HCl in the prevention of migraine headaches. Headache Quarterly 1995;5:50–3.
47. Freitag FG, Collins SD, Carlson HA, et al. A randomized trial of divalproex sodium extended-release tablets in migraine prophylaxis. For the Depakote ER Migraine Study Group. Neurology 2003;58:1652–9.
48. Hering R, Kuritzky A. Sodium valproate in the prophylactic treatment of migraine: a double-blind study versus placebo. Cephalalgia 1992;12:81–4.
49. Jensen R, Brinck T, Olesen J. Sodium valproate has prophylactic effect in migraine without aura: a triple-blind, placebo-controlled crossover study. Neurology 1994;44:241–4.
50. Pellock JM, Willmore LJ. A rational guide to routine blood monitoring in patients receiving antiepileptic drugs. Neurology 1991;41:961–4.
51. Silberstein SD. Divalproex sodium in headache—literature review and clinical guidelines. Headache 1996;36:547–55.
52. Vainionpaa LK, Rattya J, Knip M, et al. Valproate-induced hyperandrogenism during pubertal maturation in girls with epilepsy. Ann Neurol 1999;45:444–50.
53. Silberstein SD, Neto W, Schmitt J, et al. Topiramate in the prevention of migraine headache: a randomized, double-blind, placebo-controlled, multiple-dose study. For the MIGR-001 Study Group. Arch Neurol 2004;61:490–5.
54. Brandes JL, Saper JR, Diamond M, et al. Topiramate for migraine prevention: a randomized controlled trial. JAMA 2004;291:965–73.
55. Diener HC, Tfelt-Hansen P, Dahlof C, et al. Topiramate in migraine prophylaxis—results from a placebo-controlled trial with propranolol as an active control. J Neurol 2004;251:943–50.
56. Sachedo RC, Reife RA, Lim P, et al. Topiramate monotherapy for partial onset seizures. Epilepsia 1997;38:294–300.
57. Thomson Healthcare. Physicians' desk reference. 57th edition. Montvale (NJ): Thomson PDR; 2003.

58. Chen WT, Fuh JL, Lu SR, et al. Persistent migrainous visual phenomena might be responsive to lamotrigine. Headache 2001;41:823–5.
59. Steiner TJ, Findley LJ, Yuen AW. Lamotrigine versus placebo in the prophylaxis of migraine with and without aura. Cephalalgia 1997;17:109–12.
60. Freitag FG. Topiramate prophylaxis in patients suffering from migraine with aura: results from a randomized, double-blind, placebo-controlled trial. Advanced Studies in Medicine 2003;3:S562–4.
61. Schrader H, Stovner LJ, Helde G, et al. Prophylactic treatment of migraine with angiotensin converting enzyme inhibitor (lisinopril): randomized, placebo-controlled, crossover study. Br Med J 2001;322:19–22.
62. Tronvik E, Stovner LJ, Helde G, et al. Prophylactic treatment of migraine with an angiotensin II receptor blocker: a randomized controlled trial. JAMA 2003;289: 65–9.
63. Silberstein SD, Mathew N, Saper J, et al. Botulinum toxin type A as a migraine preventive treatment. Headache 2000;40:445–50.
64. Evers S, Vollmer-Haase J, Schwaag S, et al. Botulinum toxin A in the prophylactic treatment of migraine—a randomized, double-blind, placebo-controlled study. Cephalalgia 2004;24:838–43.
65. Elkind AH, O'Carroll P, Blumenfeld A, et al. A series of three sequential, randomized, controlled studies of repeated treatments with botulinum toxin type A for migraine prophylaxis. J Pain 2006;7:688–96.
66. Saper JR, Mathew NT, Loder EW, et al. A double-blind, randomized, placebo-controlled comparison of botulinum toxin type A injection sites and doses in the prevention of episodic migraine. Pain Med, In press.
67. Dodick DW, Mauskop A, Elkind AH, et al. Botulinum toxin type A for the prophylaxis of chronic daily headache: subgroup analysis of patients not receiving other prophylactic medications: a randomized double-blind, placebo-controlled study. Headache 2005;45:315–24.
68. Vogler BK, Pittler MH, Ernst E. Feverfew as a preventive treatment for migraine: a systematic review. Cephalalgia 1998;18:704–8.
69. Schoenen J, Jacquy J, Lenaerts M. Effectiveness of high-dose riboflavin in migraine prophylaxis. A randomized controlled trial. Neurology 1998;50:466–70.

Behavioral Medicine for Migraine

Dawn C. Buse, PhD[a,b,c,*], Frank Andrasik, PhD[d]

KEYWORDS

- Migraine • Headache • Biofeedback
- Behavioral medicine • Biobehavioral • Relaxation
- Cognitive behavioral therapy (CBT) • Biopsychosocial

"Behavioral Medicine is the interdisciplinary field concerned with the development and integration of behavioral, psychosocial, and biomedical science knowledge and techniques relevant to the understanding of health and illness, and the application of this knowledge and these techniques to prevention, diagnosis, treatment and rehabilitation."[1] The discipline of behavioral medicine is based on the biopsychosocial model, which asserts that biologic, psychologic (including behaviors and cognitive experiences, such as thoughts and emotions), and social or environmental factors all play a significant role in human functioning.[2] This model maps particularly well onto the understanding of migraine and other primary headache disorders,[3] in which data continue to amass demonstrating the complex interactions of biology, environment, behavior, cognitions, and emotions on the development, maintenance, progression, and remission of headache disorders.

Although the armamentarium of safe and effective acute and preventive pharmacologic treatments for migraine has grown significantly, nonpharmacologic treatments continue to play a very important role in providing the most comprehensive and effective treatment plan. Nonpharmacologic therapies may be offered individually or in conjunction with a medicine regimen. A combination of pharmacologic and nonpharmacologic approaches has been demonstrated to be more effective than either approach on its own[4,5] to help maintain positive outcomes[6] and to improve treatment adherence.[7,8]

Nonpharmacologic treatments for migraine can be broadly divided into the categories of behavioral treatments (cognitive behavioral therapy [CBT] and biobehavioral training; [ie, biofeedback, relaxation training, and stress management]); physical

[a] Department of Neurology, Albert Einstein College of Medicine of Yeshiva University, NY, USA
[b] Clinical Health Psychology Doctoral Program, Ferkauf Graduate School of Psychology of Yeshiva University, NY, USA
[c] Montefiore Headache Center, 1575 Blondell Avenue, Suite 225, Bronx, NY 10461, USA
[d] Department of Psychology, University of West Florida, 11000 University Parkway, Pensacola, FL 32514, USA
* Corresponding author. Montefiore Headache Center, 1575 Blondell Avenue, Suite 225, Bronx, NY 10461.
E-mail address: dbuse@montefiore.org (D.C. Buse).

Neurol Clin 27 (2009) 445–465
doi:10.1016/j.ncl.2009.01.003
0733-8619/09/$ – see front matter © 2009 Elsevier Inc. All rights reserved.

neurologic.theclinics.com

therapies; and education including lifestyle modification. This article reviews empirically supported and efficacious behavioral approaches to the treatment and management of migraine. These include strategies for both patients and health care providers (HCPs) and are essential components of a comprehensive headache management plan. Once learned, patients can benefit from the strategies throughout their lives. Migraine commonly first occurs during adolescence or early adulthood. By encouraging patients to train their physiology through biofeedback and relaxation, adopt healthy lifestyle habits, and recognize and mediate the effects of stress in their lives the physician is giving patients a set of tools that can last a lifetime. Behavioral techniques also have demonstrated efficacy with children and adolescents.[9–11]

Behavioral medicine researchers and practitioners have embraced the concept of empirically supported or evidence-based behavioral medicine, which is defined as "The conscientious, explicit and judicious use of current best evidence in making clinical decisions about the care of patients... thereby integrating individual clinical care with the best available clinical evidence."[12] Behavioral treatments with demonstrated empiric efficacy for headache management have become standard components of specialty headache centers and multidisciplinary pain management programs. Several empirically validated biobehavioral approaches to headache management are endorsed by the American Medical Association, the World Health Organization, and the National Institutes of Health, and many other professional organizations.[13]

The United States Headache Consortium developed evidence-based guidelines for the treatment and management of migraine headache based on an extensive review of the medical literature and compilation of expert consensus. Published guidelines include data and recommendations on the use of nonpharmacologic (behavioral and physical) treatments, among other issues regarding migraine diagnosis and management.[14] The United States Headache Consortium pointed out that nonpharmacologic treatments might be particularly well suited for patients who

1. Have a preference for nonpharmacologic interventions
2. Display a poor tolerance for specific pharmacologic treatments
3. Exhibit medical contraindications for specific pharmacologic treatments
4. Have insufficient or no response to pharmacologic treatment
5. Are pregnant, are planning to become pregnant, or are nursing
6. Have a history of long-term, frequent, or excessive use of analgesic or acute medications that can aggravate headache problems (or lead to decreased responsiveness to other pharmacotherapies)
7. Exhibit significant stress or deficient stress-coping skills

The United States Headache Consortium reported on the efficacy of behavioral interventions in the prevention of attacks, although some behavioral interventions may also provide relief once an attack has begun. They identified the following goals for behavioral interventions as preventive treatment for headache: (1) reduced frequency and severity of headache, (2) reduced headache-related disability, (3) reduced reliance on poorly tolerated or unwanted pharmacotherapies, (4) enhanced personal control of migraine, and (5) reduced headache-related distress and psychologic symptoms.

EVIDENCE ON EFFICACY OF BEHAVIORAL INTERVENTIONS FOR MIGRAINE

There is a large and constantly growing body of published evidence examining the use of behavioral therapies for migraine (and other forms of headache) including meta-analytic studies and evidence-based reviews.[15,16] These behavioral treatments have been found to be superior to various control conditions, and the benefits from these treatments are generally maintained over time. For example, a large meta-analysis of nonpharmacologic treatments for migraine sponsored by the US Agency for Healthcare Research and Quality[13] identified 355 studies of behavioral and physical treatments. Few of these (70 of 355) were controlled trials of behavioral treatments and fewer yet (39 of 355) met the criteria for inclusion in the meta-analysis. **Fig. 1** combines findings from the US Agency for Healthcare Research and Quality analysis with three other large meta-analyses, which included various control conditions, and a sample of efficacy rates for two prophylactic medications for comparison (see[16] for a more current review of the evidence).

Meta-analyses comparing behavioral and pharmacologic (prophylactic) treatments have shown similar efficacy between the two approaches (see **Fig. 1**).[17] These meta-analytic findings of comparable outcomes for behavioral and medication treatments are consistent with the findings from the few direct comparisons that have been conducted for migraine headache.[18,19]

In addition to meta-analyses of existing data, there are also consensus-based reviews conducted by expert panels. Evidence-based analyses for migraine and headache have been performed by the United States Headache Consortium (an expert panel composed of representative of the American Academy of Family Physicians, American Academy of Neurology, American Headache Society, American College of Emergency Physicians, American College of Physicians-American Society

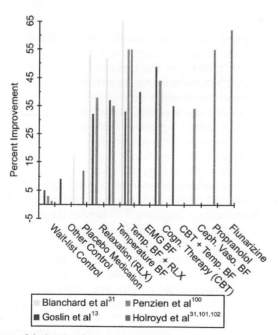

Fig. 1. Meta-analyses of behavioral and pharmacologic treatments for migraine. Percent improvement scores are reported by treatment condition. (*Data from* Andrasik F. What does the evidence show? Efficacy of behavioural treatment for recurrent headaches in adults. Neurol Sci 2007;28:S70–7; Penzien DB, Rain JC, Andrasik F. Behavioral management of recurrent headache: three decades of experience and empiricism. Appl Psychophysiol Biofeedback 2002;27:163–81.)

of Internal Medicine, American Osteopathic Association and National Headache Foundation);[14] the Cochrane collaboration;[20] the Division 12 Task Force of the American Psychological Association;[21] the Canadian Headache Society;[22] and the Association for Applied Psychophysiology and Biofeedback.[23]

The United States Headache Consortium was convened with the goal of developing "scientifically sound, clinically relevant practice guidelines on chronic headache in the primary care setting,"[14] and to "propose diagnostic and therapeutic recommendations to improve the care and satisfaction of migraine patients" based on a review of the current literature.[13] The Consortium uses a grading system based on the quality of evidence.[24] Grade A is given to multiple well-designed randomized clinical trials, directly relevant to the recommendation, that yield a consistent pattern of findings. Grade B is given where some evidence from randomized clinical trials supports the recommendation, but the scientific support is not optimal. For instance, either few randomized trials existed, the trials that did exist were somewhat inconsistent, or the trials were not directly relevant to the recommendation. An example of the last point is the case where trials were conducted using a study group that differed from the target group for the recommendation. The United Sates Headache Consortium guidelines opine the following treatments have Grade A evidence for their use: relaxation training; thermal biofeedback combined with relaxation training; electromyographic biofeedback; and CBT (for prevention of migraine). Grade B evidence is given for behavioral therapy combined with preventive drug therapy to achieve added clinical improvement for migraine.

BIOFEEDBACK

Biofeedback is a procedure that involves monitoring physiologic processes of which the patient may not be consciously aware or does not believe that he or she has voluntary control. Biofeedback training is the process of increasing awareness of and bringing those physiologic functions under the patient's voluntary control.[24–26] Literally, biologic or physiologic information is converted into a signal that is then "fed back" to the patient, usually on a computer monitor and often with audio input. Patients are typically taught various relaxation skills, such as diaphragmatic breathing or visualization, to induce the relaxation response,[27] which includes relaxation of the sympathetic nervous system and activation of the parasympathetic nervous system. Recent literature on the neurophysiology of migraine and functional MRI studies of pain networks suggest that behavioral interventions may affect neuromodulation.[28]

Early reviews demonstrated rates of improvement ranging from 40% to 65% using biofeedback for the treatment of migraine.[29,30] Similar benefits were demonstrated when behavioral interventions were combined with pharmacotherapy.[31] Several biofeedback modality options exist including peripheral skin temperature feedback or thermal biofeedback (or autogenic feedback when combined with another relaxation approach termed "autogenic training"); blood-volume-pulse feedback; electromyographic feedback; galvanic skin response training or skin conductance feedback; and electroencephalographic feedback or neuro or brain wave feedback. Grade A evidence was found for the efficacy of thermal biofeedback combined with relaxation training and electromyographic biofeedback in prevention of migraine.[14]

Thermal biofeedback involves monitoring finger temperature with a sensitive thermometer. During or preceding a headache the body may enter the "fight or flight" state (activation of the sympathetic nervous system). As sympathetic activity increases, circulation to the extremities decreases and finger temperature decreases. Conversely, as parasympathetic activity increases and the relaxation response is activated, circulation and extremity temperature increase. Finger temperature is viewed as providing an indirect measure of autonomic arousal. Patients are taught that higher finger temperature corresponds to a more relaxed state and their goal is to raise their finger temperature. It was reported that relaxation training and thermal biofeedback can produce 33% to 37% improvement in headache activity.[14]

Nestoriuc and colleagues[32] recently conducted a comprehensive efficacy ("white paper") review of all existing investigations of biofeedback for migraine and tension-type headache. The authors provided efficacy recommendations, according to the guidelines jointly established by the Association for Applied Psychophysiology and Biofeedback and the International Society for Neurofeedback and Research.[33] They examined data from two recently published meta-analyses, which included 150 outcome studies.[15,34] Ninety-four studies met rigid inclusion criteria and were analyzed for effect sizes for the treatment of the two headache types, of which only migraine is reported here. They reported medium-to-large mean effect sizes for biofeedback for the treatment of migraine in adults, and found that treatment effects were maintained over an average follow-up period of 14 months, both in completer and intention-to-treat analyses (**Fig. 2**). Nestoriuc and colleagues[32] were also able to evaluate effects for secondary variable (this is the first meta-analysis to do so). **Fig. 3** shows that biofeedback led to significant improvements in perceived self-efficacy, symptoms of depression and anxiety, and medication use (**Fig. 3** also reports findings for various pain indices). Considering the evidence examined, the authors asserted that biofeedback can be supported as an efficacious treatment option for migraine with a confidence of Level 4 evidence (efficacious) according to the Association for Applied Psychophysiology and Biofeedback and the International Society for Neurofeedback and Research criteria.

Biofeedback training generally requires several office visits (8–12) spaced 1 to several weeks apart (although research suggests biofeedback and related treatments can be delivered effectively by a reduced-contact or home-based format).[35] Providers are often psychologists who also incorporate cognitive-behavioral techniques into sessions, but biofeedback may be successfully taught by a range of properly trained medical and mental health professionals. Patients are taught techniques in the office;

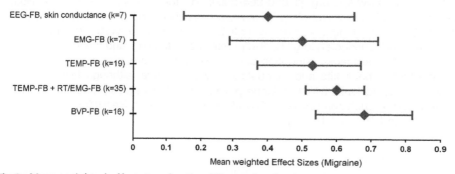

Fig. 2. Mean weighted effect sizes for the different feedback modalities in the treatment of migraine. Outcome is measured in headache pain. Mean effect sizes are displayed with their individual 95% confidence intervals (k = number of independent effect sizes). BVP-FB, blood-volume pulse feedback; EEG-FB, electroencephalographic feedback; EMG-FB, electromyographic feedback; RT, relaxation training; TEMP-FB, peripheral temperature feedback. (*From* Nestoriuc Y, Martin A, Rief W, et al. Biofeedback treatment for headache disorders: a comprehensive efficacy review. Applied Psychophysiol Biofeedback 2008;33:125–40; with permission.)

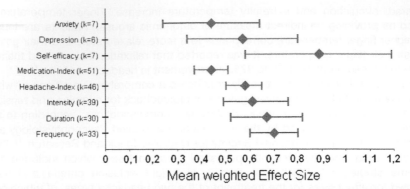

Fig. 3. Mean weighted effect sizes for the different outcome variables in the biofeedback treatment of migraine. Outcome is measured in headache pain over all biofeedback modalities. Mean effect sizes are displayed with their individual 95% confidence intervals (k = number of independent effect sizes). (*From* Nestoriuc Y, Martin A, Rief W, et al. Biofeedback treatment for headache disorders: a comprehensive efficacy review. Applied Psychophysiol Biofeedback 2008;33:125–40; with permission.)

however, home practice is also required between sessions. As the patient's ability to manipulate and control the targeted physiologic processes increases, the biofeedback device can be eliminated.

One of the biggest challenges for physicians and patients can often be locating a biofeedback practitioner.[36] The Association for Applied Psychophysiology and Biofeedback (www.aapb.org) is a professional organization of researchers and practitioners of biofeedback. The Biofeedback Certification Institute of America is an organization that certifies biofeedback providers, even though psychologists with proper training may practice biofeedback therapy without being certified or belonging to this organization. A list of certified biofeedback providers is available on their Web site (www.bcia.org/directory/membership.cfm). A list of psychologists with their specialties and location may be found at the Web sites of the American Psychological Association (www.apa.org [1-800-964-2000]) or the National Register of Health Service Providers in Psychology (www.nationalregister.org). Psychologist members of the American Headache Society can be found on their Web site: http://www.americanheadachesociety.org. To find practitioners, training, and meetings in Europe refer to the Biofeedback Foundation of Europe (www.bfe.org). Self-training and home training biofeedback kits and manuals are also available, although few have been field-tested specifically with headache patients (see the various products developed or marketed by such companies as Bio-Medical Instruments, HeartMath LLC, Helicor, InterCure, and Thought Technology).

RELAXATION TRAINING

Relaxation techniques are taught to minimize physiologic responses to stress and decrease sympathetic arousal. The United States Headache Consortium gave Grade A status to relaxation training and thermal biofeedback combined with relaxation training as treatment options for prevention of migraine.[14] Relaxation training may include a variety of techniques.[26,37] The classic procedure, progressive muscle relaxation training,[38] which was first reviewed in a publication in 1938, involves tensing and relaxing various muscle groups while taking note of the contrasting sensations. Because it is impossible to experience tension and relaxation at the same time, Wolpe[39] used progressive muscle relaxation training as part of the desensitizing procedure for treatment of phobias. Soon afterward, progressive muscle relaxation training became an essential tool in the treatment of anxiety, phobias, and other related disorders. Other traditional clinical relaxation techniques include visual or guided imagery; cue-controlled relaxation; diaphragmatic breathing; and hypnosis (therapist- or self-applied).[40,41] Patients may use any techniques or tools that quiet the mind and calm the body, however, including meditation, prayer, yoga, pleasant music, guided relaxation CDs or tapes, and any other method that a patient finds effective. Relaxation training is usually taught by clinical professionals, such as psychologists or other mental health professionals, but it can also be self-taught by patients with print or audio support materials (see the previously mentioned Web sites to locate providers). Although techniques can be learned during sessions in the office, they require regular practice to become effective automatic responses.

COGNITIVE BEHAVIORAL THERAPY

The United States Headache Consortium also found Grade A evidence for CBT for preventive treatment of migraine.[14] CBT is an empirically validated psychotherapeutic treatment comprised of cognitive and behavioral strategies. Cognitive strategies focus on identifying and challenging maladaptive or dysfunctional thoughts, beliefs, and responses to stress.[42–44] Behavioral strategies help patients identify behaviors that may precipitate, increase, or maintain headaches (including modifying triggers and promoting healthy lifestyle habits). CBT is also used to manage and reduce feelings of depression, anxiety, panic attacks, obsessive-compulsive disorder, eating disorders, sleep disorders, and common comorbidities for headache sufferers. CBT can be conducted by a licensed psychologist or other mental health provider, and patients should seek a provider with some understanding of issues related to pain. For more information about CBT refer to the Association for Behavioral and Cognitive Therapies Web site (www.abct.org). Refer to the resources listed previously to locate providers.

Specific cognitive goals of CBT for headache management include enhancing self-efficacy[45] (ie, the patient's belief in his or her ability to succeed or accomplish a certain task), and helping patients gain an internal locus of control (ie, a belief that the mechanism for change lies within oneself) as opposed to an external locus of control (ie, the belief that only the physician, medication, or medical procedures have the power for change).[46] Research has demonstrated that both poor self-efficacy and external locus of control predict poorer outcomes.[47] Cognitive therapy may also focus on changing "catastrophizing," a hopeless and overwhelming thinking pattern, which has been shown to predict poor outcome and reduced quality of life. Holroyd and colleagues[48] examined catastrophizing, comorbid anxiety, depression, quality of life, and headache characteristics among 232 migraine sufferers and found that catastrophizing and severity of associated symptoms (photophobia, phonophobia, nausea) independently predicted quality of life, demonstrating that it is not just headache severity and frequency that predict quality of life, but that patient perception is directly related to quality of life. Other targets of CBT include assertiveness training, increased coping and problem-solving skills, and cognitive restructuring.

CBT places a special emphasis on education, using headache diaries to aid in identification and avoidance of triggers and lifestyle modification. Migraineurs should be advised to maintain a regular and healthy lifestyle, especially during times when they are most vulnerable to an attack (eg, premenstrually). That includes maintaining a regular sleep-wake schedule; a regular and healthy diet; engaging in regular exercise; avoiding excessive caffeine or alcohol consumption; stopping smoking; and engaging in regular practice of stress management, relaxation techniques, and self care.

PATIENT EDUCATION

Patient education is essential to effective headache management because the patient makes most of the therapeutic decisions on his or her own and outside of the HCP's office. The patient decides which attacks to treat, when to treat them, with what to treat them, to what extent to follow medical advice, whether to make healthy lifestyle changes, and many other decisions that are central to effective management. Trials of educational interventions have demonstrated significant reductions in pain frequency, intensity, and duration; improvements in functional status and quality of life; reduced depression; and decreased service use (in terms of patient visits to both primary care providers and the emergency department).[49–52] One trial of a brief patient education procedure focusing on the proper use of abortive headache medication demonstrated improved adherence and efficacy.[53]

Education may be provided by physicians, nurses,[54] psychologists, or other team members, and may take the format of individual consultation, formal group classes, or patient self-guided learning. One such example is "ACHE," an online forum sponsored by the American Headache Society that contains useful information prepared specifically for patients. Patients must be taught the importance of their behaviors and lifestyle choices in their headache management, which helps to build self-efficacy, promote an internal locus of control, and solidify the provider-patient collaborative relationship.

Some of the most important areas to include in patient education are discussed next. The first is a basic understanding of the pathology of migraine. A patient should be informed of the expected course of this chronic disease, which is characterized by episodic manifestations, and also be reassured that the pain of migraine and primary headaches is relatively benign (once other causes have been ruled out). Patients should be made aware of potential prodromal symptoms and triggers and asked to keep a headache diary to learn their personal prodromal symptoms and triggers. Patients should be taught how migraine medications need to be used (both acute and preventative) and the reasons for these guidelines including the importance of timing and other factors. Optimal timing and maximum use of abortive and analgesic medications need addressing. Studies with other medical disorders have shown that patients who understand the therapeutic mechanism of their prescription and how it fits into their treatment plan are twice as likely to fill the prescription.[55] Patients should be educated about the potential for medication-overuse headache, potential adverse effects of medications, and possible drug interactions. Because many patients also use over-the-counter and herbal treatments, their potential effects and interactions should also be discussed. Finally, patients can be reassured that there are many effective treatment options available and new possibilities on the horizon.

The degree to which information has been understood by the patient and whether the patient agrees with his or her treatment plan should be assessed by asking the patient for feedback and using communication strategies (discussed later). Rains and colleagues[8] provided the following additional recommendations for effective education: (1) limit instructions to three or four major points during each discussion; (2) use simple, everyday language, especially when explaining diagnoses and treatment instructions (model or demonstrate, when possible); (3) supplement oral instructions with written materials; (4) involve the patient's family members or significant others; (5) ask patients to restate recommendations back to you; and (6) repeat and reinforce the concepts that were discussed.

SUPPORT GROUPS

Social support, whether obtained through informal conversation in the doctor's waiting room, the Internet, or organized support groups, can be valuable to patients.[56,57] Patients often appreciate talking with someone else who "truly understands" and having the opportunity to speak with others outside of their family and regular social circle about how headaches affect their lives. Many countries and states have national headache associations that sponsor support groups. These organizations can provide useful advice on how to cope with headache and put patients in contact with other headache sufferers in their area.

MIGRAINE AND PSYCHOLOGIC COMORBIDITIES, HEALTH-RELATED QUALITY OF LIFE, AND PRODUCTIVITY

Migraine is associated with an increase in comorbid psychiatric conditions, functional impairment across all aspects of life, and reduced health-related quality of life (HRQoL). Migraine sufferers have been demonstrated to experience increased rates of comorbidity for depression, anxiety, panic disorder, obsessive-compulsive disorder, and suicide attempts than controls.[58,59] Migraine and depression are bidirectional and place those who experience one at a higher risk for the other.[58] Anxiety and depression are correlated with greater impairment in functional ability and HRQoL in migraineurs and lowered HRQoL is associated with increased migraine-related-disability.[60]

In a cross-sectional analysis, the gender-adjusted odds ratios for migraineurs for these disorders ranged from 2.6 for phobia to 6.6 for panic disorder. In a longitudinal, follow-up study, researchers found that migraineurs were more likely to experience future depressive and anxiety disorders.[58] Similar results of increased comorbidity rates between migraine and certain psychiatric disorders were found in the 2002 Canadian Community Health Survey.[59] Major depressive disorder, bipolar disorder, panic disorder, and social phobia were more than twice as common in migraineurs as in controls. Health-related outcomes, such as HRQoL, restriction of activities, and mental health care use, were poorest in those subjects who had both migraine and a psychiatric disorder.

Screening, assessment, referral, and education about common psychiatric comorbidities should be included in routine headache care. Brief screening instruments can be used to assess depression and anxiety.[61] The PHQ-2 is a two-item screening instrument that has been empirically shown to detect the presence of depression with two questions.[62] The PHQ-9 can be used to conduct a more thorough depression assessment and assign a diagnosis based on *Diagnostic and Statistical Manual of Mental Disorders-IV* criteria.[63] Anxiety that is clinically significant can be evaluated using the Generalized Anxiety Disorder-7, a seven-item, self-administered questionnaire.[64] Once these questionnaires are completed, the health care professional can review them with the patient during the visit; they may facilitate discussion about other areas of concern and further inform treatment decisions, which may include a multidisciplinary and multimodal approach.[49] Questionnaires may also be used at every visit to track progress or changes over time.

Migraine also negatively impacts HRQoL and many aspects of sufferers' lives. Lipton and colleagues[65] examined HRQoL between 200 migraineurs and 200 controls in a population-based, case-control study in England and found that migraineurs scored significantly lower (ie, worse) in eight of the nine HRQoL domains and the two summary scores of the SF-36. They also found that migraine-related disability was inversely correlated with HRQoL. Dueland and colleagues[66] used a telephone survey to study the impact of migraine on work, family, and leisure activities among 1810 women aged 18 to 35 years living in Israel and eight European countries. Most respondents reported an inability to function fully at work or school during the prior 6 months because of migraine (74%); one or more instances of being unable to spend time with family or friends because of migraine (62%); and one or more instances of being unable to enjoy recreational or leisure activities because of migraine (67%).

Migraine can place a significant burden on sufferers' lives, both during attacks and also interictally. Buse and colleagues[67] found that migraine sufferers with high levels of interictal-headache–related burden experienced higher rates of psychologic disorders than those with lower levels of interictal burden. Of those respondents who experienced "severe" levels of interictal burden, 44% met criteria for an anxiety disorder, 47% for panic disorder, and 46% for a depressive disorder, compared with 20%, 23%, and 25%, respectively, of those individuals who had headaches with low or no interictal disability, and 3% (anxiety), 2% (panic), and 7% of women and 3% of men (depression) in the general population. Moderate negative correlations were noted between the level of interictal burden and HRQoL and moderate positive correlations were noted between interictal burden and measures of workplace productivity.

In addition to completing a thorough medical and headache history, the practitioner also needs to obtain a thorough qualitative understanding of the patient's experience and beliefs, headache-related disability and impairment in all areas of life, quality of life, level of self-efficacy, and information about related comorbidities. When information is gathered about headache-related disability, this leads to a more accurate recognition of the severity of the effect of migraine on the patient's life, which in turn tends to result in treatment plans that are more aggressive and comprehensive.[68]

RISK FACTORS FOR PROGRESSION

Biobehavioral techniques can be used to reduce the risk of progression of migraine from episodic to chronic or transformed migraine. Migraine can be conceptualized as a chronic disorder with episodic manifestations.[69] Patients with migraine may spontaneously remit for unknown reasons, they may continue to have intermittent attacks for many decades, or they may develop a clinically progressive disorder characterized by attacks of increasing frequency at times leading to headaches on more days than not. As defined by the second edition of the International Classification of Headache Disorders,[70] chronic migraine is a diagnosis given for 15 or more headache days per month over the past 3 months, of which at least 8 headache days per month meet criteria for migraine without aura or respond to migraine-specific treatment.

Recent research has identified risk factors for progression,[71] of which some are nonremediable (gender, age, race) and some can be modified including frequency of migraine attacks, obesity, acute medication overuse, caffeine overuse, stressful life events, depression, and sleep disorders. These modifiable risk factors are important targets for behavioral intervention.

COMPLIANCE AND ADHERENCE

Compliance refers to the degree to which patients follow medical recommendations of their HCPs.[7,72] Adherence refers to an active and collaborative involvement by the patient in the implementation of a therapeutic regimen. These terms are often used interchangeably. The term "adherence" is used here to emphasize the importance of the patient's participation in effective treatment. Nonadherence can pose a significant barrier to effective headache management in many ways. Common adherence problem areas in headache treatment include misuse of medication (including unfilled, overused, underused, incorrectly used, and nonadvised discontinuation of prescribed medications or treatments); appointment keeping; record keeping (diaries); and unwillingness or inability to follow clinical suggestions. Improper medication use may not only limit relief but may also aggravate the primary headache condition (eg, lead to medication overuse or rebound headache).[7]

Adherence declines with more frequent and complex dosing regimens,[73] increased side effects,[74] and increased costs,[75] and is worse in chronic conditions compared with acute conditions.[76] Most of these conditions apply to headache care. In addition, rates of adherence with behavioral recommendations, such as dietary modifications, weight loss, exercise, smoking cessation, and treatment for alcohol or substance use (some of the primary components of behavioral headache management), are even lower than rates of adherence with prescribed medication regimens.[74] Further, sociodemographic factors play a role in predicting adherence, but even more important is a patient's perceived level of self-efficacy.

One study of 1160 severe headache sufferers found that 11% chose not to fill a prescription for headache medication and 71% had delayed or avoided taking a prescription medication for headache.[77] Commonly cited reasons for not filling a prescription were high cost (33%) and concerns about tolerability and side effects (30%). Several studies have also reported problems with appointment keeping, with approximately 40% of patients not keeping follow-up appointments after the initial consultation and 24% not keeping subsequent appointments.[78,79] The reasons for not keeping appointments included administrative issues, dissatisfaction with clinician and clinical care, change in headache or medical status, and problems associated with the treatment regimen.

ENHANCING ADHERENCE AND MOTIVATION

Bandura[80] developed social learning theory to help explain human behavior and change. The theory posits that two components predict and mediate behavior: self-efficacy, or confidence in one's ability to perform an action; and outcome efficacy, or the belief that a behavior or set of behaviors will have a desirable result.[45] Several other models have been developed to explain and influence health-related behaviors.[81,82] In general they share the hypothesis that health-related behavior change and motivation are based on three basic components: (1) the patient's readiness for change, (2) self-efficacy, and (3) outcome efficacy.[83] Following this line of reasoning, skills or knowledge alone are not sufficient to ensure behavior change. Rather, the patient must want to change, believe that he or she can change, and believe that the necessary actions will accomplish the desired goals.

To operationalize these concepts, Miller and colleagues[83,84] developed the technique of Motivational Interviewing (MI) to assess and enhance patients' motivation for change. MI was based upon Prochaska's transtheoretical model which was originally developed for the treatment of substance abuse.[85] The transtheoretical model proposes that patients' readiness and motivation for change can be categorized into one of five stages: (1) precontemplation (the patient is not thinking about changing behavior and does not recognize the need or a problem); (2) contemplation (the patient recognizes a need or problem and begins to think about changing behavior and may be developing a plan, but has not taken any action); (3) preparation (the patient has done research, developed a plan, and may begin making minor changes or actions); (4) action (the patient is actively engaged in the behavior change or new actions); and (5) maintenance (the patient is continuing behaviors necessary to maintain changes). When the patient reaches the maintenance stage, behaviors and actions may be performed habitually and automatically. Relapse may occur at any point in the process, and should be considered a challenge from which the patient needs to return to the steps of a previous stage and move through the sequence again. Relapse is not considered a failure or a permanent state, and it is understood that patients may move forward and backward or even jump from one stage to another over time. Indeed, the model prefers the term "lapse" when referring to slips as opposed to "relapse."

HCPs should consider a patient's stage of readiness for change and tailor their interventions, clinical advice, and education accordingly. For example, in the case of weight loss or smoking cessation, a patient in the precontemplation stage should be educated about the general health risks and negative consequences on the patient's headache condition. A patient in an action stage of readiness already knows and believes the consequences and benefits from concrete advice and solutions (eg, a prescription for a nicotine patch or referral to a weight loss and exercise program).

Motivational interviewing focuses on the patient's stage of readiness and explores the patients' beliefs, concerns, perspective, and ambivalence about behavior change. The goal of the HCP is to help the patient realize the importance of change while maintaining an empathic, supportive, and nonjudgmental approach. Motivation for change is increased when patients examine the pros and cons of change and make decisions themselves rather than being passive recipients of instructions from their HCPs. HCPs can encourage patients to explore their ambivalence toward changing the identified behavior. According to behavior theory,[86] humans perform behaviors for which they are rewarded; to facilitate change the existing reward must be identified and recognized and then replaced with a more appropriate reward. Identifying conflicting rewards helps give the patient and the health care provider a better understanding of the challenges that must be met to identify effective solutions. Rains and colleagues[7] recommend several behavioral strategies to enhance patient adherence and maximize efficacy of treatment in headache care based on a review of the adherence literature (**Box 1**).

COMMUNICATION

Effective communication is essential for effective medical care. Communication between HCPs and patients is the basis of the therapeutic relationship, and is directly related to patient satisfaction,[87–90] medication adherence and treatment adherence,[91] and medical outcomes.[92,93] Improved communication also decreases the risk of malpractice,[94] HCP burnout, and HCP work-related stress.[95] Effective communication is especially important in managing headache disorders, a condition where diagnosis is based almost entirely on a patient's report of symptoms and degree of impairment, and where treatment success is largely dependent on a patient's level of adherence to medication and behavioral recommendations.[96,97] The degree to which communication is successful depends, in large part, on the communication strategies and interpersonal skills of the HCP. Models of effective communication emphasize the importance of both the physical and psychologic well-being of the patient, involve and empower the patient in decision making, and place attention and value on the relationship and interactions between the HCP and patient. These models incorporate the elements of effective communication to convey a sense of partnership and caring toward the patient.

Box 1

Empirically based compliance-enhancing strategies

I. Administrative

- Scheduling regular contacts of sufficient duration for complete assessment and rapport-building
- Recalling missed appointments
- Clinic orientation
- Verbal and written recommendations
- Screen for psychiatric comorbidities
- Assess and track compliance (multimodal assessment preferred, such as interview, patient monitoring, pill counts, pharmacy records)
- Encourage participation of key significant others
- Assess and treat psychiatric comorbidities (eg, depression, anxiety)

II. Psychoeducational

- Patient education by provider, staff, computer (prophylactic versus acute, abortive, overuse consequences)
- Printed materials for increased retention
- Involve patient in treatment planning (elicit discussion of barriers [eg, cost, side effects])
- Education on adherence and health behavior change

III. Behavioral

- Simplify regimen
- Self-monitor compliance
- Stimulus control (medication reminder systems, cue-dose training)
- Medication contracts
- Enhance self-efficacy
- Reinforcement for successful adherence

IV. Social support

- Provider communication and rapport skills (conducive environment, active listening, empathy, adjust language, nonverbal behavior, cultural sensitivity)
- Collaborative therapeutic alliance (negotiated rather than dictated plan)
- Spouse and family support

From Rains JC, Lipchik GL, Penzien DB. Behavioral facilitation of medical treatment for headache – Part I: Review of headache treatment compliance. Headache 2006;46:1387–94; with permission.

The American Migraine Communication Studies I and II (AMCS) evaluated HCP-patient communication in headache care and tested a simple educational intervention. The AMCS-I[98] was an observational study of actual discussions and diagnoses of migraine in clinical practice. Analyses of patient visits in AMCS-I revealed several key problematic issues. The average migraine discussion lasted 12 minutes, during which HCPs asked an average of 13 questions, of which 91% were closed-ended or short-answer questions focused on frequency (primarily number of attacks per month), severity, headache symptoms, triggers, and other similar features. Questions regarding headache-related impairment and quality of life were infrequent. Researchers interviewed the health care professionals and their patients immediately following the visit to assess understanding and found high levels of disagreement on migraine frequency and impairment. Fifty-five percent of health care professional and patient pairs did not report matching information regarding frequency, and 51% did not agree on impairment. Researchers noted that asking about migraine attacks versus migraine days led HCPs to underestimate the number of headache days per month and relying almost exclusively on closed-ended questions limited patients to "yes or no" responses or short answers, which impaired their ability to communicate the effect of migraine on their lives.

In response to these findings, researchers developed and tested a brief educational intervention designed to address the identified problem areas. In the AMCS-II,[99] 15 HCPs who participated in AMCS-I participated in an audio-interactive, 90-minute, Internet-based training session that reviewed the results of AMCS-I and provided two communication strategies: the patient-centered "ask-tell-ask" strategy to assess headache frequency and the use of open-ended questions to assess migraine-related impairment.[31,96,100–102] The "ask-tell-ask" strategy is based on the theory that effective education requires assessing what the patient already knows and believes, then building on (or correcting when necessary) that understanding. The "ask-tell-ask" strategy can be used for any medical communication, but in this study it was used primarily to ensure optimal communication about migraine frequency in headache days. This strategy is based on three simple steps. (1) Step 1: "ask" the patient to explain or restate the issue, problem, or treatment in his or her own words. This step, which allows the HCP to assess the patient's personal beliefs, emotional responses, and understanding of the situation, helps guide the HCP in furthering effective communication. (2) Step 2: "tell" the patient the relevant facts, diagnosis, or treatment plan, using language at a level that he or she understands. This provides opportunities to correct any misunderstanding or incorrect information communicated by the patient in response to the first question and to reinforce and validate the correct information that the patient shared. (3) Step 3: again "ask" the patient to rephrase the information given in Step 2 ("tell") in his or her own words. This allows the HCP to reassess the patient's level of understanding and gives the patient an opportunity to ask questions and express concerns (for more detailed information and a vignette using this strategy, see).[103]

Such strategies as the use of open-ended questions, the "ask-tell-ask" technique, active listening, and "being fully present" with the patient can significantly improve the quality of the medical relationship, with positive and more satisfying outcomes for both patient and health care provider. Use of the "ask-tell-ask" strategy led to a more accurate picture of the patients' migraine frequency and impairment during and between attacks, more frequent discussion and prescription of preventive therapy, greater satisfaction with office visits on the part of the health care professionals and their patients, and more frequent discussion and prescription of appropriate migraine therapies. Although 79% of HCP participants expressed a concern that using the "ask-tell-ask" strategy would significantly increase the length of the interview, the average visit length was actually 90 seconds shorter than visits without the intervention (AMCS-I).

SUMMARY

Behavioral medicine is based on the biopsychosocial model, which points out that biologic, psychologic, and social or environmental factors all play a significant role in human functioning. This is especially evident in the care of patients with primary headache disorders, where factors of biology, environment, behaviors, and beliefs are interwoven with the development, maintenance, progression, and remission of headache disorders. The application of behavioral medicine to the management of migraine calls for increased reliance on evidence-based nonpharmacologic treatments, which can be broadly divided into the categories of behavioral treatments (CBT and biobehavioral training [biofeedback, relaxation training, and stress management]), physical therapies, and education including and lifestyle modification, techniques that have demonstrated clinical efficacy when practiced correctly. They may be used individually or in conjunction with pharmacologic and other interventions and may augment the effectiveness of other treatments, or minimize the need for their use. A combination of pharmacologic and nonpharmacologic approaches has been demonstrated to be superior to either approach on its own, to help maintain positive outcomes and to improve treatment adherence.

Biobehavioral tools should be used prophylactically and practiced on a regular basis to maintain homeostasis and manage stress so that the patient does not trigger a headache attack in the first place. Patients should be educated about times and situations in which they may be most vulnerable to an attack. During this time period they need to be especially aware of potential triggers and need to avoid stress, engage in relaxing and nurturing activities, and maintain a very regular and healthy lifestyle. Some patients have the benefit of fairly predictable migraine attacks. For these patients, particular triggers, time periods, and prodromal symptoms provide windows of opportunity in which to use behavioral tools as a way to stop or slow the process of migraine early, even before headache onset. It is important for patients to use a diary to note associations. Some triggers cannot be changed or avoided, such as the menstrual cycle, in which case patients should be aware of their vulnerability to headache during this time and protect themselves by following a very healthy lifestyle. By doing so they may reduce the number of headache attacks, although it is unlikely that they will disappear altogether. Patients also may be able to modify or eliminate other triggers.

Patients can be taught ways to modify thoughts, feelings, and behavior with CBT. CBT interventions aid in headache management by making patients more aware of triggers including the relationship between stress and headache, and by identifying and challenging counterproductive or self-defeating beliefs and ideas. They can be taught to manage the physiologic effects of stress with biofeedback and relaxation training.

Stress, depression, anxiety, and other psychologic and emotional factors are all related to migraine and many psychologic conditions have elevated rates of comorbidity with migraine. Patients should be routinely assessed and appropriately treated or referred for psychologic comorbidities. Improvements in psychologic comorbidities may translate into improvements in headache status, and vice versa.

Effective communication is essential for effective medical care. Communication between HCPs and patients is the basis of the therapeutic relationship, and can help or hinder medication and treatment adherence, outcomes, and both patient and provider satisfaction. Strategies for enhancing communication include active listening, such as the "ask-tell-ask" model; demonstration of empathy; and attention given to headache-related impairment, mood, and quality of life.

Some behavioral techniques can be incorporated by HCPs during an appointment (eg, communication strategies, education, diaphragmatic breathing, and guided imagery); some can be self-taught and practiced by the patient (eg, relaxation practice and stress management); and some require a referral to an appropriately trained professional (eg, biofeedback training, CBT). HCPs can use these strategies with their patients on a daily basis, whether by helping a patient gain a more realistic understanding of their illness; helping a patient recognize the effort and contribution that they themselves must make in their treatment (ie, enhancing self-efficacy and encouraging an internal locus of control); or instructing a patient to maintain a headache diary to facilitate assessment and treatment planning. The patient should be encouraged to adopt an internal locus of control and consider his or her treatment a collaborative process. The strategies reviewed in this article can help build feelings of self-efficacy and encourage patients actively to participate in the management of their migraines.

REFERENCES

1. Society of Behavioral Medicine Web Site. Available at: http://www.sbm.org. Accessed July 16, 2008.
2. Engel GL. The need for a new medical model: a challenge for biomedicine. Science 1977;196:129–36.
3. Andrasik F, Flor H, Turk DC. An expanded view of psychological aspects in head pain: the biopsychosocial model. Neurol Sci 2005;26(Suppl 2) S87–91.
4. Holroyd KA, O'Donnell FJ, Stensland M, et al. Management of chronic tension-type headache with tricyclic antidepressant medication, stress management therapy, and their combination: a randomized controlled trial. JAMA 2001;285:2208–15.
5. Holroyd KA, France JL, Cordingley GE, et al. Enhancing the effectiveness of relaxation-thermal biofeedback training with propranolol hydrochloride. J Consult Clin Psychol 1995;63:327–30.
6. Grazzi L, Andrasik F, D'Amico D, et al. Behavioral and pharmacologic treatment of transformed migraine with analgesic overuse: outcome at three years. Headache 2002;42:483–90.
7. Rains JC, Lipchik GL, Penzien DB. Behavioral facilitation of medical treatment for headache – Part I: Review of headache treatment compliance. Headache 2006; 46:1387–94.
8. Rains JC, Penzien DB, Lipchik GL. Behavioral facilitation of medical treatment for headache – Part II: Theoretical models and behavioral strategies for improving adherence. Headache 2006;46:1395–403.
9. Hermann C, Kim M, Blanchard EB. Behavioral and prophylactic pharmacological intervention studies of pediatric migraine: an exploratory meta-analysis. Pain 1995;20:239–56.
10. Holden EW, Deichmann MM, Levy JD. Empirically supported treatments in pediatric psychology: recurrent pediatric headache. J Pediatr Psychol 1999;24:91–109.
11. Hermann C, Blanchard EB. Biofeedback in the treatment of headache and other childhood pain. Appl Psychophysiol Biofeedback 2002;27:143–62.
12. Eddy DM. Evidence-based clinical improvements. Presentations at "Directions for success: Evidence-based health care symposium" sponsored by Group Health Cooperative, May 7–9, 2001. Tucson (AZ).
13. Goslin RE, Gray RN, McCrory DC, et al. Behavioral and physical treatments for migraine headache. Technical review 2.2 February 1999. Prepared for the Agency for Health Care Policy and Research under Contract No. 290-94-2025. Available at: http://www.clinpol.mc.due.edu. Accessed July 25, 2008.
14. Campbell JK, Penzien DB, Wall FM. Evidence-based guidelines for migraine headache: behavioral and physical treatments. US Headache Consortium 2000. Available at: http://www.aan.com. Accessed July 16, 2008.

15. Nestoriuc Y, Martin A. Efficacy of biofeedback for migraine: a meta-analysis. Pain 2007;128:111–27.
16. Andrasik F. What does the evidence show? Efficacy of behavioural treatment for recurrent headaches in adults. Neurol Sci 2007;28:S70–7.
17. Penzien DB, Johnson CA, Carpenter DE, et al. Drug vs. behavioral treatment of migraine: long-acting propranolol vs. home-based self-management training. Headache 1990;30:300.
18. Mathew NT. Prophylaxis of migraine and mixed headache: a randomized controlled study. Headache 1981;21:105–9.
19. Holroyd KA, Holm JE, Hursey KG, et al. Recurrent vascular headache: home-based behavioral treatment vs. abortive pharmacological treatment. J Consult Clin Psychol 1988;56:218–23.
20. Nicholson R, Penzien D, McCrory DC. Behavioral therapies for migraine. (Protocol) Cochrane Database Syst Rev 2004 (1) Art. No.: CD004601. DOI:10.1002/14651858.CD004601.
21. Task Force on Promotion and Dissemination of Psychological Procedures. Training in and dissemination of empirically validated psychological treatments: report and recommendations. Clin Psychol 1995;48:3–23.
22. Pryse-Phillips WE, Dodick DW, Edmeads JG, et al. Guidelines for the nonpharmacologic management of migraine in clinical practice. Canadian Headache Society. CMAJ 1998;159:47–54.
23. Yucha C, Gilbert C. Evidence-based practice in biofeedback and neurotherapy. Wheat Ridge (CO): Association for Applied Psychophysiology and Biofeedback; 2004.
24. Fiore M, Bailey W, Cohen S, et al. Smoking cessation clinical practice guideline no. 18. Rockville (MD): Agency for Health Care Policy and Research, US Department of Health and Human Services; 1996.
25. Schwartz MS, Andrasik F, Headache. In: Schwartz MS, Andrasik F, editors. Biofeedback: a practitioner's guide. 3rd edition. New York: The Guilford Press; 2003. p. 275–346.
26. Penzien DB, Holroyd KA. Psychosocial interventions in the management of recurrent headache disorders—II: Description of treatment techniques. Behav Med 1994;20:64–73.
27. Benson H. The relaxation response. New York: William Morrow; 1975.
28. Andrasik F, Rime C. Can behavioural therapy influence neuromodulation? Neurol Sci 2007;28:S124–9.
29. Blanchard EB, Andrasik F. Biofeedback treatment of vascular headache. In: Hatch JP, Fisher JG, Rugh JD, editors. Biofeedback: studies in clinical efficacy. New York: Plenum; 1987. p. 1–79.
30. Blanchard EB, Andrasik F, Ahles TA, et al. Migraine and tension headache: a meta-analytic review. Behav Ther 1980;14:613–31.
31. Holroyd KA, Penzien DB. Pharmacological versus non-pharmacological prophylaxis of recurrent migraine headache: a meta-analytic review of clinical trials. Pain 1990;42:1–13.
32. Nestoriuc Y, Martin A, Rief W, et al. Biofeedback treatment for headache disorders: a comprehensive efficacy review. Appl Psychophysiol Biofeedback 2008; 33:125–40.
33. LaVaque TJ, Hammond DC, Trudeau D, et al. Template for developing guidelines for the evaluation of the clinical efficacy of psychophysiological interventions. Efficacy Task Force. Appl Psychophysiol Biofeedback 2002; 27:273–81.

34. Nestoriuc Y, Rief W, Martin A. Meta-analysis of biofeedback for tension-type headache: efficacy, specificity, and treatment moderators. J Consult Clin Psychol 2008;76:379–96.

35. Haddock CK, Rowan AB, Andrasik F, et al. Home-based behavioral treatments for chronic benign headache: a meta-analysis of controlled trials. Cephalalgia 1997;17:113–8.

36. Andrasik F, Oyama ON, Packard RC. Biofeedback therapy for migraine. In: Diamond S, editor. Migraine headache prevention and management. New York: Marcel Dekker; 1990. p. 213–38.

37. Bernstein DA, Borkovec TD, Hazlett-Stevens H. New directions in progressive relaxation training: a guidebook for helping professions. Westport (CT): Praeger Publishers; 2000.

38. Jacobson E. Progressive relaxation. Chicago: University of Chicago Press; 1938.

39. Wolpe J. Psychotherapy by reciprocal inhibition. Stanford (CA): Stanford University Press; 1958.

40. Andrasik F, Rime C, Biofeedback. In: Waldman SD, editor, Pain management, vol. 2. Philadelphia: Saunders/Elsevier; 2007. p. 1010–24.

41. Hall H. Hypnosis. In: Waldman SD, editor, Pain management, vol. 2. Philadelphia: Saunders/Elsevier; 2007. p. 1025–32.

42. Beck AT, Rush AJ, Shaw BF, et al. Cognitive therapy of depression. New York: Guilford Press; 1979.

43. Holroyd KA, Andrasik F. A cognitive-behavioral approach to recurrent tension and migraine headache. In: Kendall PC, editor, Advances in cognitive-behavioral research and therapy, vol. 1. New York: Academic; 1982. p. 275–320.

44. McCarran MS, Andrasik F. Migraine and tension headaches. In: Michelson L, Ascher M, editors. Anxiety and stress disorders: cognitive-behavioral assessment and treatment. New York: Guilford; 1987. p. 465–83.

45. Bandura A. Self-efficacy: toward a unifying theory of behavioral change. Psychol Rev 1977;84:191–215.

46. Heath RL, Saliba M, Mahmassani O, et al. Locus of control moderates the relationship between headache pain and depression. J Headache Pain 2008;9(5): 301–8.

47. French DJ, Holroyd KA, Pinell C, et al. Perceived self-efficacy and headache-related disability. Headache 2000;40:647–56.

48. Holroyd KA, Drew JB, Cottrell CK, et al. Impaired functioning and quality of life in severe migraine: the role of catastrophizing and associated symptoms. Cephalalgia 2007;27(10):1156–65.

49. Lemstra M, Stewart B, Olszynski W. Effectiveness of multidisciplinary intervention in the treatment of migraine: a randomized clinical trial. Headache 2002;42:845–54.

50. Harpole L, Samsa G, Jurgelski A, et al. Headache management program improves outcome for chronic headache. Headache 2003;43:715–24.

51. Blumenfeld A, Tischio M. Center of excellence for headache care: group model at Kaiser Permanente. Headache 2003;43:431–40.

52. Rothrock JF, Parada VA, Sims C, et al. The impact of intensive patient education on clinical outcome in a clinic-based migraine population. Headache 2006;46: 726–31.

53. Holroyd KA, Cordingley GE, Pingel JD, et al. Enhancing the effectiveness of abortive therapy: a controlled evaluation of self-management training. Headache 1989;29:148–53.

54. Cady R, Farmer K, Beach ME, et al. Nurse-based education: an office-based comparative model for education of migraine patients. Headache 2007;48(4): 564–9.
55. Cameron C. Patient compliance: recognition of factors involved and suggestions for promoting compliance with therapeutic regimens. J Adv Nurs 1996;24: 244–50.
56. Alemi F, Mosavel M, Stephens RC, et al. Electronic self-help and support groups. Med Care 1996;34:OS32–44.
57. Klapper J, Stanton J, Seawell M. The development of a support group organization for headache sufferers. Headache 1992;32:193–6.
58. Breslau N, Davis GC. Migraine, physical health and psychiatric disorder: a prospective epidemiologic study in young adults. J Psychiatr Res 1993; 27(2):211–21.
59. Jette N, Patten S, Williams J, et al. Comorbidity of migraine and psychiatric disorders: a national population-based study. Headache 2008;48(4): 501–16.
60. Lanteri-Minet M, Radat F, Chautard M-H, et al. Anxiety and depression associated with migraine: influence on migraine subjects' disability and quality of life, and acute migraine management. Pain 2005;118(3):319–26.
61. Maizels M, Smitherman TA, Penzien DB. A review of screening tools for psychiatric comorbidity in headache patients. Headache 2006;46(Suppl 3):S98–109.
62. Whooley MA, Avins AL, Miranda J, et al. Case-finding instruments for depression: two questions are as good as many. J Gen Intern Med 1997;12:439–45.
63. American Psychiatric Association. Diagnostic and statistical manual of mental disorders. 4th edition. Washington, DC: American Psychiatric Press; 2000.
64. Spitzer RL, Kroenke K, Williams JB, et al. A brief measure for assessing generalized anxiety disorder: the GAD-7. Arch Intern Med 2006;166(10):1092–7.
65. Lipton RB, Liberman JN, Kolodner KB, et al. Migraine headache disability and health-related quality-of-life: a population-based case-control study from England. Cephalalgia 2003;23(6):441–50.
66. Dueland AN, Leira R, Burke TA, et al. The impact of migraine on work, family, and leisure among young women: a multinational study. Curr Med Res Opin 2004; 20(10):1595–604.
67. Buse DC, Bigal ME, Rupnow MFT, et al. The Migraine Interictal Burden Scale (MIBS): results of a population-based validation study. Headache 2007;47(5):778.
68. Holmes WF, MacGregor EA, Sawyer JP, et al. Information about migraine disability influences physicians' perceptions of illness severity and treatment needs. Headache 2001;41:343–50.
69. Haut SR, Bigal ME, Lipton RB. Chronic disorders with episodic manifestations: focus on epilepsy and migraine. Lancet Neurol 2006;5:148–57.
70. Headache Classification Subcommittee of the International Headache Society. The International Classification of Headache Disorders: 2nd edition. Cephalalgia 2004;24(suppl 1):1–160.
71. Bigal ME, Lipton RB. Modifiable risk factors for migraine progression. Headache 2006;46(9):1334–43.
72. Urquhart J. Patient non-compliance with drug regimens: measurement, clinical correlates, economic impact. Eur Heart J 1996;17(suppl A):8–15.
73. Claxton AJ, Cramer J, Pierce C. A systematic review of the associations between dose regimens and medication compliance. Clin Ther 2001;23:1296–310.
74. Dunbar-Jacob J, Erlen JA, Schlenk EA, et al. Adherence in chronic disease. Annu Rev Nurs Res 2000;18:48–90.

75. Motheral BR, Henderson R. The effect of copay increase on pharmaceutical utilization, expenditures, and treatment continuation. Am J Manag Care 1999;5: 1383–94.

76. Dunbar-Jacob J, Mortimer-Stephens MK. Treatment adherence in chronic disease. J Clin Epidemiol 2001;54(suppl 1):S57–60.

77. Gallagher RM, Kunkel R. Migraine medication attributes important for patient compliance: concerns about side effects may delay treatment. Headache 2003;43:36–43.

78. Edmeads J, Findlay H, Tugwell P, et al. Impact of migraine and tension-type headache on life-style, consulting behaviour, and medication use: a Canadian population survey. Can J Neurol Sci 1993;20:131–7.

79. Spierings EL, Miree LF. Non-compliance with follow-up and improvement after treatment at a headache center. Headache 1993;33:205–9.

80. Bandura A. Social foundations of thought and action: a social cognitive theory. Englewood Cliffs (NJ): Prentice Hall; 1986.

81. Elder JP, Ayala GX, Harris S. Theories and intervention approaches to health-behavior change in primary care. Am J Prev Med 1999;17:275–84.

82. Jensen MP. Enhancing motivations to change in pain treatment. In: Turk DC, Gatchel RJ, editors. Psychological approaches to pain management: a practitioner's handbook. 2nd edition. New York: The Guilford Press; 2002. p. 71–93.

83. Miller WR, Rollnick S. Motivational interviewing: preparing people for change. 2nd edition. New York: The Guilford Press; 2002.

84. Miller WR. Motivational interviewing: research, practice, and puzzles. Addict Behav 1996;21:835–42.

85. Prochaska JO, Redding A, Evers KE. The transtheoretical model and stages of change. In: Glanz K, Lewis FM, Rimer BK, editors. Health behavior and health education. San Francisco (CA): Jossey-Bass; 1997. p. 60–84.

86. Skinner BF. Behavior of organisms. Acton (MA): Copley Pub Group; 1991.

87. Hulsman RL, Ros WJ, Winnubst JA, et al. Teaching clinically experienced physicians communication skills: a review of evaluation studies. Med Educ 1999;33:655–68.

88. Hall JA, Irish JT, Roter DL, et al. Satisfaction, gender, and communication in medical visits. Med Care 1994;32:1216–31.

89. Frederikson LG. Exploring information-exchange in consultation: the patients' view of performance and outcomes. Patient Educ Couns 1995;25:237–46.

90. Hall JA, Roter DL, Katz NR. Meta-analysis of correlates of provider behavior in medical encounters. Med Care 1988;26:657–75.

91. Stevenson F, Cox K, Britten N, et al. A systematic review of the research on communication between patients and health care professionals about medicines: the consequences for concordance. Health Expect 2004;7(3):235–45.

92. Stewart M, Meredith L, Brown JB, et al. The influence of older patient-physician communication on health and health-related outcomes. Clin Geriatr Med 2000; 16:25–36.

93. Stewart MA. Effective physician-patient communication and health outcomes: a review. CMAJ 1995;152:1423–33.

94. Cole SA. Reducing malpractice risk through more effective communication. Am J Manag Care 1997;3:649–53.

95. Graham J, Potts HW, Ramirez AJ. Stress and burnout in doctors. Lancet 2002; 360:1975–6.

96. Hahn SR. Communication in the care of the headache patient. In: Silberstein SD, Lipton RL, Dodick DW, editors. Wolff's headache and other head pain. New York: Oxford University Press; 2008. p. 805–24.

97. Buse DC, Lipton RB. Facilitating communication with patients for improved migraine outcomes. Curr Pain Headache Rep 2008;12(3):230–6.
98. Lipton RB, Hahn SR, Cady RK, et al. In-office discussions of migraine: results from the American Migraine Communication Study. J Gen Intern Med 2008; 23(8):1145–51.
99. Hahn SR, Lipton RB, Sheftell FD, et al. Healthcare provider-patient communication and migraine assessment: results of the American Migraine Communication Study (AMCS) Phase II. Curr Med Res Opin 2008;24(6):1711–8.
100. Penzien DB, Holroyd KA, Holm JE, et al. Behavioral management of migraine: results from five-dozen group outcome studies. Headache 1985;25:162.
101. Holroyd KA, Penzien DB, Cordingley GE. Propranolol in the management of recurrent migraine: a meta-analytic review. Headache 1991;3:333–40.
102. Holroyd KA, Penzien DB, Rokicki LA, et al. Flunarizine vs. propranolol: a meta-analysis of clinical trials. Headache 1992;32:256.
103. Penzien DB, Rain JC, Andrasik F. Behavioral management of recurrent headache: three decades of experience and empiricism. Appl Psychophysiol Biofeedback 2002;27:163–81.

The Face of Chronic Migraine: Epidemiology, Demographics, and Treatment Strategies

Bert B. Vargas, MD[a],*, David W. Dodick, MD[b]

KEYWORDS

- Chronic migraine • Transformed migraine
- Chronic daily headache • Chronic migraine treatment
- Chronic daily headache epidemiology

Chronic daily headache (CDH) has a worldwide prevalence of approximately 4% according to epidemiologic studies.[1,2] By definition, CDH occurs with a frequency of at least 15 headache days per month for greater than 3 months duration.[3] Chronic migraine (CM) makes up a subset of this population along with other primary headache disorders such as chronic tension-type headache (CTTH) and new daily persistent headache. It is estimated that the prevalence of CM is approximately 2% of the population.[2]

Although the phenomenon of CM is not new, it was not until the second edition of the *International Classification of Headache Disorders* (ICHD) was published that a set of criteria was established by which to define its presence. Since that time, these criteria have been tested against other definitions of CM, some with more restrictive and others with more liberal criteria. Field-testing these criteria ultimately yielded a more workable definition for CM, which is presented in the appendix of the ICHD.[4]

Although the exact mechanism by which episodic migraine (EM) transforms into a more aggressive phenotype is unknown, numerous theories exist and seem to center around the concept of central sensitization as a means by which the threshold for peripheral transmission and central processing of nociceptive input becomes significantly reduced.[5] Additionally, there appear to be numerous risk factors that have been identified that portend the transition from EM to CM including female sex, Caucasian race, lower socioeconomic status,[6] habitual snoring,[7] and increased

[a] Center for Neurosciences, 2450 East River Road, Tucson, AZ 85718, USA
[b] Department of Neurology, Mayo Clinic Arizona, 5777 East Mayo Boulevard, Phoenix, AZ 85054, USA
* Corresponding author.
E-mail address: bvargas@neurotucson.com (B.B. Vargas).

Neurol Clin 27 (2009) 467–479
doi:10.1016/j.ncl.2009.01.001
0733-8619/09/$ – see front matter © 2009 Elsevier Inc. All rights reserved.

neurologic.theclinics.com

caffeine consumption.[8] Obesity has also been identified as a risk factor,[6,9,10] especially when comorbid with depression or anxiety.[11] Moreover, the excessive consumption of analgesic medications leading to medication overuse headache (MOH) frequently can complicate the diagnosis of CM.[6]

Investigations into potential therapeutic options are numerous and range from nonpharmacologic and drug treatments to invasive surgical interventions with modalities such as occipital[12,13] and vagal nerve stimulation.[14] The only pharmacologic options that have been tested in randomized, double-blind, placebo-controlled studies or active comparator-controlled trials include amitriptyline, topiramate, gabapentin, tizanidine, fluoxetine, and botulinum toxin type-A (BoNT-A).[15]

Overall, the prognosis seems favorable for improvement provided that potential secondary causes are excluded, the diagnosis is accurate, and appropriate interventions are implemented and address not only the need for treatment with prophylactic medications, but also the management of modifiable risk factors such as the overuse of analgesic medications and comorbid conditions such as obesity, sleep disorders, and depression.[5]

CHRONIC MIGRAINE DEFINED

CDH, transformed migraine (TM), and CM are frequently used terms to describe the population of individuals who have a previous diagnosis of migraine and headache that occurs on more than half the days of the month. Recognizing that TM implies the presence of a specific time or set of circumstances marking a transition from EM to TM, the use of these terms was not preferred by the classification committee.[4] The term CM was introduced in 2004 within the second edition of the ICHD along with newly established diagnostic criteria for its diagnosis. Required for the diagnosis of CM is the presence of headache that meets criteria for migraine without aura (MO) for at least15 days per month for greater than 3 months.[3] Given the fact that patients who have CM may exhibit a great deal of phenotypic variability, it was determined that many individuals who had CM were not being identified in the clinic setting.

Additionally, when tested alongside the criteria for TM according to the original Silberstein-Lipton criteria, the definition for CM again appeared to be too restrictive. Bigal and colleagues[16] noted a significant discrepancy between TM and ICHD-defined CM in that only 5.6% of patients meeting criteria for TM without medication overuse met criteria for the diagnosis of CM. Additionally, taking into account the overuse of analgesic medications, only 10.2% of patients who had TM with medication overuse met criteria for probable CM with probable MOH.[16] Alternative criteria investigated included at least 15 headache days per month meeting criteria for migraine or probable migraine, at least 15 headache days per month with at least 50% of the days meeting ICHD criteria for MO, and at least 15 headache days per month with at least 8 headache days meeting criteria for MO or probable migraine.[16] These alternative criteria captured 48.7%, 88%, and 94.9% of individuals who had TM, respectively, suggesting that the appendix criteria were the most reflective of true CM.[16]

The criteria for CM is among the most frequently contested issues within the ICHD in that not only did it appear to be too restrictive, but the term chronic appeared to have multiple implications depending on the primary headache disorder.[4] The criteria were revised to address these issues, and a more liberal definition was included in the appendix to the ICHD pending further evaluation and field testing. The revised criteria specified that within the 15 or more headache days, in the absence of MOH, at least 8 days should be characterized by headache that meets criteria for MO or responds to migraine-specific treatment before it can develop characteristics allowing it to meet criteria for MO.[4,17]

Alternative criteria proposed included a less restrictive definition of CM as at least 4 migraine days and at least 15 total headache days, in contrast to the more conservative definition of CM as at least 50% of headache days meeting criteria for migraine with at least 15 headache days per month. Zeeberg and colleagues[18] field- tested these alternative criteria against the current ICHD criteria for CM and the appendix criteria for CM. Among a population of 685 patients from the Danish Headache Center without MOH, 3% met current ICHD criteria for CM in contrast to 7% who met appendix criteria.[18] Fourteen percent of patients met the more liberal alternative criteria allowing for at least 4 migraine days, and 4% met the more conservative criteria requiring at least 50% migraine days.[18] It was suggested that the findings support the appendix criteria as being neither too restrictive nor too inclusive and worthy of inclusion in the main body of the ICHD upon its next revision.[18]

EPIDEMIOLOGY OF CHRONIC MIGRAINE

The estimated prevalence of CDH as defined by presence of headache at least 15 days per month is approximately 4%.[1,2] Within the United States, the most common subsets of individuals suffering CDH are nearly equally distributed among CTTH and CM with the latter exerting the greatest impact on quality of life as defined by increased headache duration, increased absenteeism from school or work, and more frequent consultation with physicians.[2,5]

In a study that was designed to identify possible risk factors that predict CDH onset or remission, Scher and colleagues[6] noted that 3% of individuals who have EM develop CDH over 1 year. This finding was corroborated by Bigal and colleagues[19] in a recent study of 8219 individuals who had EM, 2.5% of whom progressed to TM over the course of 1 year. Risk factors associated with CDH were female sex, history of being unmarried because of divorce, separation, or death of a spouse, and Caucasian race.[6] Additionally, associations have been made between lower socioeconomic status[6,20] and an increased risk for the development of CDH. These findings appear to be consistent on a more global scale, as countries with economic hardships have a higher prevalence of chronic headache compared with Europe and the United States.[17] Habitual (daily) snoring also appears to be a modest risk factor, as it is more common in CDH sufferers even after adjustment for risk factors associated with sleep-related breathing disorders such as hypertension, body mass index (BMI), gender, and alcohol consumption.[7] When compared with individuals who have episodic headache, CDH sufferers are also more likely to have been in the upper quartile of dietary caffeine consumers (311 mg/d or approximately three 8 oz cups of coffee per day) or to have used caffeine-containing analgesics as the preferred means of headache treatment before the onset of CDH.[8]

Additionally, there appears to be an association between obesity and risk for the development of CDH and TM[6,9,10] and increased frequency and severity of migraine attacks.[21,22] Several potential mechanisms by which obesity is linked to CM have been proposed by Bigal and colleagues,[9] including the possibility that either condition may have direct causal influences on the development and progression of the other (ie, migraines may condemn their sufferers to more sedentary lifestyles and the consumption of more medications that increase weight) versus the presence of biologic factors that may be influential in the progression of obesity and migraine. Specifically, calcitonin gene-related peptide (CGRP), a neuropeptide that has been implicated in the pathogenesis of migraine, is elevated in obese individuals and is elevated further after the consumption of fat. Interestingly, CGRP levels remain stable even after weight loss, suggesting a genetic predisposition toward increased levels.

Other neuropeptides such as orexins, which are responsible for the modulation of appetite and feeding through circadian-dependent mechanisms, also have been found to modulate nociceptive input at the level of the hypothalamus and exert an analgesic effect comparable to morphine when given parenterally or intrathecally. Adiponectin, which is an adipocytokine secreted from adipocytes, has an important modulatory effect on glycemic control and fatty acid catabolism and has been implicated to play a role in obesity. Additionally, adiponectin levels are inversely proportional to BMI and appear to have an anti-inflammatory effect through the induction of anti-inflammatory cytokines and the potential to induce a proinflammatory state when present in low levels as they correlate to high levels of C-reactive protein, interleukin-6, and tumor necrosis factor α.[9]

In a cross-sectional, multicenter survey of migraineurs conducted by Tietjen and colleagues[11] (n = 721), the impact of obesity on migraine frequency and headache-related disability was found to be increased further when comorbid with depression or anxiety. The Headache Impact Test (HIT-6), Patient Health Questionnaire (PHQ-9), and Beck's Anxiety Inventory (BAI) were used to assess headache impact, current depression, and current anxiety, respectively. Responses to the questionnaires then were compared with each subject's calculated BMI, with individuals obtaining scores of at least 30 kg/m^2 classified as obese. A significantly increased prevalence of depression and anxiety was found among the obese individuals who had higher BMIs correlating to increased PHQ-9 (r = 0.14, P<.001) and BAI scores (r = 0.13, P<.001). Furthermore, obesity correlated to severity of depression (odds ratio [OR] = 1.86; 95% CI, 1.25 to 2.78) and anxiety (OR = 1.58; 95% CI, 1.12 to 2.22). Correlations also were made between BMI and headache frequency (r = 0.12, P = .002) and headache frequency and depression scores (r = 0.29, P<.0001). Logistic regression analysis indicated that depression and anxiety have significant influences on the strength of relationship between elevated BMI and increased headache frequency, with obese migraineurs with depression being over four times more likely to have a higher headache frequency (OR = 4.16; 95% CI, 1.92 to 8.99) and those with anxiety nearly twice as likely to have higher headache frequency (OR = 1.96; 95% CI, 1.07 to 3.61). HIT-6 scores also were elevated significantly in obese migraineurs who had depression (OR = 7.10; 95% CI 2.69 to 18.77) and anxiety (OR = 3.59; 95% CI, 1.64 to 7.86), suggesting an increased proclivity toward headache-related disability.[11]

Vieira and colleagues also noted an association between CM and idiopathic intracranial hypertension without papilledema (IIHWOP), with a significant number of these cases noted in patients who had comorbid obesity and intractable headache. Of 62 patients who had CM enrolled in the study, six were found to have an elevated opening cerebrospinal fluid (CSF) pressure, five of whom had a BMI greater than 25, each without papilledema or abnormalities on magnetic resonance venography.[19]

In another study on CSF in chronic migraineurs, Peres and colleagues[23] investigated CSF glutamate levels in 20 patients who had CM compared with normal controls. The subjects who had CM were stratified further into those with comorbid fibromyalgia and those without. Elevated glutamate levels were correlated positively with the presence of CM and elevated pain scores and were found to be elevated even further in the population with both CM and fibromyalgia.[23] The authors postulated that their findings had implications for treatment, suggesting that medications acting on glutamate receptors such as topiramate and lamotrigine may be more likely to exert a meaningful benefit.[23]

In another study investigating progression of EM to CDH, Katsarava and colleagues[24] followed a population of 532 patients who had less than 15 hoadache days over the course of 1 year. A strong correlation between headache frequency and progression to CDH over 1 year was found as the OR of developing headache greater than or equal to 15 days was 20.1 in individuals suffering 10 to 14 headache days per month compared with those suffering less than 5 headache days per month.[24] Moreover, individuals suffering 6 to 9 headache days per month had an OR of 6.2 of developing CDH compared with the less than 5 headache days per month group.[24] Headache frequency also was noted to be a risk factor for progression to TM by Bigal and colleagues.[19] The Katsarava study additionally identified an OR of 19.4 for development of CDH among patients who had medication overuse.[24] Furthermore, Bigal and colleagues[19] noted no significant increased risk for transition to TM among individuals overusing triptans, and a seemingly protective effect with overuse of NSAIDs (in those with a low frequency of headache) with individuals overusing acetaminophen used as the reference group. Overuse of barbiturate-containing compounds and opiates was associated with a statistically significant twofold increased risk of developing TM over the course of 1 year.[19]

With migraine and CM more prevalent among women of childbearing age, it is noted that menstrual-related migraine (MRM) is frequently comorbid with CM and MOH.[25] Calhoun and colleagues[25] sought to address the question of whether MRM and its treatment have an impact on remission of CM and MOH. In this study, 229 women who had MRM were enrolled, 92% of whom had CM, and 72% of whom had MOH. Treatment with hormonal medications for prophylaxis of MRM was initiated, resulting in resolution of MRM in 81% of subjects, 59% of whom also noted a remission of CM to a pattern of EM.[25] Additionally, 54% noted a resolution of MOH, suggesting that addressing MRM and the use of hormonal medications may have a role in the treatment of CM and MOH.[25]

TREATMENT STRATEGIES FOR CHRONIC MIGRAINE

One of the most important benefits to a workable definition for CM is the ability for these patients to have a defined set of inclusion criteria for their diagnosis, making possible the standardization of clinical trials aimed at the treatment of CM.[4] Because of the relatively recent definition of CM, there is a paucity of good evidence-based therapeutic options available for treating CM. Treatments that have been investigated for managing CDH range from pharmacologic interventions to invasive surgical options such as occipital and vagus nerve stimulation.

PHARMACOLOGIC MANAGEMENT
Amitriptyline

Krymchantowski and colleagues[26] investigated the efficacy and tolerability of amitriptyline alone versus combination treatment with amitriptyline and fluoxetine in 27 patients who had TM. The product of severity and intensity of headaches (headache index) was used as a measure of efficacy before and after treatment, and both groups were found to have a significant improvement in their overall response to treatment. There was not a significant difference between the two groups, however, suggesting that amitriptyline monotherapy is an effective treatment for TM.[26]

Among the therapeutic considerations with the use of amitriptyline is the frequent occurrence of adverse effects that may interfere with patient compliance while awaiting therapeutic levels.[26] Among the 13 patients randomized to the amitriptyline monotherapy arm, the most common adverse effects reported were dry mouth (46%), weight gain (30.8%), and heartburn (30.8%). Amitriptyline is thought to act by increasing the amount of synaptic amines (norepinephrine and serotonin), thereby enhancing the descending modulation of nociception within the trigeminal nucleus caudalis and spinal dorsal horn, and by enhancing the action of endogenous opiate receptors.[26,27] Additionally, amitriptyline has been shown to inhibit cortical spreading depression in rat models.[28]

Fluoxetine

In a double-blind placebo-controlled study involving 64 patients who had CDH (at least16 headaches per month for at least 3 previous months), fluoxetine was shown to be moderately effective for managing CDH.[29] Patients in the fluoxetine group noted significant improvement in headache frequency and mood ratings, but not headache severity.[29] Of note, improvement in mood was noted in the beginning of the second month of treatment, with improvements in headache not noted until the end of the third month. Moreover, patients who had improvements in mood were more likely to report improvement in headache. These findings led the authors to conclude that the efficacy of fluoxetine is likely linked to its effect on mood symptoms and not directly on the headache itself. The most common adverse effects experienced by the fluoxetine group included sleep disturbances (28%), tremors (20%), and stomach pain (13%).[29]

Tizanidine

Saper and colleagues[30] investigated the efficacy of tizanidine for the adjunctive treatment of CDH in a double-blind placebo-controlled trial. Forty-four patients randomized to the tizanidine group completed 12 weeks of treatment and were included in the final analysis. Tizanidine was shown to be superior to placebo in significantly reducing headache index (headache frequency times headache severity), mean headache days per week, number of severe headache days, mean headache intensity, and mean headache duration.[30] Most commonly reported adverse events reported by the tizanidine group included somnolence (47%), dizziness (24%), dry mouth (23%), and weakness (19%).[30] Of particular note, the authors state that tizanidine does not seem to exert its effect through the relaxation of skeletal muscle, but acts through its effect on noradrenergic a2-receptors in the brainstem.[30]

Gabapentin

Spira and colleagues[31] evaluated the efficacy of gabapentin for treating CDH in a randomized, placebo-controlled, multicenter crossover study. The study enrolled 133 patients enrolled to receive either 2400 mg/d of gabapentin or placebo. After a 4-week baseline period, a 2-week titration was initiated to reach the goal dose, followed by a 6-week treatment period. A 1-week washout period then was undertaken, followed by a crossover a reinitiation of another 2-week titration and 6-week maintenance period.

At the end of the study period, 95 patients were included in the final analysis, with the gabapentin group exhibiting a 9.1% difference in headache-free rates over placebo.[31] Gabapentin also proved to be significantly superior to placebo with regard to number of headache-free days per month, headache severity, visual analog scale scores, decreased associated features such as nausea and photophobia/phonophobia, disability affecting routine activity, and number of attacks requiring bed rest.[31] Most common adverse effects experienced by the gabapentin group included dizziness (21%), somnolence (18%), ataxia (8%), and nausea (7%).[31] Gabapentin is thought to act by enhancing GABAergic neurotransmission and inhibition of voltage-gated calcium and sodium channels, decreasing glutaminergic neurotransmission.[32]

Topiramate

A small-scale (n = 28) double-blind, placebo-controlled trial by Silvestrini and colleagues[33] demonstrated that low-dose topiramate (50 mg/d) may be effective in reducing headache frequency in patients who were experiencing CM with acute MO. During the last 4 weeks of the maintenance phase (8 weeks), topiramate-treated patients reported significantly lower headache frequencies compared with those treated with placebo (mean number of days with headache (plus or minus SD): 8.1 plus or minus 8.1 versus 20.6 plus or minus 3.4, $P<.0007$). They reported a 71% responder rate (greater than or equal to 50% improvement in monthly headache frequency) for topiramate-treated patients versus a 7% placebo response rate.

Siberstein and colleagues[34] conducted a recent randomized, double-blind, placebo-controlled, multicenter trial investigating the efficacy and safety of topiramate 100 mg/d for treating CM. In this study, patients in the topiramate group were treated with 25 mg/d with a weekly titration by 25 mg/d to a goal dose of 100 mg/d or to the highest dose tolerated. The use of abortive headache medications was limited to 4 days per week. Three hundred twenty-eight patients were randomized, from which an intent-to-treat (ITT) population of 306 individuals was obtained. CM was operationally defined as the presence of at least 15 headache days per 28 days, of which at least 50% were migraine or migrainous headache (Silberstein-Lipton criteria for transformed migraine with additional qualifications regarding the frequency of headaches possessing migraine features). These diagnostic criteria are similar (but not identical) to those recently adopted by the ICHD-II. The ITT population consisted of a total of 306 patients (n = 153 [topiramate], n = 153 [placebo]).[34]

The mean maintenance dose of topiramate was 86.0 mg/d, and mean duration of treatment was 91.7 days for the topiramate group and 90.6 days for the placebo group. The key clinical efficacy results included a significant reduction in mean (plus or minus SD) monthly rate of migraine/migrainous days in patients receiving topiramate treatment (6.4 plus or minus 5.8 days) compared with placebo (4.7 plus or minus 6.1 days, $P = .010$), and a mean reduction from baseline of 5.6 (plus or minus 6.0) migraine days per month compared with 4.1 (plus or minus 6.1) days for the placebo group ($P = .032$). The most common topiramate-associated adverse events (AEs) were paresthesia (28.8% versus placebo 7.5%), upper respiratory tract infection (13.8% versus 12.4% placebo) and fatigue (11.9% versus placebo 9.9%). Treatment-emergent AEs were mild to moderate in severity and were consistent with those observed in previous topiramate clinical trials. No serious AE was reported in either treatment group, and 10.9% of patients in the topiramate group discontinued their participation in the trial because of adverse events.[34] Diener and colleagues[35] recently reported results from a randomized, double-blind, placebo-controlled, parallel-group, multicenter study consisting of 16 weeks of double-blind treatment. CM was defined as those patients experiencing at least15 monthly migraine days for at least 3 months before trial entry, regardless of whether they were overusing acute medications (ICHD-II). Patients were included if they had at least 12 migraine days during the 4-week (28-day) baseline phase. The ITT population included 59 patients (n = 32 [topiramate], n = 27 [placebo]). The primary efficacy variable was the change in the mean number of monthly migraine days from baseline to the last 4 weeks of the double-blind phase. Treatment with topiramate resulted in a significant reduction in mean monthly migraine days (-3.5 days) compared with placebo (0.2 days, $P = .02$). Topiramate treatment also significantly reduced the mean number of migraine days, periods, and attacks at all time points during the double-blind phase (except week 8), compared with placebo. A key difference between the Silberstein and Diener trials was that patients were allowed to take acute rescue medication as usual in the Diener trial. Interestingly, the benefits of topiramate treatment extended to the subgroup of patients overusing acute medications (topiramate, n = 23; placebo, n = 23) as demonstrated by significant reductions in mean monthly migraine days (-3.5 days) compared with placebo (0.8 days, P = .03).[35]

Botulinum Toxin Type A

The use of BoNT-A for CDH has been the subject of two large double-blind, placebo-controlled, multicenter trials.[36,37] These two trials represent two of the largest among numerous open-label and smaller placebo-controlled studies.[15]

Mathew and colleagues[36] investigated BoNT-A in an 11-month study on patients who had CDH as defined by greater than 15 headache days per month at 13 study sites across North America. Headache phenotypes permitted in the study included any combination of migraine with or without aura, probable migraine, migrainous headache, episodic tension-type headache, and CTTH. Patients were assessed during a 30-day baseline period to evaluate headache characteristics and determine eligibility for the study, after which a 30-day single-blind placebo response period was initiated. Placebo responders were defined as individuals whose headache frequency fell below 16 headache days within the placebo month, or whose headaches were reduced by 30% of their original frequency. Three hundred fifty-five patients including 76 (21%) placebo responders and 279 (79%) placebo nonresponders were randomized into either the placebo group or the BoNT-A group, receiving between 105 and 260 units of BoNT-A.[36] Follow-up was conducted every 30 days, and additional treatments were repeated in 90-day intervals for four treatments.

At day 180 after the two blinded study injections, there was no significant difference for the primary endpoint of an increase in headache free-days between the two groups.[36] A significant improvement was noted, however, in the percentage of BoNT-A treated patients, with a 50% or more decrease in number of headache days per month (32.7%) as compared with the placebo group (15.0%) at treatment day 180. Additionally, a significant improvement was noted in the mean change in frequency of headaches per month in the BoNT-A group (-6.1) compared with the placebo group (-3.1).[36]

Among the 173 BoNT-A treated patients, the most commonly reported adverse events were muscular weakness (22.0%), neck pain (13.3%), headache (6.9%), and blepharoptosis (6.9%).[31] Most of the adverse events were described as mild to moderate, and only four patients (2.3%) discontinued their participation in the study because of adverse events.[36]

Silberstien and colleagues,[37] in a separate randomized, double-blind, placebo-controlled study, sought to evaluate the efficacy of three different doses of BoNT-A in a population of patients who had CDH. This was an 11-month study with a 30-day screening period, followed by a 30-day single-blind placebo period, followed by four double-blind treatment periods every 90 days. Patient data were collected every 30 days.

Of 702 patients enrolled into the single-blind placebo run-in period, 538 (76.6%) were determined to be placebo nonresponders, and 164 (23.4%) to be placebo responders.[37] Individuals within each group were randomized to receive 225, 150, or 75 units of BoNT-A or placebo. There was no significant difference between the two groups for the primary endpoint of a change in the number of headache-free days at 180 days after randomization.

Most commonly reported adverse events in the Silberstein[37] study among the 225, 150, and 75 unit groups were muscular weakness at the injection site (30.8%, 26.2%,

16.7%), neck pain (22.5%, 22.0%, 17.2%), neck rigidity (14.8%, 8.3%, 8.0%), and hypertonia (7.1%, 8.9%, 7.5%). BoNT-A is a neurotoxin that inhibits the release of acetylcholine at the neuromuscular junction and also is thought to act, in disorders such as headache, by inhibiting the release of nociceptive neurotransmitters such as substance P, calcitonin gene-related peptide, and glutamate.[38–40]

In a recent double-blind placebo-controlled randomized trial of BoNT-A 100 units administered in a fixed-dose and -site paradigm, 41 patients were treated with the study medication or placebo.[41] BoNT-A was statistically superior to placebo for the primary endpoint of reduction in migraine headache episodes. Six patients on BoNT-A compared with three patients on placebo had at least a 50% reduction in their migraine episodes. Active treatment was superior to placebo for the secondary endpoints of total headache days, headache index, and quality-of-life measures.

Based on the mixed results of the BoNT-A studies, the results of two large, pivotal phase 3 randomized controlled studies evaluating the safety and efficacy of BoNT-A for the preventive treatment of chronic daily headache in subjects with migraine have been conducted and will be completed soon.

DIVALPROEX SODIUM

In a retrospective chart review (n = 138), 67% of patients who had CDH taking divalproex sodium for migraine preventive treatment experienced at least 50% reductions in monthly migraine frequency.[42] The efficacy of extended-release divalproex sodium in patients who had probable CM and probable MO was evaluated in a prospective case series that included 15 patients who had migraine from a headache clinic population that fulfilled the ICHD-2 criteria for CM with MO.[43] Divalproex sodium was initiated at 500 mg taken daily at bedtime and increased to 1000 mg daily at bedtime after 2 weeks. The total treatment period was 2 months. Treatment with extended-release divalproex sodium resulted in a significant reduction in mean headache days, from 21.6 at baseline to 10.4 at month 1 and 8.9 at month 2 (P<.0001 versus baseline for both months).

NONPHARMACOLOGICAL MANAGEMENT OF CHRONIC DAILY HEADACHE

Behavioral therapy (eg, biofeedback, relaxation, cognitive behavioral therapy) is effective for managing primary headaches such as migraine and also may help in the management of CM. Unfortunately, only a few studies have tested this hypothesis, and most did not isolate components when reporting outcome, making it difficult to assess the contribution of the nonpharmacological therapy to treatment success. Grazzi and colleagues conducted an investigation to more clearly determine the role of behavioral therapy in managing CDH associated with medication overuse. In a 3-year follow-up, prospective study, 61 patients who had CDH and analgesic overuse received either pharmacologic therapy alone or pharmacologic therapy supplemented with biofeedback-assisted relaxation. Both treatment groups achieved similar levels of improvement for up to 1 year following treatment. At the 3-year follow-up point, however, patients who had received biofeedback-assisted relaxation in addition to pharmacologic therapy had greater sustained improvement on two out of three outcome measures (ie, fewer headache days and reduced intake of analgesic medications) and fewer relapses.[44]

Procedural and Surgical Options

Greater occipital nerve blockade

Greater occipital nerve blockade (GONB) has been shown to be effective for treating primary headache disorders such as CDH including TM, cluster, and chronic cluster headache with the mechanism of action thought to be the result of the anatomic overlap of the trigeminal nucleus caudalis and the C2 nerve roots that supply the greater occipital nerves.[45–47] Noting the presence of suboccipital pain in many migraineurs, Afridi and colleagues[45] sought to investigate the response of 54 chronic migraineurs to greater occipital nerve blockade with 3 mL of 2% lidocaine and 80 mg of methylprednisolone. Overall, 26 migraineurs had at least a partial response as defined by greater than 30% reduction in frequency or frequency of their headaches after 4 weeks. Nine patients reported a complete response and were pain-free at the 4-week follow-up assessment.[45] Tenderness over the greater occipital nerves was predictive of a positive response in contrast to the presence or absence of medication overuse and the presence of local anesthesia after the procedure, which was not predictive of outcome.[45]

The need for steroid in combination with local anesthetics for GONB for the treatment of TM was investigated further by Ashkenazi and colleagues.[47] In this study, patients who had TM were randomized to receive GONB with 2% lidocaine and 0.5% bupivacaine and either saline or triamcinolone. There were no statistically significant differences between the two groups with regard to reduction in pain severity or reduction in number of headache days after 4 weeks.[47]

Occipital nerve stimulation

There is evidence that greater occipital nerve stimulation (GONS) may exert some benefit in chronic migraine that is unresponsive to pharmacologic treatment.[12,13] The mechanisms by which GONS is effective for medically refractive primary headache disorders is unclear; however, stimulation of the greater occipital nerve is thought to suppress nociceptive input through small c-fiber and a-delta fiber afferents.[12,13] More recent findings suggest centrally mediated antinociceptive mechanisms may be responsible for the efficacy of GONS in CM.[13,48]

Schwedt and colleagues reported a series of 15 patients, consisting of eight patients with CM who were treated with GONS and followed for a mean of 19 months. Although the results were not stratified by primary headache diagnosis, a significant improvement was seen among the entire subject population with regard to headache frequency and severity, Migraine Disability Assessment (MIDAS), Headache Impact Test-6 (HIT-6), and Beck Depression Inventory (BDI).[12]

Recently, a multicenter, prospective, randomized, single-blind, controlled feasibility study evaluating the safety and efficacy of GONS in 110 patients who had CM was reported. Subjects met ICHD-II criteria for chronic migraine and were randomized 2:1:1 to adjustable stimulation (AS), preset stimulation (PS), or a medically managed (MM) control group. The PS group received predetermined stimulation and served as an implanted control. All subjects received diagnostic occipital nerve block (ONB) before randomization. The first eight who failed ONB formed an ancillary group (AG) and were offered AS. There was no significant difference at 3 months between the AS and PS groups with regards to the primary endpoint of a change in the number of headache days. The responder rate (greater than 50% reduction in frequency or severity) in the AS group, however, was 39% compared with 6% in the PS group ($P = .032$) and 0% ($P = .003$) in the MM group. This feasibility study suggests that ONS may be a promising treatment for some patients who have medically refractory CM, but further randomized controlled trials are required. The data also suggested that GONB might not be predictive of response to GONS. The most common adverse device-related event was lead migration, which occurred in 12 of 51 (24%) implanted subjects.[49]

Vagal nerve stimulation

Additionally, observations made in studies investigating vagus nerve stimulation (VNS) in epilepsy suggested that it might play a role in treatment of medically refractive headache. Through its effect on neurotransmitters, brain metabolism, and cerebral blood flow, VNS is thought to exert its influence on the parasympathetic dysfunction, which is thought to occur in primary headache disorders such as migraine and cluster as well as suppress nociceptive input.[14] Mauskop published a series of case reports of patients with primary headache disorders who underwent VNS implantation. Of the three patients who had CM, two had an excellent response to VNS, and one had an initially good response with a return to his baseline frequency of headache the following month.[14] This treatment modality, however, has not undergone formal randomized studies.

SUMMARY

The relatively low prevalence of CDH and CM is disproportionate to the significant degree of disability they exert on patients who suffer from these disorders. Given the degree of nociceptive bombardment of the nervous system resulting in peripheral and central sensitization, and the ensuing tendency to overuse analgesic medications, CDH represents a therapeutic challenge for many clinicians.

Treatment strategies should be aimed at correctly identifying the presence of CDH armed with the knowledge that many patients who have chronic headache may fail to report headaches that they feel to be manageable focusing only on their bad headache days. In addition, an effective prophylactic regimen should be initiated; the presence of medication overuse must be addressed, and the offending medication being overused must be discontinued. Aside from analgesic overuse, other modifiable risk factors associated with the development of CM and CDH and their likelihood for remission must be addressed including obesity and caffeine use and the effective management of comorbid conditions such as depression, anxiety, and sleep-related breathing disorders.

REFERENCES

1. Castillo J, Munoz P, Guitera V, et al. Epidemiology of chronic daily headache in the general population. Headache 1999;39:190–6.
2. Scher AI, Stewart WF, Liberman J, et al. Prevalence of frequent headache in a population sample. Headache 1998;38:497–506.
3. Headache Classification Committee of the International Headache Society. The international classification of headache disorders. Cephalalgia 2004;24:1–160.
4. Olesen J, Bousser M-G, Diener H-C, et al. Headache Classification Committee. New appendix criteria open for a broader concept of chronic migraine. Cephalalgia 2006;26:742–6.
5. Dodick DW. Chronic daily headache. N Engl J Med 2006;354:158–65.
6. Scher AI, Stewart WF, Ricci JA, et al. Factors associated with the onset and remission of chronic daily headache in a population-based study. Pain 2003;106:81–9.
7. Scher AI, Lipton RB, Stewart WF. Habitual snoring as a risk factor for chronic daily headache. Neurology 2003;60:1366–8.
8. Scher AI, Stweart WF, Lipton RB. Caffeine as a risk factor for chronic daily headache: a population-based study. Neurology 2004;63:2022–7.
9. Bigal ME, Lipton RB, Holland PR, et al. Obesity, migraine, and chronic migraine: possible mechanisms of interaction. Neurology 2007;68:1851–61.

10. Bigal ME, Lipton RB. Obesity is a risk factor for transformed migraine but not chronic tension-type headache. Neurology 2006;67:252–7.
11. Tietjen GE, Peterlin BL, Brandes JL, et al. Depression and anxiety: effect on the migraine–obesity relationship. Headache 2007;47:866–75.
12. Schwedt TJ, Dodick DW, Hentz J, et al. Occipital nerve stimulation for chronic headache—long-term safety and efficacy. Cephalalgia 2007;27:153–7.
13. Goadsby PJ, Bartsch T, Dodick DW. Occipital nerve stimulation for headache: mechanisms and efficacy. Headache 2008;48:313–8.
14. Mauskop A. Vagus nerve stimulation relieves chronic refractory migraine and cluster headaches. Cephalalgia 2005;25:82–6.
15. Mathew NT. The prophylactic treatment of chronic daily headache. Headache 2006;46:1552–64.
16. Bigal ME, Tepper SJ, Sheftell FD, et al. Field testing alternative criteria for chronic migraine. Cephalalgia 2006;26:477–82.
17. Silberstein S, Diener H-C, Lipton R, et al. Epidemiology, risk factors, and treatment of chronic migraine: a focus on Topiramate. Headache 2008;48:1087–95.
18. Zeeberg P, Olesen J, Jensen R. Medication overuse headache and chronic migraine in a specialized headache center: field-testing proposed new appendix criteria. Cephalalgia 2009;29:214–20.
19. Bigal ME, Serrano D, Buse D, et al. Acute migraine medications and evolution from episodic to chronic migraine: a longitudinal population-based study. Headache 2008;48:1157–68.
20. Hagen K, Vatten L, Stovner LJ, et al. Low socioeconomic status is associated with increased risk of frequent headache: a prospective study of 22,718 adults in Norway. Cephalalgia 2002;22:672–9.
21. Bigal ME, Liberman JN, Lipton RB. Obesity and migraine: a population study. Neurology 2006;66:545–50.
22. Vieira DSS, Masruha MR, Gonçalves AL, et al. Idiopathic intracranial hypertension with and without papilloedema in a consecutive series of patients with chronic migraine. Cephalalgia 2008;28:609–13.
23. Peres MFP, Zukerman E, Senne Soares CA, et al. Cerebrospinal fluid glutamate levels in chronic migraine. Cephalalgia 2004;24:735–9.
24. Katsarava Z, Schneeweiss S, Kurth T, et al. Incidence and predictors for chronicity of headache in patients with episodic migraine. Neurology 2004;62:788–90.
25. Calhoun A, Ford S. Elimination of menstrual-related migraine beneficially impacts chronification and medication overuse. Headache 2008;48:1186–93.
26. Krymchantowski AV, Silva MT, Barbosa JS, et al. Amitriptyline versus amitriptyline combined with fluoxetine in the preventive treatment of transformed migraine: a double-blind study. Headache 2002;42:510–4.
27. Casucci G, Villani V, Frediani F. Central mechanism of action of antimigraine prophylactic drugs. Neurol Sci 2008;29:S123–6.
28. Ayata C, Jin H, Kudo C, et al. Suppressing cortical spreading depression in migraine prophylaxis. Ann Neurol 2006;59:652–61.
29. Saper JR, Silberstien SD, Lake AE III, et al. Double-blind trial of fluoxetine: chronic daily headache and migraine. Headache 1994;34:497–502.
30. Saper JR, Lake AE III, Cantrell DT. Chronic daily headache prophylaxis with tizanidine: a double-blind, placebo-controlled, multicenter outcome study. Headache 2002;42:470–82.
31. Spira PJ, Beran RG. Australian Gabapentin Chronic Daily Headache Group. Gabapentin in the prophylaxis of chronic daily headache: a randomized, placebo-controlled study. Neurology 2003;61:1753–9.

32. Landmark CJ. Antiepileptic drugs in nonepileptic disorders: relations between mechanisms of action and clinical efficacy. CNS Drugs 2008;22:27–47.
33. Silvestrini M, Bartolini M, Coccia M, et al. Topiramate in the treatment of chronic migraine. Cephalalgia 2003;23:820–4.
34. Silberstein SD, Lipton RB, Dodick DW. Efficacy and safety of topiramate for the treatment of chronic migraine: a randomized, double-blind, placebo-controlled trial. Headache 2007;47:170–80.
35. Diener HC, Bussone G, Van Oene JC, et al. TOPMAT-MIG-201(TOP-CHROME) Study Group. Topiramate reduces headache days in chronic migraine: a randomized, double-blind, placebo-controlled study. Cephalalgia 2007;27(7):814–23.
36. Mathew NT, Frishberg BM, Gawel M, et al. Botulinum toxin type A (BOTOX) for the prophylactic treatment of chronic daily headache: a randomized, double-blind, placebo-controlled trial. Headache 2005;45:293–307.
37. Silberstein SD, Stark SR, Lucas SM, et al. Botulinum toxin type A for the prophylactic treatment of chronic daily headache: a randomized, double-blind, placebo-controlled trial. Mayo Clin Proc 2005;80:1126–37.
38. Cui M, Khanijou S, Rubino J, et al. Subcutaneous administration of botulinum toxin type A reduces formalin-induced pain. Pain 2004;107:125–33.
39. Durham PL, Cady R, Cady R. Regulation of calcitonin gene-related peptide secretion from trigeminal nerve cells by botulinum toxin type A: implications for migraine therapy. Headache 2004;44:35–43.
40. Aoki KR. Evidence for antinociceptive activity of botulinum toxin type A in pain management. Headache 2003;43(Suppl 1):S9–15.
41. Freitag FG, Diamond S, Diamond M, et al. Botulinum toxin type A in the treatment of chronic migraine without medication overuse. Headache 2008;48:201–9.
42. Freitag FG, Diamond S, Diamond ML, et al. Divalproex in the long-term treatment of chronic daily headache. Headache 2001;41:271–8.
43. Landy SH, Baker JD. Divalproex ER prophylaxis in migraineurs with probable chronic migraine and probable medication overuse headache: a case series. Pain Pract 2004;4:292–4.
44. Grazzi L, Andrasik F, D'Amico D, et al. Behavioral and pharmacologic treatment of transformed migraine with analgesic overuse: outcome at 3 years. Headache 2002;42:483–90.
45. Afridi SK, Shields KG, Bhola R, et al. Greater occipital nerve injection in primary headache syndromes—prolonged effects from a single injection. Pain 2006;122: 126–9.
46. Ambrosini A, Vandenheede, Rossi P, et al. Suboccipital injection with a mixture of rapid- and long-acting steroids in cluster headache: a double-blind placeb-controlled study. Pain 2005;118:92–6.
47. Ashkenazi A, Matro R, Shaw JW, et al. Greater occipital nerve block using local anesthetics alone or with triamcinolone for transformed migraine: a randomized comparative study. J Neurol Neurosurg Psychiatr 2008;79:415–7.
48. Marathu MS, Bartsch T, Ward N, et al. Central neuromodulation in chronic migraine patients with suboccipital stimulators: a PET study. Brain 2004;127: 220–30.
49. Saper JR. Occipital nerve stimulation (ONS) for treatment of intractable migraine headache: 3 month results from the ONSTIM feasibility study. Presented at the American Headache Society Meeting; Boston, June, 2008.

Pediatric Migraine

Donald W. Lewis, MD

KEYWORDS

• Migraine • Headache • Children • Adolescents

Migraine is a chronic, progressive, and debilitating disorder that has an impact on the lives of millions of individuals. The origins of the disability can be traced into childhood and adolescence for most adult migraine sufferers.[1] Accurate diagnosis and aggressive treatment interventions during childhood and adolescence are essential to prevent the decades of suffering and diminished quality of life that are directly attributable to migraine. Adequately addressing migraine during adolescence has as much importance on the patient's overall well-being as providing immunizations and weight management.

Diagnosing migraine in children can be a particular challenge. The clinical manifestations of migraine vary widely through childhood because the disorder may be expressed differently or incompletely. Mimickers of migraine also emerge during childhood to complicate the diagnostic landscape. Such entities as mitochondrial or metabolic disorders, epilepsy syndromes, vascular disorders, and congenital malformations may present with episodic symptoms, including headache. In addition, the medical history can be limited by the child's inability to articulate the symptoms, coupled with parental interpretation, distortion, and editorial. Furthermore, children are often brought for medical evaluation at the onset of transient neurologic, autonomic, gastrointestinal, or visual symptoms, before the characteristic recurrent pattern is established, and, curiously, headache may not be the primary symptom. The key aspect to recognizing the spectrum of migraine in children is to appreciate that migraine is an episodic disorder separated by symptom-free intervals.

The purpose of this article is to review the clinical manifestations and management options for migraine in children and adolescents, with an emphasis on those entities peculiar to young children. All pharmacologic comment is "off-label."

EPIDEMIOLOGY

Headaches are common during childhood. Bille's landmark epidemiologic survey conducted in the 1950s in Sweden of 6000 school children found that the prevalence of generic "headache" ranged from 37% to 51% in 7-year-old children and gradually

---

The author has received research grant support from Ortho McNeil Neurologics, Abbott Laboratories, Glaxo Smith Kline, Merck, Astra Zeneca, and American Home Products.

Department of Pediatrics, Children's Hospital of The King's Daughters, Eastern Virginia Medical School, 601 Children's Lane, Norfolk, VA 23507, USA

E-mail address: dlewis@chkd.org

Neurol Clin 27 (2009) 481–501

doi:10.1016/j.ncl.2008.11.003

rose to 57% to 82% by adolescence.[2] Frequent or recurring patterns of headache, of which migraine represents a significant subset, occurred in 2.5% of 7-year-olds and in up to 15% of 15-year-olds.

Subsequent epidemiologic studies have found that the prevalence of migraine headache steadily increases through childhood, peaking in adolescence. Depending on the diagnostic criteria used, the prevalence increases from 3% in the preschool years, to 4% to 11% by the elementary school years, and then up to 8% to 23% during the high school years. Before puberty, boys have more headaches than girls, but after puberty, migraine headaches occur more frequently in girls.[3–5]

The incidence of migraine peaks earlier in boys than in girls.[6] The mean age of onset of migraine is 7 years for boys and 11 years for girls; the gender ratio also shifts during the adolescent years (**Table 1**). The incidence of migraine with aura peaks earlier than the incidence of migraine without aura.[5–13]

Classification of Pediatric Migraine

The International Classification of Headache Disorders for migraine is shown in **Box 1** and is available on-line ([14]).

There are three primary groups:

1. Migraine without aura (formerly common migraine)
2. Migraine with aura (formerly classic migraine)
3. Childhood "periodic syndromes" that are commonly precursors of migraine

Notably absent in the 2004 classification system are several clinical entities peculiar to childhood, such as "Alice in Wonderland" syndrome, benign paroxysmal torticollis, confusional migraine, and ophthalmoplegic migraine (OM), which are discussed for completeness.

MIGRAINE WITHOUT AURA

This is the most frequent form of migraine in children and adolescents (60%–85% of cases). The diagnostic criteria are shown in **Box 2** and include three modifications to increase sensitivity of diagnosis for children: brief duration (1–72 hours), bilateral or bifrontal location (age <15 years), and the inference of photophobia and phonophobia by behavioral response rather than verbal report.

The key feature of migraine with aura in children is episodes of intense disabling headache separated by symptom-free intervals. The criteria require at least five distinct attacks lasting 1 to 72 hours and permit attacks to be briefer than in adults (range: 4–72 hours). The location of the pain may be unilateral or, in children younger than 15 years of age, bilateral (bifrontal or bitemporal). The quality of pain is typically pulsing or throbbing, a symptom that may require specific questioning in young children. By definition, the pain is moderate to intense and aggravated by routine physical activity, such as walking or climbing stairs. The accompanying associated autonomic

Table 1			
Prevalence of migraine headache through childhood			
	Age		
	3–7 Years	7–11 Years	15 Years
Prevalence	1.2%–3.2%	4%–11%	8%–23%
Gender ratio	Boys > girls	Boys = girls	Girls > boys

Box 1
Migraine classification

Migraine without aura

Migraine with aura

Typical aura with migraine headache

Typical aura with nonmigraine headache

Typical aura without headache

Familial hemiplegic migraine

Sporadic hemiplegic migraine

Basilar-type migraine

Childhood periodic syndromes that are commonly precursors of migraine

Cyclic vomiting

Abdominal migraine

Benign paroxysmal vertigo of childhood

Retinal migraine

Complications of migraine

Chronic migraine

Status migraine

Persistent aura without infarction

Migrainous infarction

Probable migraine

Box 2
Diagnostic criteria for pediatric migraine without aura

A. At least five attacks fulfilling criteria B through D

B. Headache attacks lasting 1 to 72 hours

C. Headache has at least two of the following characteristics:

   1. Unilateral location, which may be bilateral or frontotemporal (not occipital)

   2. Pulsing quality

   3. Moderate or severe pain intensity

   4. Aggravation by or causing avoidance of routine physical activity (eg, walking, climbing stairs)

D. During the headache, at least one of the following:

   1. Nausea or vomiting

   2. Photophobia and phonophobia, which may be inferred from a child's behavior

E. Not attributed to another disorder

features (nausea, vomiting, photophobia, and phonophobia) may be as disabling as the pain. The latter two features may be inferred by the patient's behavior if the child withdraws to a quiet dark place during the attack. The International Headache Society (IHS) criteria wisely also state that the headache must "not attributed to another disorder," implying that the prudent physician should carefully consider other possible causes for the recurrent headaches.

MIGRAINE WITH AURA

The disorders within the migraine with aura spectrum reflect the concept that the focal symptoms, such as visual disruptions, hemiparesis, and aphasia, are manifestations of the regional neuronal depolarization and oligemia caused by cortical spreading depression (CSD). Clinical entities of childhood with focal neurologic symptoms, previously termed *migraine variants*, such as hemiplegic and basilar type, now are included within this category of migraine with aura.

Approximately 15% to 30% of children and adolescents who have migraine report visual disturbances, distortions, or obscurations before, or as, the headache begins. The visual symptoms begin gradually and last for several minutes (typical aura). The most frequent forms are binocular visual impairment with scotoma (77%), distortion or hallucinations (16%), and monocular visual impairment or scotoma (7%).[15] Formed illusions (eg, spots, balloons, colors, rainbows) or other bizarre visual distortions (eg, Alice in Wonderland syndrome) may be described, albeit infrequently.

Sudden images and complicated visual perceptions should prompt consideration of benign occipital epilepsy, specifically Panayiotopoulos syndrome.[16] Transient visual obscurations may also be described with idiopathic intracranial hypertension; thus, not all visual symptoms with headache are attributable to migraine with aura.

BASILAR-TYPE MIGRAINE

Basilar-type migraine (BM) represents 3% to 19% of childhood migraine and has a mean age onset of 7 years. Attacks are characterized by episodes of dizziness, vertigo, visual disturbances, ataxia, or diplopia as the aura, followed by the headache phase. The pain of BM may be occipital in location, unlike the usual frontal or bitemporal pain of typical migraine. The diagnostic criteria require two or more symptoms and emphasize bulbar and bilateral sensorimotor features (**Box 3**). Familiar forms of BM linked to the same genes as familial hemiplegic migraine (FHM), types 1 and 2, have recently been reported.[17]

FAMILIAL HEMIPLEGIC MIGRAINE

No form of migraine has yielded more information about the underlying molecular genetics of migraine than FHM. FHM, type 1, is an uncommon autosomal dominant form of migraine with aura caused by a missense mutation in the calcium channel gene (CACNA1A) linked to chromosome 19p13. Clinically, FHM is a migraine headache heralded by an aura that has "stroke-like" qualities, producing some degree of hemiparesis (**Box 4**). The transient episodes of focal neurologic deficits precede the headache phase by 30 to 60 minutes but, occasionally, extend well beyond the headache itself (hours to days). The location of headache is often (but not invariably) contralateral to the focal deficits. Many children and adolescents report transient somatosensory symptoms heralding an attack with focal paresthesias around the mouth and hand (eg, chiro-oral) without weakness; this does not fulfill the criteria for hemiplegic migraine. Genetic testing is commercially available for FHM type 1.

Box 3

Diagnostic criteria for basilar-type migraine

A. Fulfills criteria for migraine with aura

B. Accompanied by two or more of the following types of symptoms:

1. Dysarthria

2. Vertigo

3. Tinnitus

4. Hypacusia

5. Diplopia

6. Visual phenomena in the temporal and nasal fields of both eyes

7. Ataxia

8. Decreased level of consciousness

9. Decreased hearing

10. Double vision

11. Simultaneous bilateral paresthesias

C. At least one of the following:

1. At least one aura symptom develops gradually over 5 minutes or more, and different aura symptoms occur in succession over 5 minutes or more.

2. Each aura symptoms lasts more than 5 minutes and 60 minutes or less.

D. Headache-fulfilling criteria: migraine without aura begins during the aura or follows aura within 60 minutes.

Box 4

Diagnostic criteria for familial hemiplegic migraine

A. Fulfills criteria for migraine with aura

B. Aura consisting of fully reversible motor weakness and at least one of the following:

1. Fully reversible visual symptoms, including positive features (eg, flickering lights, spots, lines) or negative features (eg, loss of vision)

2. Fully reversible sensory symptoms, including positive features (eg, pins and needles)

3. Fully reversible dysphasic speech disturbance

C. At least two of the following:

1. At least one aura symptom develops gradually over more than 5 minutes

2. Aura symptom lasts more than 5 minutes and less than 24 hours

3. Headache that fulfills criteria for migraine without aura begins during the aura or follows the onset of aura within 60 minutes

D. At least one first-degree or second-degree relative has had an attack

E. At least one of the following:

1. History and physical and neurologic examinations not suggesting any organic disorder

2. History or physical or neurologic examination suggesting such a disorder, which is ruled out by appropriate investigations

FHM types 2 and 3 are clinically quite similar but have distinctly different molecular mechanisms: FHM type 2 attributable to point mutation of the α_2-subunit of the sodium-potassium pump (ATP1A2) gene on chromosome 1q21 to 23 and FHM type 3 attributable to sodium channel gene mutation (SCN1A).[18,19]

Sporadic hemiplegic migraine includes those patients who present with the abrupt onset of focal neurologic signs or repetitive episodes of focal neurologic symptoms without a family history.

PERIODIC SYNDROMES OF CHILDHOOD THAT REPRESENT PRECURSORS OF MIGRAINE

The term *migraine variants* was formerly applied to this grouping of migraine precursors and some of the forms of migraine with aura; however, today, they are more appropriately categorized according to IHS criteria. Three childhood conditions are included in the category of periodic syndromes: benign paroxysmal vertigo, cyclic (or cyclical) vomiting syndrome (CVS), and abdominal migraine. A fourth, benign paroxysmal torticollis, is discussed in this section, because recent molecular genetic information has demonstrated linkage to migraine.

Benign paroxysmal vertigo occurs in young children with abrupt episodes of unsteadiness or ataxia. The child may appear startled or frightened by the sudden loss of balance. Witnesses may report nystagmus or pallor. Verbal children may describe dizziness and nausea. The spells may occur in clusters that typically resolve with sleep. In series of patients available for long-term follow-up, many evolve to BM. The diagnosis of benign paroxysmal vertigo is based on a characteristic clinical history, but caution must be exercised to exclude seizure disorders (eg, benign occipital epilepsy), otologic pathologic conditions, posterior fossa lesions, cervical spine abnormalities, or metabolic disorders.

A pattern of cycling episodes of vomiting may be seen with a variety of gastrointestinal, neurologic, and metabolic disorders, but a significant subset of children with stereotyped episodes of vomiting have a migrainous basis for their symptoms, which represent CVS. The key clinical feature of CVS is recurrent episodes of severe vomiting with interval wellness (**Box 5**).

The episodes occur on a regular, often predictable, basis every 2 to 4 weeks, lasting 1 to 2 days, and commencing in the early morning hours. The age of onset is approximately 5 years, and boys and girls are affected equally. The age of diagnosis is approximately 8 years, and most children "outgrow" their symptoms by the age of 10 years; however, a significant proportion of patients have symptoms through adolescence and even as young adults.

After a complete diagnostic investigation has excluded other causes of the cyclic vomiting pattern, a comprehensive treatment plan, including acute and prophylactic measures, may be instituted. For acute treatment of attacks, aggressive hydration, sedation, and an antiemetic agent represent the mainstays. Oral or intravenous hydration with a glucose-containing solution is essential. Antiemetic choices include the following:

Ondansetron (0.3–0.4 mg/kg administered intravenously or 4–8 mg administered as an oral disintegrating form or tablet)
Promethazine (0.25–0.5 mg/kg per dose administered intravenously or orally)
Metoclopramide (1–2 mg/kg up to 10 mg twice a day administered intravenously or orally)
Prochlorperazine (2.5–5 mg twice a day administered intravenously)

During an attack, sedation with a benzodiazepine (lorazepam, 0.05–0.1 mg/kg up to 5 mg) or diphenhydramine (0.25–1 mg/kg) is often necessary. Cautious enthusiasm for

---

Box 5
Diagnostic criteria for cyclic vomiting syndrome

Recurrent episodic attacks, usually stereotypical in the individual patient, of vomiting and intense nausea. Attacks are associated with pallor and lethargy. There is complete resolution of symptoms between attacks.

Diagnostic criteria

A. At least five attacks fulfilling criteria B and C

B. Episodic attacks, stereotypical in the individual patient, of intense nausea and vomiting lasting 1 to 5 days

C. Vomiting during attacks occurs at least five times per hour for at least 1 hour

D. Symptom-free between attacks

E. Not attributed to another disorder and history and physical examination do not show signs of gastrointestinal disease

---

use of nasal (5 mg) or subcutaneous (~0.07 mg/kg) sumatriptan preparations is growing as field experience mounts, although none of the triptan preparations have been subjected to blind clinical trials for CVS and none are yet approved by the US Food and Drug Administration (FDA).

Initiation of a migraine prophylactic agent for CVS should be strongly considered because CVS is an extraordinarily disabling condition for the child and the family. Options include the following:

Cyproheptadine (2–4 mg/d)
Amitriptyline (5–25 mg/d)
Anticonvulsants
    Valproate (~10–14 mg/kg/d)
    Topiramate (1–10 mg/kg/d)
Beta-blockers (eg, propranolol)
Calcium channel blockers (eg, verapamil).

Abdominal migraine is characterized by episodic vague, midline, or periumbilical abdominal pain (**Box 6**). Abdominal migraine includes a subset of patients with chronic recurrent abdominal pain who have features that overlap with those of migraine without aura. Abdominal migraine generally occurs in school-aged children, who report recurrent attacks of midline or upper abdominal pain that is dull in nature and generally lasts for hours.

As with CVS, the key to this entity is to recognize the recurrent pattern of symptoms and to exclude other gastrointestinal or renal diseases by appropriate investigations. An up-to-date reference list for CVS and abdominal migraine is available on-line ([20]).

Benign paroxysmal torticollis is a rare paroxysmal dyskinesia characterized by attacks of head tilt alone or tilt accompanied by vomiting and ataxia that may last hours to days. Other tortional or dystonic features, including truncal or pelvic posturing, may be seen. Attacks first manifest during infancy between 2 and 8 months of age.

Paroxysmal torticollis is likely an early-onset variant of basilar migraine, but the differential diagnosis must include gastroesophogeal reflux (Sandifer syndrome), idiopathic torsional dystonia, and complex partial seizure. Particular attention must be paid to the posterior fossa and craniocervical junction, however, where congenital or acquired lesions may produce torticollis. Once the diagnosis is established and the benign nature is confirmed, there may be no requirement for treatment beyond reassurance.

Box 6
Diagnostic criteria for abdominal migraine description

An idiopathic recurrent disorder seen mainly in children and characterized by episodic midline abdominal pain manifesting in attacks lasting 1 to 72 hours with normality between episodes. The pain is of moderate to severe intensity and is associated with vasomotor symptoms, nausea, and vomiting.

Diagnostic criteria

A. At least five attacks fulfilling criteria B through D

B. Attacks of abdominal pain lasting 1 to 72 hours

C. Abdominal pain has all the following characteristics:

　　1. Midline location, periumbilical or poorly localized

　　2. Dull or "just sore" quality

　　3. Moderate or severe intensity

D. During abdominal pain, at least two of the following:

　　1. Anorexia

　　2. Nausea

　　3. Vomiting

　　4. Pallor

E. Not attributed to another disorder; history and physical examination do not show signs of gastrointestinal or renal disease, or such disease has been ruled out by appropriate investigations

---

OTHER UNUSUAL FORMS OF MIGRAINE IN CHILDHOOD

Alice in Wonderland syndrome represents the spectrum of migraine with aura, but the visual aura is quite atypical and may include bizarre visual illusions and spatial distortions preceding an otherwise nondescript headache. Affected patients describe distorted visual perceptions, such as micropsia, macropsia, metamorphopsia, teleopsia, and macro- or microsomatognopsia. The visual symptoms likely represent CSD and oligemia involving the parieto-occipital region heralding the headache.

Confusional migraine has perceptual distortions as a cardinal feature. Affected patients, usually boys, abruptly become agitated, restless, disoriented, and occasionally combative. The confusion phase may last minutes to hours. Later, once consciousness returns to baseline, the patients describe an inability to communicate, frustration, confusion, and loss of orientation to time, and they may not recall a headache phase at all. Confusional migraine often occurs after seemingly innocuous head injury occurring in sports (eg, soccer, football, skating). Clearly, any sudden unexplained alteration of consciousness after head injury warrants investigation for intracranial hemorrhage, drug intoxication, metabolic derangements, or epilepsy.

Clinically, confusional migraine most likely represents an overlap between hemiplegic migraine and BM. Patients who present with unilateral weakness or language disorders should be classified as having hemiplegic migraine, and patients with vertiginous or ataxic patterns should be classified as having BM.

Ophthalmoplegic migraine (OM) has been removed from the migraine spectrum into the group of "cranial neuralgias" as a result of elegant neuroimaging evidence demonstrating an underlying demyelinating-remyelinating mechanism. The key clinical feature is painful ophthalmoparesis. The pain may be a nondescript ocular or retro-ocular discomfort. Ptosis, limited adduction, and vertical displacement (eg, cranial nerve III) are the most common objective findings. The oculomotor symptoms and signs may appear well into the headache phase rather than heralding the headache, contrary to the sequence of typical migraine. The signs may persist for days or even weeks after the headache has resolved. Because OM is no longer viewed as migraine, eventually, the term *ophthalmoplegic migraine* is likely to evolve to *ophthalmoplegic neuralgia* or *neuralgiform disorder*.

The migraine precursors and these unusual forms of migraine with aura are unique to pediatrics and represent a challenging group of disorders characterized by the abrupt onset of focal neurologic signs and symptoms (eg, hemiparesis, altered consciousness nystagmus, ophthalmoparesis) followed by headache. Frequently, these ominous neurologic signs initially point the clinician in the direction of epileptic, cerebrovascular, traumatic, or metabolic disorders, and the migraine diagnosis become apparent only after thorough neurodiagnostic testing. Some of these entities occur in infants and young children, in whom a history is limited. Only after obtaining a careful history and performing a physical examination and appropriate neurodiagnostic studies can these diagnoses be comfortably entertained. All represent diagnoses of exclusion.

MANAGEMENT

Once the diagnosis of migraine is established, a balanced, flexible, and individually tailored treatment plan can be put in place. It is important to educate the patient and the family about the diagnosis of migraine and to provide reassurance about the absence of other life-threatening disorders. This essential explanation and reassurance can get the family "on board" with the treatment regimen; otherwise, all subsequent efforts are likely to be fruitless.

When developing the treatment plan, the first step is to appreciate the degree of disability imposed by the patient's headache. Understanding the impact of the headache on the quality of life can guide the decisions regarding the most appropriate therapeutic course.[21,22]

The fundamental goals of long-term migraine treatment have been established:[23]

1. Reduction of headache frequency, severity, duration, and disability
2. Reduction of reliance on poorly tolerated, ineffective, or unwanted acute pharmacotherapies
3. Improvement in the quality of life
4. Avoidance of acute headache medication escalation
5. Education and enablement of patients to manage their disease to enhance personal control of their migraine
6. Reduction of headache-related distress and psychologic symptoms

To achieve these goals, the treatment regimen must balance biobehavioral strategies and pharmacologic measures. Biobehavioral treatments include biofeedback, stress management, sleep hygiene, exercise, and dietary modifications (**Box 7**). The value of these interventions cannot be overstated. Virtually all migraine sufferers can benefit from review of these measures; however, certainly, in patients who have more frequent attacks, even daily migraine, and a greater degree of disability, there is a greater need to reinforce the following measures. Biofeedback and stress management, which are underused therapies, have been subjected to controlled trials and have been reviewed recently.[24]

Box 7
Biobehavioral therapies for pediatric migraine

Identification of migraine triggers

Biobehavioral

Biofeedback

Electromyographic biofeedback

Electroencephalography

Thermal hand warming

Galvanic skin resistance feedback

Relaxation therapy

Progressive muscle relaxation

Autogenic training

Meditation

Passive relaxation

Self-hypnosis

Cognitive therapy/stress management

Cognitive control

Guided imagery

Dietary measures

"Avoidance diets"

Caffeine moderation

Herbs

Butterbur root

Feverfew (*Tanacetum parthenium*)

Ginkgo

Valerian root

Minerals

Magnesium

Vitamins

Riboflavin

Acupuncture

Aroma therapy

The basic recommendations given to migraine sufferers include regular sleep and exercise, moderation of caffeine intake, and adequate hydration. The role of diet remains controversial.[25] Somewhere between 7% and 44% of patients report that a particular food or drink can precipitate a migraine attack.[26,27] In children, the principal dietary triggers are cheese, chocolates, and citrus fruits. Wholesale dietary elimination of a list of foods is, however, not recommended. Elimination diets are excessive and set the stage for a battleground at home when parents attempt to enforce a restrictive diet on an unwilling resistant adolescent. The ensuing family friction may ultimately heightened tensions at home, worsening the headache pattern. A more reasonable approach is to review the list of foods thought to be linked to migraine and encourage the patient to keep a headache diary to see if a temporal relation exists between ingestion of one or more of those foods and the development of headache. If a link is discovered, common sense dictates avoidance of the offending food substance.

Within **Box 7** are included some of the complementary and alternative treatment measures for pediatric and adult migraine. Few have been subjected to controlled trials in children, but they have become commonly used and recommended on patient education Web sites. Magnesium ($\sim$400–800 mg/d) and riboflavin ($\sim$400 mg/d) have demonstrated efficacy in controlled prophylaxis trials and are currently recommended for the prevention of migraine in adults.[28] Data regarding other herbal remedies are limited in children. Butterbur root, for example, was compared with placebo and music therapy, and only music therapy showed superiority compared with placebo during the trial period; however, during extended follow-up, music therapy and butterbur root showed value.[29]

An intriguing study was conducted by Hershey and colleagues[30] to explore the value of coenzyme Q10 (CoQ10) in the management of migraine. These researchers measured the levels of CoQ10 in 1550 children and found that 33% had values less than the reference range. These patients were supplemented with CoQ10 at a rate of 1 to 3 mg/kg/d, and in follow-up, their headache frequency improved from 19 ($\pm$10) to 12 ($\pm$11) per month (P<.001). These investigators proposed that CoQ10 deficiency may be a common phenomenon in children with frequent migraine.[30] This clearly warrants further study.

Overuse of "over-the-counter" analgesics (more than five times per week) can be a contributing factor to frequent, even daily, headache patterns. When recognized, patients who are overusing analgesics must be educated to discontinue the practice. Retrospective studies have suggested that this recommendation alone can decrease headache frequency.[31,32]

The pharmacologic management of pediatric migraine has been subjected to thorough review, but controlled data are, unfortunately, limited; therefore, recommendations are all "off-label."[33–37]

Acute treatments represent the mainstay of migraine management. The patient should be offered several acute treatment options to explore after the initial office visit so that he or she may determine what works most effectively. Regardless of the acute treatment selected, there are several basic guidelines regarding the use of acute treatments that must be included as part of the patient's educational process. The essential message is to give enough and to give it early.

1. Take the medicine as soon as possible when the headache begins (within 20–30 minutes).
2. Take the appropriate dose; do not "baby" the headache.
3. Have the medicine available at the location where the patient usually has his or her headaches (eg, school), and complete the school medicine forms.
4. Avoid analgesic overuse (more than three doses of analgesic per week).

For the acute treatment of migraine, the most rigorously studied agents are ibuprofen, acetaminophen, and selected "triptans" (eg, rizatriptan and almotriptan tablets, sumatriptan and zolmitriptan nasal sprays), which have shown safety and efficacy in controlled trials (**Table 2**). Although the triptans have revolutionized acute migraine treatment for adults, none have been approved by the FDA for use in children and adolescents, even though multiple studies have demonstrated the safety of their use in children.[38,39]

Table 2
Evidence summary for treatment of acute attacks of migraine in children and adolescents

Drug	Class	Study Design	n	Age (Years)	Primary End Point	Efficacy	Placebo Response	Clinical Impression of Effect[a]	Adverse Effects	Reference
NSAIDs and nonopiate analgesics										
Ibuprofen	II	DBPC	88	4–16	HA response	68%	37%	+++	Infrequent	45
	II	DBPC	84	6–12	HA response	76%	53%	+++	Infrequent	46
	II	DBPCCO	32	10–17	HA relief	69%	28%	+++		63
Acetaminophen	II	DBPC	88	4–16	HA response	54%	37%	++	Infrequent	45
Triptans (serotonin$_{1B/1D}$ receptor agonists)										
Nasal spray	II	OL	58	4–11	HA relief	78%	—	++	Occasional to frequent	64
Sumatriptan	III	DBPC	14	6–10	HA response	86%	43%	+++		41
Zolmitriptan	I	DBPC	510	12–17	2-hour HA response	63%–66%	53%	+++		39
	I	SB-DBPC	171	12–17	1-hour HA response	58%	43%	+++		42
Oral triptans										
Naratriptan	I	DBPC	300	12–17	4-hour HA relief	64%–72%	65%	O	Occasional	65
Rizatriptan	I	DBPC	296	12–17	2-hour pain relief	66%	56%	++	Occasional	66
	I	DBPC	96	6–17	2-hour HA relief	74%	36%			43
Sumatriptan	I	DBPC	302	12–17	2-hour pain relief	NA	NA	0	Occasional	68
Sumatriptan	II	DBPCCO	23	8–16	2 hour >50% decrease	34%	21%	0	Occasional	67
Zolmitriptan	IV	OL	38	12–17	HA improvement	88%	—	+	Occasional	69
	II	DBPCCO	32	11–17	2-hour pain relief	62%	28%	++		63
	I	DBPC	850	12–17	2-hour HA response	53%–57%	58%	0		70
Eletriptan	II	DBPC	267	12–17	2-hour HA response	57%	57%	0	Occasional	71
Almotriptan	IV	OL	15	11–17	HA reduction	85%	—	+	Occasional	72
	I	DBPC	866	12–17	2-hour pain relief	67%	55%	++		44
Sumatriptan	IV	OL	17	6–16	HA response	64%	—	+	Occasional	73
Subcutaneous	IV	OL	50	6–18	HA response	78%	—	+	Frequent 80%	74

Abbreviations: DBPC, double blind placebo-controlled; DBPCCO, double blind placebo-controlled crossover; HA, headache; IV, intravenous; NSAID, nonsteroidal anti-inflammatory drug; OL, open-label; SB, single blind.

[a] Clinical impression of effect: O, ineffective: most patients get no improvement; +, somewhat effective: few patients get clinically significant improvement; ++, effective, some patients get clinically significant improvement; +++, very effective: most patients get clinically significant improvement.

Data from Refs. 63–74.

Only sumatriptan (5 and 20 mg) and zolmitriptan (5 mg) in the nasal spray form and rizatriptan (5 and 10 mg) and almotriptan (6.25, 12.5, and 25 mg) in the tablet form have demonstrated safety and efficacy in controlled trials in adolescents 12 to 17 years of age.[40–45] For young children less than 12 years of age, ibuprofen (7.5–10 mg/kg) and acetaminophen (15 mg/kg) have demonstrated efficacy and safety for the acute treatment of migraine.[46,47] Combination agents, such as sumatriptan, 85 mg, plus naproxen, 550 mg, have demonstrated efficacy in adults, but their utility in adolescents has not yet been demonstrated.[48]

A diverse group of medications is used to prevent attacks of migraine, and it is useful to become comfortable with a few of these agents. Their use should, however, be limited to those patients whose headaches occur with sufficient frequency or severity as to warrant a daily treatment program. Most clinical studies require a minimum of three headaches per month to justify a daily agent. A clear sense of functional disability must be established before committing to a course of daily medication. It is also useful to identify the presence of "comorbid conditions" (eg, depression, obesity), which may suggest the relative benefit of one agent over another.

Once preventive treatment is initiated, patience must be encouraged to permit enough time for the beneficial effects to be appreciated. Generally, an 8- to 12-week course is necessary before success or failure can be determined. This point must be emphasized at the time the prescriptions are provided, because many impatient families expect immediate effects after the first days of treatment. The author sees many patients in his practice who have "failed" multiple prophylactic courses, only to find that the therapeutic trials lasted for only a few days each.

The duration of treatment is controversial. In recognition of the cyclic nature of migraine, the daily agents should be used for a finite period. The general recommendation is to provide treatment through the calendar school year and then to eliminate daily agents gradually during summer vacation. Another option in younger children is to use a shorter course (eg, 6–8 weeks), followed by slow weaning off the medicine.

For preventive or prophylactic treatment in the population of children and adolescents who have frequent disabling migraine, flunarizine, unavailable in the United States, has established and reproducible efficacy data, but encouraging data are emerging regarding several antiepileptic agents, such as topiramate, disodium valproate, and levetiracetam, in addition to the antihistamine cyproheptadine and the antidepressant amitriptyline (**Table 3**).[49–51]

For children younger than the age of 10 years who do not have problems related to being overweight, cyproheptadine at a starting dose of 2 to 4 mg as a single bedtime dose is a simple and safe strategy. The dose may gradually be elevated to two or even three times a day; however, in the author's experience, most children become too sedated at doses much higher than 4 to 8 mg/d.

Amitriptyline has never been assessed in controlled fashion but remains one of the most widely used agents. Starting doses of 5 to 10 mg at bedtime may gradually be increased toward 1 mg/kg/d. Controversy exists as to whether or not a pretreatment electrocardiogram (ECG) is warranted, but the author generally does not order an ECG for children on low doses (10–25 mg).

Topiramate is gaining wide acceptance, and mounting evidence, based on well-designed controlled trials, supports its use. A 26-week trial of 50-, 100-, and 200-mg doses of topiramate found a reduction in monthly migraine frequency of 46%, 63%, and 65%, respectively, versus 16% with placebo.[52] A second trial evenly randomized 44 children to receive 100 mg divided twice a day versus placebo and found a reduction in the mean monthly migraine attacks from 16 per month to 4 per month in the treatment group versus 13 per month to 8 per month in the placebo group ($P = .025$).[53] In that study,

Table 3
Summary of evidence for the preventive therapies for migraine in children and adolescents

Drug	Class	Study Design	n	Age (Years)	Primary End Point	Efficacy	Placebo Response	Clinical Impression of Effect[a]	Adverse Effects	Reference
Antiepileptics										
Divalproex sodium/ sodium valproate	IV	OL	42	7–16	HA/month	81%	—	+	Occasional to frequent	55
	IV	OL	10	9–17	HA/month	83%	—	+		75
	IV	OL	23	7–17	HA/month	65% > 50% reduction	—	+		76
Gabapentin	IV	Retrospect OL	18	6–17	HA freq/month	83% > 50% reduction	—	++	Occasional to frequent	77
Topiramate	II	DBPC	44	9–17	HA/month	75%	38%	++	Occasional to frequent	53
	I	DBPC	51	12–17	HA/month	54%–67%	42%	+++		52
	I	DBPC	85	12–17	HA/month	76%	45%	+++		54
Levetiracetam	IV	OL	20	6–17	HA/month	90%	—	+	Occasional to frequent	56
	IV	OL	19	Mean 12	HA/month	67%	—	+		57
Zonisamide	IV	OL	12	Mean 13	HA/month	75%	—	+	Occasional	58
Antidepressants										
Trazodone	II	DBPC	35	7–18	HA freq	45%	40%	0	Occasional to frequent	78
Pizotifen	II	DBPCCO	47	7–14	HA/month	15%	16%	0	Occasional to frequent	91
Tricyclic antidepressants										
Amitriptyline	IV	OL	192	9–15	HA freq/month	84%	—	++	Occasional to frequent	79
	IV	OL	73	3–18	HA freq/month	89%	—	++		80
Antihistamines										
Cyproheptadine	II	DBPC	68[a]	17–53	% improve	75%	—	++	Occasional to frequent	81
	IV	Retrospective	30	3–18	HA/month	62%	—	++		80

Calcium channel blockers										
Flunarezine	II	DBPC	42	7–14	>50% improve HA/month	76%	19%	+++	Occasional	82
		DBPCCO	63	5–11		67%	33%	+++		83
Nimodipine	II	DBPCCO	37	7–18	HA/month	15%	16%	O	Occasional	92
Antihypertensive agents										
Propranolol	II	DBPC	39	3–12	HA freq	58%	55%	O	Occasional to frequent	84
	II	DBCO	28	7–16	HA freq	71%	10%	++		85
	II	DBPC	28	6–12	HA freq	NS	NS	O		86
Timolol	II	DBPCCO	19	6–13	HA/month	38%	40%	O	Occasional	87
Clonidine	II	DBPC	43	7–14	HA/6 weeks	NS	NS	O	Occasional to frequent	88
	II	DBPC	54	<15	HA/month	40%	65%	O		89
NSAIDs										
Naproxen sodium	III	DBPC	10	6–17	HA freq	60%	40%	+	Occasional	90

Abbreviations: DBPC, double blind placebo-controlled; DBPCCO, double blind placebo-controlled crossover; freq, frequency; HA, headache; IV intravenous; NSAID, nonsteroidal anti-inflammatory drug; OL, open-label; NS, not significant.

[a] Clinical impression of effect: O, ineffective: most patients get no improvement; +, somewhat effective: few patients get clinically significant improvement; ++, effective: some patients get clinically significant improvement; +++, very effective: most patients get clinically significant improvement.

Data from Refs. [75–92]

there was a significant reduction in overall disability and school absenteeism. A third recent report comparing 50 mg/d versus 100 mg/d versus matched placebo found a statistically significant improvement from the prospective baseline period in migraine frequency with the 100-mg dose (75% decrease in monthly migraines) but not with the 50-mg dose (46% decrease in monthly migraines) or in the placebo group (45%) ($P = .016$). The most benefit was appreciated in 100-mg group (50 mg administered orally twice a day), in which it was observed that more than 80% of patients experienced a greater than 50% reduction in headache burden after approximately 8 weeks of treatment.[54]

Typically, for teenagers, a 15- to 25-mg dose of topiramate is initiated as a single bedtime dose and then gradually titrated toward 50 mg twice a day incrementally on a weekly or every-other-week basis. Clinical experience has demonstrated that many patients respond to doses as low as 25 mg given at bedtime; thus, it is valuable to "titrate to effect." Cognitive effects must be monitored quite carefully, and more evidence is needed to assess the educational impact of topiramate for prevention of adolescent migraine. It is counterproductive to reduce the headache burden at the expense of academic performance.

Divalproex sodium has strong efficacy data in adults and is approved for use as a migraine preventative agent, but no controlled trials exist in children or adults. Open-label trials have had success. In one study of 42 children (aged 7–16 years, mean age = 11.3 years), a 50% headache reduction was seen in 78.5%, a 75% headache reduction was seen in 14.2%, and 9.5% of patients became headache-free. These open-label results indicated that divalproex sodium was an effective and well-tolerated treatment for the prophylaxis of migraine in children.[55]

Likewise, levetiracetam has open-label data from 19 patients (mean age = 11.9 years) whose mean migraine frequency fell from 6.3 migraines per month to 1.7 per month at doses of 125 to 250 mg given twice a day. Ten patients (52.6%) had complete resolution of headache. The investigators concluded that levetiracetam seemed to be a promising candidate for well-controlled clinical trials of pediatric patients who have migraine.[56] A second open-label trial of 20 patients found that 18 of 20 patients had a 50% or greater reduction in monthly migraine frequency and had lowered disability scale scores at doses of approximately 20 mg/kg/d.[57]

In one small open-label study in children (10–17 years of age) with mixed refractory headache conditions (50% migraine), the children were treated with zonisamide at an average dose of 6 mg/kg/d.[58] Two thirds of the children had a greater than 50% reduction in headache frequency from baseline.

PROGNOSIS

The long-term prognosis of adolescents who have migraine has not been well studied. Five- to 7-year follow-up studies revealed that 20% to 25% of adolescents originally diagnosed with migraine have remission of symptoms, 50% to 60% have persistence of their migraine with aura, and 25% convert to tension-type headache (TTH). Twenty percent who originally had TTH converted to migraine.[59,60] Monastero and colleagues[61] evaluated 55 adolescents with migraine who were available for 10 years of follow-up and found that 42% had persistent migraine, 38% had experienced remission, and 20% had transformed to TTH. Interestingly, only migraine without aura persisted through the 10-year follow-up period, whereas other migrainous disorders and nonclassifiable headaches did not. The longest follow-up available came from Brna and colleagues,[62] with 20-year information on 60 members of an original cohort of 95 from 1983. Of the 60, 27% were headache-free, 33% had TTH, 17%

had migraine, and 23% had TTH and migraine. Of those with persistent headache, 80% described their headaches as moderate to severe, although an overall improvement was described in 66%. TTH was more likely to remit. Headache severity at diagnosis was the most predictive of headache outcome at 20 years. These data indicate that female gender, migraine severity at diagnosis, and longer duration from time of onset of headache until time of initial medical examination tended toward an unfavorable prognosis. Given our current understanding of the long-term neuropathologic and psychosocial consequences of persistent frequent migraine, further longitudinal epidemiologic study of the evolution of adolescent migraine is imperative.

SUMMARY

Migraine is a common disorder in children and adolescents. There is a wide spectrum of clinical forms, but the most frequent form is migraine without aura, which is characterized by attacks of frontal or bitemporal pounding and nauseating headache lasting 1 to 72 hours. A fascinating and challenging subset known as migraine with aura and the periodic syndromes can be associated with frightening focal neurologic disturbances and may require careful consideration for the possibility of neoplastic, vascular, metabolic, or toxic disorders.

Migraine treatment philosophy now embraces a balanced approach with biobehavioral interventions and pharmacologic measures. Treatment decisions must be based on the disability produced by the headaches, the headache burden. A growing body of controlled pediatric data is beginning to emerge regarding the acute and preventative agents, lessening our dependence on extrapolated adult data.

In the near future, we anticipate further advances in understanding the molecular genetics of migraine, advances that should translate to improved care of the pediatric patient who has migraine headache. Furthermore, therapeutic energy expended for our pediatric patients should translate to decreased disability as our patients progress into adulthood, lessening the lifespan burden of migraine.

APPENDIX

Box A1

American Academy of Neurology evidence classification scheme for a therapeutic article and linkage to level of recommendation (2003 version)

Rating of therapeutic article

Class I: prospective, randomized controlled, clinical trial with masked outcome assessment, in a representative population

Class II: prospective matched group cohort study in a representative population with masked outcome assessment that meets a through d or a randomized clinical trial in a representative population that lacks one criterion

Class III: all other controlled trials in a representative population, in which outcome is independently assessed or independently derived by objective outcome measurement

Class IV: evidence from uncontrolled studies, case series, case reports, or expert opinion

In exceptional cases, one convincing class I study may suffice for an "A" recommendation if (1) all criteria are met, (2) there is a magnitude of effect of 5 or greater, and (3) there are narrow confidence intervals (lower limit >2).

REFERENCES

1. Bigal ME, Lipton RB. The prognosis of migraine. Curr Opin Neurol 2008;21:301–8.
2. Bille B. Migraine in school children. Acta Paediatr 1962;136(51 Suppl):1–151.
3. Deubner DC. An epidemiologic study of migraine and headache in 10–20 year olds. Headache 1977;17:173–80.
4. Sillanpaa M. Changes in the prevalence of migraine and other headache during the first seven school years. Headache 1983;23:15–9.
5. Dalsgaard-Nielsen T. Some aspects of the epidemiology of migraine in Denmark. Headache 1970;10:14–23.
6. Laurell K, Larsson B, Eeg-Olofsson O. Prevalence of headache in Swedish school-children, with a focus on tension-type headache. Cephalalgia 2004;24:380–8.
7. Lipton RB, Silberstein SD, Stewart WF. An update on the epidemiology of migraine. Headache 1994;34:319–28.
8. Mortimer MJ, Kay J, Jaron A. Epidemiology of headache and childhood migraine in an urban general practice using ad hoc, Vahlquist and IHS criteria. Dev Med Child Neurol 1992;34:1095–101.
9. Valquist B. Migraine in children. Int Arch Allergy 1955;7:348–55.
10. Small P, Waters WE. Headache and migraine in a comprehensive school. In: Waters WE, editor. The epidemiology of migraine. Bracknell-Berkshire, England: Boehringer Ingel-helm, Ltd; 1974. p. 56–67.
11. Sillanpaa M. Prevalence of migraine and other headache in Finnish children starting school. Headache 1976;15:288–90.
12. Stewart WF, Linet MS, Celentano DD, et al. Age and sex-specific incidence rates of migraine with and without visual aura. Am J Epidemiol 1991;34:1111–20.
13. Stewart WF, Lipton RB, Celentano DD, et al. Prevalence of migraine headache in the United States. JAMA 1992;267:64–9.
14. Available at: www.i.h.s.org. Accessed January 12, 2009.
15. Hachinski VC, Porchawka J, Steele JC, et al. Visual symptoms in the migraine syndrome. Neurol 1973;23:570–9.
16. Parisi P, villa MP, Pelliccia A, et al. Panayiotopoulos syndrome: diagnosis and management. Neurol Sci 2007;28:72–9.
17. Kirchmann M, Thomsen LL, Olesen J. Basilar-type migraine; clinical, epidemio-logic, and genetic features. Neurology 2006;66:880–6.
18. DeFusco M, Marconi R, Silvestri L, et al. Haploinsufficiency of ATP1A2 encoding Na+/K+ pump alpha-2 subunit associated familial hemiplegic migraine, type 2. Nat Genet 2003;33:192–6.
19. Dichgans M, Freilinger T, Eckstein G, et al. Mutation in the neuronal voltage-gated sodium channel SCN1A in familial hemiplegic migraine. Lancet 2005;366:371–7.
20. Available at: www.cvsaonline.org. Accessed January 12, 2009.
21. Powers S, Patton S, Hommel K, et al. Quality of life in childhood migraine: clinical aspects and comparison to other chronic illness. Pediatrics 2003;112:e1–5.
22. Powers S, Patton S, Hommell K, et al. Quality of life in paediatric migraine: charac-terization of age-related effects using PedsQL 4.0. Cephalalgia 2004;24:120–7.
23. Silberstein SD. Practice parameter: evidence-based guidelines for migraine headache (an evidence-based review). Neurology 2000;55:754–62.
24. Trautmann E, Lackschewitz H, Kröner-Herwig B. Psychological treatment of recurrent headache in children and adolescents–a meta-analysis. Cephalalgia 2006;26(12):1411–26.
25. Millichap J, Yee M. The diet factor in pediatric and adolescent migraine. Pediatr Neurosci 2003;28:9–15.

26. Stang P, Yanagihar P, Swanson J, et al. Incidence of migraine headache: a population based study in Olmsted Country, Minnesota. Neurology 1992;42:1657–62.
27. Van den Bergh V, Amery W, Waelkens J. Trigger factors in migraine: a study conducted by the Belgian Migraine Society. Headache 1987;27:191–6.
28. Schurks M, Diener HC, Goadsby P. Update on the prophylaxis of migraine. Curr Treat Options Neurol 2008;10:20–9.
29. Oelker A. Butterbur root extract and music therapy in the prevention of childhood migraine: an explorative study. Eur J Pain 2008;12:301–13.
30. Hershey AD, Powers SW, Vockell AL, et al. Coenzyme Q10 deficiency and response to supplementation in pediatric and adolescent migraine. Headache 2007;47:73–80.
31. Reimschisel T. Breaking the cycle of medication overuse headache. Contemp Pediatr 2003;20:101–14.
32. Rothner A, Guo Y. An analysis of headache types, over-the-counter (OTC) medication overuse and school absences in a pediatric/adolescent headache clinic. Headache 2004;44:490.
33. Lewis D, Ashwal S, Hershey A, et al. Practice parameter: pharmacological treatment of migraine headache in children and adolescents. Neurology 2004;63:2215–24.
34. Victor S, Ryan S. Drugs for preventing migraine headaches in children. Cochrane Database Syst Rev 2003;4:CD002761.
35. Lewis DW, Yonker M, Winner P, et al. The treatment of pediatric migraine. Pediatr Ann 2005;34:448–60.
36. Hamalainen ML. Migraine in children and adolescents; a guide to drug treatment. CNS Drugs 2006;20:813–20.
37. Gunner KB, Smith HD, Ferguson LE. Practice guideline for the diagnosis and management of migraine headaches in children and adolescents: part two. J Pediatr Health Care 2008;22:52–9.
38. Major P, Grubisa H, Thie N. Triptans for the treatment of acute pediatric migraine: a systematic literature review. Pediatric Neurology 2003;29:425–9.
39. Silver S, Gano D, Gerretsen P. Acute treatment of paediatric migraine; a meta-analysis of efficacy. J Paediatr Child Health 2008;44:3–9.
40. Winner P, Rothner AD, Saper J, et al. A randomized, double-blind, placebo-controlled study of sumatriptan nasal spray in the treatment of acute migraine in adolescents. Pediatrics 2000;106:989–97.
41. Ahonen K, Hamalainen ML, Rantala H, et al. Nasal sumatriptan is effective in the treatment of migraine attacks in children. Neurology 2004;62:883–7.
42. Ueberall M. Sumatriptan in paediatric and adolescent migraine. Cephalalgia 2001;21(Suppl 1):21–4.
43. Lewis DW, Winner P, Hershey AD, et al. Efficacy of zolmitriptan nasal spray in adolescent migraine. Pediatrics 2007;120:390–6.
44. Ahonen K, Hämäläinen ML, Eerola M, et al. A randomized trial of rizatriptan in migraine attacks in children. Neurology 2006;67:1135–40.
45. Linder SL, Mathew NT, Cady RK, et al. Efficacy and tolerability of almotriptan in adolescents; a randomized, double-blind, placebo-controlled trial. Headache 2008;48:1326–36.
46. Hamalainen ML, Hoppu K, Valkeila E, et al. Ibuprofen or acetaminophen for the acute treatment of migraine in children: a double-blind, randomized, placebo-controlled, crossover study. Neurology 1997;48:102–7.
47. Lewis DW, Kellstein D, Burke B, et al. Children's ibuprofen suspension for the acute treatment of pediatric migraine headache. Headache 2002;42:780–6.

48. Brandes JL, Kudrow D, Stark SR, et al. Sumatriptan-naproxen for acute treatment of migraine: a randomized trial. JAMA 2007;297:1443–54.
49. Hershey AD, Powers SW, Vockell AL, et al. Effectiveness of topiramate in the prevention of childhood headache. Headache 2002;42:810–8.
50. Serdaroglu G, Erhan E, Tekgul H, et al. Sodium valproate prophylaxis in childhood migraine. Headache 2002;42:819–22.
51. Eiland LS, Jenkins LS, Durham SH. Pediatric migraine; pharmacological agents for prophylaxis. Ann Pharmacother 2007;41:1181–90.
52. Damen L, Bruijn J, Verhagen AP, et al. Prophylactic treatment of migraine in children. A systematic review of pharmacological trials. Cephalalgia 2006;26: 497–505.
53. Winner P, Gendolla A, Stayer C, et al. Topiramate for migraine prevention in adolescents: a pooled analysis of efficacy and safety. Headache 2006;46:1503–10.
54. Lakshmi CV, Singhi P, Malhi P, et al. Topiramate in the prophylaxis of pediatric migraine; a double-blind placebo-controlled trial. J Child Neurol 2007;22:829–35.
55. Lewis D, Winner P, Saper J, et al. A randomized, double-blind, placebo-controlled study to evaluate the efficacy and safety of topiramate for migraine prevention in pediatric subjects 12 to 17 years of age. Headache 2008; 48(suppl 1):S8–9.
56. Caruso JM, Brown WD, Exil G, et al. The efficacy of divalproex sodium in the prophylactic treatment of children with migraine. Headache 2000;40:672–6.
57. Miller GS. Efficacy and safety of levetiracetam in pediatric migraine. Headache 2004;44:238–43.
58. Pakalnis A, Kring D, Meier L. Levetiracetam prophylaxis in pediatric migraine—an open label study. Headache 2007;47:427–30.
59. Pakalnis A, Kring D. Zonisamide prophylaxis in refractory pediatric headache. Headache 2006;46:804–7.
60. Camarda R, Monastero R, Santangela G, et al. Migraine headaches in adolescents: a five year follow up study. Headache 2002;42:1000–5.
61. Kienbacher C, Wober C, Zesch HE, et al. Clinical features, classification and prognosis of migraine and tension-type headache in children and adolescents: a long term follow up study. Cephalalgia 2006;26:820–30.
62. Monastero R, Camarda C, Pipia C, et al. Prognosis of migraine headaches in adolescents; a 10 year follow-up study. Neurology 2006;67:1353–6.
63. Brna P, Dooley J, Gordon K, et al. The prognosis of childhood headache; a 20 year follow up study. Arch Pediatr Adolesc Med. 2005;158:1157–60.
64. Evers S, Rahmann A, Kraemer C, et al. Treatment of childhood migraine attacks with oral zolmitriptan and ibuprofen. Neurol 2006;67:497–9.
65. Ueberal MA, Wenzel D. Intranasal sumatriptan for the acute treatment of migraine in children. Neurol 1999;52:1507–10.
66. Rothner A, Edwards K, Kerr L, et al. Efficacy and safety of naratriptan tablets in adolescent migraine. J Neurol Sci 1997;150:S106.
67. Winner P, Lewis D, Visser H, et al. Rizatriptan 5 mg for the acute treatment of migraine in adolescents; a randomized double blind placebo controlled study. Headache 2002;42:49–55.
68. Hamalainen M, Hoppu K, Santavuori P. Sumatriptan for migraine attacks in children: a randomized placebo controlled study. Neurol 1997;48:1100–3.
69. Winner P, Prensky A, Linder S, et al. Adolescent migraine: efficacy and safety of sumatriptan tablets. J Neurol Sci 1997;150(Suppl):S172.
70. Linder S, Dowson A. Zolmitriptan provides effective migraine relief in adolescents. Int J Clin Pract 2000;54:466–9.

71. Rothner A, Wasiewski W, Winner P, et al. Zolmitriptan oral tablets in migraine treatment; high placebo response responses in adolescents. Headache 2006;46: 101–9.
72. Winner P, Linder S, Lipton R, et al. Eletriptan for the acute treatment of migraine in adolescents: results of a double blind, placebo controlled trial. Headache 2007; 47:511–8.
73. Charles J. Almotriptan in the acute treatment of migraine in patients 12–17 years old; an open label pilot study of efficacy and safety. J Headache Pain 2006;7:95–7.
74. MacDonald JT. Treatment of juvenile migraine with subcutaneous sumatriptan. Headache 1994;34:581–2.
75. Linder S. Subcutaneous sumatriptan in the clinical setting: the first 50 consecutive patients with acute migraine in the pediatric neurology office practice. Headache 1996;36:419–22.
76. Pakalnis A, Greenberg G, Drake ME, et al. Pediatric migraine prophylaxis with divalproex. J Child Neurol 2001;16:731–4.
77. Belman A, Milazo M, Savatic M. Gabapentin for migraine prophylaxis in children. Ann Neurol 2001;50(suppl 1):s109.
78. Battistella P, Ruffilli R, Baldin L, et al. Trazodone nella profilassi farmacologica dell'emicrania in eta evolutiva. Giorn Neuropsich Eta Evol 1993;13:179–86.
79. Hershey AD, Powers SW, Bentti AL, et al. Effectiveness of amitriptyline in the prophylactic management of childhood headaches. Headache 2000;40:539–49.
80. Lewis D, Diamond S, Scott D, et al. Prophylactic treatment of pediatric migraine. Headache 2004;44:230–7.
81. Rao BS, Das DG, Taraknath VR, et al. A double blind controlled study of propranolol and cyproheptadine in migraine prophylaxis. Neurol India 2000;48:223–6.
82. Sorge F, Marano E. Flunarizine v. placebo in childhood migraine. A double-blind study. Cephalalgia 1985;5(suppl 2):145–8.
83. Sorge F, DeSimone R, Marano E, et al. Flunarizine in prophylaxis of childhood migraine. Cephalalgia 1988;8:1–6.
84. Forsythe W, Gillies D, Sills M. Propranolol in the treatment of childhood migraine. Dev Med Child Neuroll 1984;26:737–41.
85. Ludvigsson J. Propranolol used in prophylaxis of migraine in children. Acta Neurol Scand 1974;50:109–15.
86. Olness K, MacDonald JT, Uden DL. Comparison of self-hypnosis and propranolol in the treatment of juvenile classic migraine. Pediatr 1987;79:593–7.
87. Noronha MJ. Double blind randomized cross-over trial of timolol in migraine prophylaxis in children. Cephalalgia 1985;5(suppl 3):174–5.
88. Sills M, Congdon P, Forsythe I. Clonidine and childhood migraine; a pilot and double blind study. Dev Med Child Neurol 1982;24:837–41.
89. Sillanpaa M. Clonidine prophylaxis of childhood migraine and other vascular headache. A double blind study of 57 children. Headache 1977;17:28–31.
90. Lewis D, Middlebrook M, Deline C. Naproxen sodium for chemoprophylaxis of adolescent migraine. Ann Neurol 1994;36:542.
91. Gillies D, Sills M, Forsythe I. Pizotifen in childhood migraine. A double blind controlled trial. Eur Neurol 1986;25:32–5.
92. Battistella P, Ruffilli R, Moro R, et al. A placebo controlled trial of nimodipine in pediatric migraine. Headache 1990;30:264–8.

Migraine in Women

Christine L. Lay, MD[a],*, Susan W. Broner, MD[b]

KEYWORDS

- Women • Migraine • Menstrual migraine • Hormonal
- Management

As noted, after puberty there is an emerging female predominance in migraineurs, and thus adolescence can be a time of troublesome headaches, with an overall estimate of 5% to 10% of children being afflicted with migraine. Many practitioners miss the diagnosis of migraine at this stage in a young woman's life. As women grow older, and headache patterns become more established, migraine may be more identifiable and more accurately diagnosed, but yet still not treated adequately. Changes in the hormonal milieu can impact migraine in women, and these hormonal changes occur not only monthly, triggering menstrual migraine, but there are also numerous other times in a woman's life when endogenous or exogenous changes in estrogen will impact her migraines. These changes in estrogen may be more predictable as in pregnancy or quite unpredictable as in the chaotic changes in estrogen levels occurring in puberty or in the years leading to menopause. Because gender is a risk factor for chronification of headache, with women more commonly affected with chronic daily headache than men, educational efforts, accurate diagnosis, and appropriate intervention are critical.

MENSTRUAL MIGRAINE

As early as 1666, menstrual migraine (MM) was described by Johannis Van der Linden,[1] who wrote about a one-sided headache associated with nausea and vomiting, occurring monthly during the menstrual flow of the Marchioness of Brandenburg. In modern times, close to 60% of women migraneurs experience menstrually related migraines.[2] MM develops most frequently in the second decade of life, around the onset of menarche, and prevalence peaks around age forty; as menopause approaches prevalence declines.[3] Migraine attacks may occur before, during, or after menstruation, but attacks associated with menstruation are often more severe, of longer duration, and less responsive to both acute and prophylactic treatment than migraines occurring at other times of the cycle.[4–6]

Pure menstrual migraine (PPM) affects 10% to 14% of women with migraine and refers to attacks occurring exclusively on days 1 ± 2 (ie, days -2 to +3 of menstruation)

[a] Department of Medicine, Division of Neurology, Centre For Headache, Women's College Hospital, 76 Grenville Street, Toronto, Ontario, Canada M5S 1B2
[b] Department of Neurology, St. Luke's-Roosevelt Hospital, 1000 Tenth Avenue, Suite 1C-10, New York, NY 10019, USA
* Corresponding author.
E-mail address: christine.lay@wchospital.ca (C.L. Lay).

Neurol Clin 27 (2009) 503–511
doi:10.1016/j.ncl.2009.01.002
0733-8619/09/$ – see front matter © 2009 Elsevier Inc. All rights reserved.

in at least two out of three cycles and at no other time of the month.[7–9] Menstrually related migraine (MRM) affects over 50% of women who have migraine and by definition migraines occur not only in the perimenstrual period as described, but also at other times of the month. By definition, menstrual migraine (both PMM and MRM) is migraine without aura, although a patient who have MRM may experience aura during migraine attacks outside the menstrual period.[7,8] Both MRM and PMM typically occur from 2 days before, through the first 3 days of the cycle, with an increased severity and prevalence of nausea and vomiting. The highest risk of migraine is during the first three days of the cycle.[4] It is important to distinguish premenstrual headache from MM. Premenstrual headache occurs earlier in the cycle, typically 2 to 7 days before the onset of menses and may be part of premenstrual syndrome (PMS). Whereas MM begins around the onset of menses, headache associated with PMS usually resolves with the onset of menstruation.[10]

Pathophysiology of Menstrual Migraine

Throughout a woman's life, from puberty through menopause, there is a constant cycling of ovarian function under the influence of hypothalamic-secreted gonadotropin-releasing hormone (GnRH), pituitary-secreted luteinizing hormone (LH), and follicle- stimulating hormone (FSH), leading to the ovarian secretion of estrogen and progesterone. The luteal phase is key in triggering migraine, when, in the event of a lack of fertilization and implantation, there is an abrupt drop in both estrogen and progesterone levels, heralding menstruation. This drop in estrogen is felt to be an important trigger in MM.[11,12] This fall in estrogen may in some yet-to-be described fashion prime blood vessels to be more susceptible to other factors. One of these factors may be the prostaglandins (PGs), which are fatty acid derivatives of arachidonic acid believed to promote neurogenic inflammation and inhibit norepinepherine release. PGs may play a role in MM, given that there is a threefold increase in prostaglandin levels by the luteal phase, with a further increase during menstruation.[8] Additionally, PG inhibitors, such as the nonsteroidal anti-inflammatory drugs (NSAIDs), have been found to be effective in treating and preventing MM in some women.

Treatment of Menstrual Migraine

Treatment of MM is often challenging, because acute treatments may suffice for some women, while others may require prophylactic therapy, either hormonal or nonhormonal. Effective treatment of MM, however, can lead to a reduction in headache burden.[13] A critical first step in the management process is to have the patient keep a headache diary for 3 months to determine whether there is indeed a link between her headaches and her period. Both nonpharmacologic methods (including avoidance of known triggers, regular exercise, sleep hygiene, good hydration, and biofeedback) and pharmacologic approaches should be explored, and most women will require both approaches. It can be frustrating for women to determine triggers, because certain triggers may be critically important during a MM attack, and yet be insufficient to trigger a migraine at another time of the month. Other than the migraine-specific triptans that have shown clear benefit, pharmacologic agents are chosen based upon comorbid conditions, previous successes or failures, and the adverse effect profiles of the various medications. Patients must be advised to use adequate birth control methods, because many of the drugs used in the treatment of migraine are contraindicated in pregnancy and should be avoided in a woman who is attempting to conceive.

Acute therapy of MM employs migraine-specific agents often in conjunction with gastrokinetic antiemetics such as metoclopramide or prochloperazine, or NSAIDs may be required. Choice of the seven available triptans is made on patient's prior success or failure, speed of onset, associated nausea/vomiting, and personal preference. Preventative therapy should be considered for women experiencing three to four or more debilitating headaches per month, or in whom MM is unresponsive to abortive medications. The goal of prevention is to reduce the frequency, duration, and intensity of the migraine headaches. Unfortunately, as previously noted, MM can be very difficult to treat, and even with preventative therapy, a woman may continue to experience MM, despite relief of headache at all other times of the month. Daily preventatives are used for those experiencing MRM and frequent migraine at other times, and miniprophylaxis is used for the patient who has PMM or MRM and few other migraine attacks. Miniprophylactic therapy requires that the timing of the migraine can be predicted either by a regular menstrual cycle or by associated features heralding its occurrence.

In miniprophylaxis, both hormonal and nonhormonal prophylactic options are available. In nonhormonal prophylaxis, standard migraine prophylactic agents and some abortive medications are used perimenstrually. One class of abortive agents is the NSAIDs. Naproxen sodium (550 mg twice daily) or mefenamic acid (500 mg TID) may be used effectively 2-4 days before the MM and continued through day 3 of menstrual flow.[14,15] As response is variable, it is important to try different classes of NSAIDs, because a lack of response to one type of NSAID does not rule out a response to an alternate NSAID.

Triptans have been studied as preventative agents for MM, and sumatriptan (25 mg three times daily), naratriptan (1 mg twice daily), frovatriptan (2.5 mg twice daily), and zolmitriptan (2.5 mg two or three times daily) have been found to be effective.[16–19] Dosing of the triptan begins 2 days before the onset of the MM and is continued for a total of 5 to 6 days. Ergotamine derivatives may be used for short-term prophylaxis without risk of developing ergot dependence provided they are used only during the vulnerable period.[20] Effective regimens include ergotamine tartrate one tablet twice daily or 0.5 suppository taken every night over the vulnerable perimenstrual time period. Dihydroergotamine (DHE) has shown effectiveness in its various forms and in a double-blind cross-over trial, DHE nasal spray given every 8 hours for a 6 days was effective,[20] as was intermittent prophylaxis with a timed-release formulation of DHE.[21] Triptans and ergot preparations must be avoided in women who have uncontrolled hypertension, or other risk factors for vascular disease.

Standard migraine prophylactic medications, including anticonvulsants, β-blockers, calcium channel blockers, and antidepressants may be used for 5 to 7 days before the onset of menses and continued through to the end of menses or vulnerable time for migraine. For women who are taking preventative agents, transiently increasing the dose during the perimenstrual period may reduce or eliminate the MM.

Hormonal prophylaxis attempts to counteract or prevent the luteal phase drop in estrogen and may be considered for refractory MM provided there are no contraindications to estrogen therapy, including a history of migraine with aura, blood clotting disorders, and risk factors for arterial disease such as diabetes, hypertension and tobacco use. Any patient who develops an aura while on hormones, or in whom there is a change from simple aura, should discontinue its use. Hormonal intervention has variable effect on migraine (headaches may improve, worsen, or remain unchanged), and this should be communicated to patients.[22]

The lowest effective dose should be used when attempting to stabilize estrogen levels and percutaneous and transdermal methods are preferred to oral supplementation; the latter has more variable absorption and can lead to unstable plasma levels, resulting in reduced efficacy. Most women, however, prefer oral contraceptives. If there are no contraindications, the patient could be switched to periodic noncycling of the oral contraceptive pill to eliminate three of every four cycles and therefore in theory, three of every four MRM attacks.

Using 1.5 mg percutaneous estradiol daily for the 3 days before menses and continued for 6 days has shown efficacy in two studies.[23,24] When using transdermal estradiol, a 100 µg patch is placed 3 days before menses, then replaced 1 day before menses and replaced again on day 2 after menses begins. In either case, when using an estrogen supplement, it is advisable to check progesterone levels to ensure that there is adequate endometrial protection.

For refractory cases, it is best to discuss this with the patient's gynecologist. Both the synthetic androgen, danazol acting as an estrogen antagonist, and the antiestrogen tamoxifen have shown efficacy in miniprophylaxis.[25,26] The dopamine receptor agonist bromocriptine, an inhibitor of prolactin release, given three times daily during the luteal phase, has also showed moderate effect.[27] GnRH analogs, which induce a medical menopause, also have been effective; however, they generally are limited to short (6 month) courses.[28,29] None of these methods have been subjected to clinical trials and therefore are not recommended universally for therapy of MM. Additionally, these drugs often cause unpleasant or intolerable adverse effects.

No long-term or controlled studies have been undertaken evaluating hysterectomy or oophorectomy for treating MM. In one study, two thirds of patients undergoing surgical menopause reported a worsening of their headaches.[30] Anecdotal reports of success are complicated by the postoperative use of daily estrogen replacement, which may account for the positive results.[31] As such, there is no role for hysterectomy or oophorectomy for managing MM.

ORAL CONTRACEPTIVE USE

For millions of women, oral contraceptive pills (OC) are the birth control method of choice; however, their use in migraineurs requires careful thought, as their effect is unpredictable. Because most women who have migraine are afflicted during their childbearing and peak productive years, the question of birth control invariably will arise whether in the adolescent girl or in the young through older-aged premenopausal woman. Thus, one must be aware of the risks and benefits of the use of the birth control pill to accurately council patients who have migraine. When a woman who has migraine begins OC therapy, the migraine may improve, worsen, remain stable, or occur for the first time.[32] In women who experience a worsening of their migraines, it is typically during the placebo week. Generally speaking, OC use is considered safe in women who experience migraine without aura or migraine with simple aura and in whom there is an absence of vascular risk factors.[33] If after beginning an OC the aura pattern changes or develops for the first time, the OC should be discontinued because of increased stroke risk.[34] As estrogen levels tend to fluctuate more with oral dosing, a patch or vaginal insert contraceptive may provide more steady-state levels and be less likely to impact migraine. Because the patch provides very high levels of estrogen, however, it may be relatively contraindicated due to potential stroke risks.

When choosing an OC. it is best to choose a low-dose, monophasic pill, rather than a mid- or high-dose pill. Biphasic and triphasic pills, while commonly prescribed, are not generally the best choice in migraineurs because of the fluctuating levels of estrogen. As previously noted, in women who have MRM, adding on estrogen during the placebo week can be helpful, as can noncycling of an OC, as it reduces the number of menstrual cycles and thus the number of MRMs.

PREGNANCY AND THE POSTPARTUM PERIOD

As previously noted, most migraine patients are women in their childbearing years; thus there is inevitably potential for the unintentional administration of acute migraine therapy in early pregnancy.[35] Given this, and the fact that perhaps more than 50% of pregnancies are unplanned, it is advisable to discuss migraine treatment and pregnancy issues with all female patients. In retrospective studies, 60% to 70% of pregnant migraineurs reportedly improve and in a more recent prospective study, up to 87% improved.[36] This improvement in or alleviation of migraine typically occurs during the second and third trimesters, although migraine often persists during the first trimester.[37,38] Improvement in pregnancy is more likely in women who have migraine without aura and in women who previously experienced MRM.[36] Migraine beginning for the first time in pregnancy is more often migraine with aura.[39] In addition to the hormonal changes of pregnancy, disrupted sleep, nausea, dehydration, and stress likely contribute to headache.

In pregnant women who have a prior history of migraine and an uneventful pregnancy, the challenge faced by the clinician is not usually diagnostic, but rather therapeutic. Given the unpredictable nature of migraine symptoms, however, management during pregnancy should begin by ruling out underlying pathology with new-onset headaches and then selecting a treatment to maximize benefit to the woman while minimizing risk to the fetus. The greatest concern regarding treatment of migraine during pregnancy of course relates to the potential teratogenicity of drug therapy. Reassurance, rest, ice packs, acupuncture, biofeedback, and avoidance of known triggers are often beneficial and may help the pregnant patient get through the first trimester, after which migraine may improve. No increased risk of major or minor abnormalities in infants born to women with migraine has been found.[40,41]

In the early stages of pregnancy, small doses of caffeine and acetaminophen are considered safe. Several NSAIDs are category B in pregnancy and include diclofenac, flurbiprofen, ibuprofen, ketoprofen, naproxen, piroxicam, and indomethacin; however, they are all category D in the third trimester. Some narcotics, meperidine and morphine, are category B, except in the third trimester when their use is cautioned. Codeine, while often used in pregnancy, has been associated with cardiac, respiratory, and cleft defects, but the relationships may not be causal. After the first trimester, category B antiemetics include dimenhydrinate, diphenhydramine, pyridoxine, and Emetrol. In suppository form, prochlorperazine, metoclopramide, and promethazine are generally considered safe. If steroids are required, prednisone often is preferred to dexamethasone, because the latter crosses the placenta more easily. Clearly more data are needed to guide clinicians in the safe use of therapeutic options in the pregnant migraineur.[42]

Triptans, ergots, and aspirin should be avoided. Pregnancy registries have been established for several of the triptans to monitor women (and their pregnancy outcomes) who inadvertently took these medications while pregnant. No evidence for any specific effect of sumatriptan on pregnancy outcome has been found.[43,44] Proof of absence of any risk is never absolute, however, and as such, it is not recommended to prescribe a triptan to a pregnant migraineur without clear indication.

For pregnant women who have severe, intractable migraine (often accompanied by nausea, vomiting and dehydration), medical therapy may be indicated, because this could pose a risk to the developing fetus greater than the risk of medication. For severe attacks, intravenous fluids and an intravenous antiemetic often are indicated. When migraine is frequent and disabling (three to four prolonged, severe migraines per month), preventative therapy may be required but should be undertaken with the full consent of both the patient and her partner, because most preventatives are category C or higher. Commonly employed agents include labetolol, propranolol, and occasionally amitriptyline or fluoxetine. Migraine often recurs in the postpartum period, presumably related to the rapid fall in estrogen levels.

PERIMENOPAUSE AND MENOPAUSE

Migraine tends to improve with age, and in women who have a history of menstrually related migraine, there may be improvement following menopause. On average, menopause is reached around age 50 years, with most women completing menopause by age 55 years. However, in the years preceding menopause, the perimenopause, many women notice a worsening of their migraines, and unfortunately, this stage in a woman's hormonal life may last several years. This is a transitional phase, which may begin in the mid- to late thirties and may last 10 years or more. During this time, episodic fluctuations in hormone levels occur, along with an overall decline in absolute levels, culminating in the symptoms of perimenopause, which may include fatigue, insomnia, irritability, irregular periods, night sweats, hot flashes, forgetfulness, a drop in libido, and difficulty concentrating.

In a woman who has migraine, worsening headaches may herald the onset of perimenopause. The chaotic, often unpredictable hormonal fluctuations of this time may even contribute to the new onset or return of previously abated migraines. In women who have MRM, a worsening in both the severity and frequency of migraines may occur, and monthly menstruation can become an important and predictable trigger for migraine. When irregular cycles set in and make migraine attacks unpredictable, treatment is more challenging. The other symptoms of perimenopause such as poor sleep from hot flashes and insomnia also contribute to worsening headaches. Although hormone levels can be measured, their absolute results are unlikely to sway the diagnosis and treatment plan significantly. In some women, the symptoms of perimenopause are managed with hormone replacement therapy (HRT).

Depending on the route of administration, type of estrogen, and cyclical versus continuous use, HRT has varying effects on a woman's migraines.[45-48] For women experiencing the ill effects of the fluctuating hormones of perimenopause, HRT on a short-term basis to stabilize estrogen levels may prove beneficial. For others, HRT may worsen migraine and consequently, strategies will need to be considered. In women migraineurs, the type of estrogen used and its method of delivery can impact migraine significantly.

To cope with worsening migraine, numerous strategies may be employed including reducing the dose of HRT, using a noncycling method, switching from conjugated estrogens to pure estradiol or from synthetic to bioidentical estrogen.[46] Switching from oral to transdermal is also beneficial, because with oral estrogen replacement, serum levels rise rapidly and thereafter decline until the next dose. The amount of estrogen absorbed also can vary with each dose. These fluctuations may be a trigger for migraine, especially because a woman's own endogenous estrogen levels also are fluctuating.[47,49] Transdermal estrogens, in contrast, provide more stable physiologic estrogen levels. If adjustments in the estrogenic component of the HRT are unsatisfactory with respect to improving migraine, then manipulation of the progesterone component can be considered.

SUMMARY

Migraine affects women from the preadolescent through the postmenopausal years. As such, clinicians involved in managing migraine need to be aware of the particular issues facing women migraineurs. The effect of hormonal fluctuations, whether endogenously or exogenously induced, is often unpredictable, and thus careful thought must be given to the various treatment options. Additionally, the potential for pregnancy always must be considered. With perseverance, effective migraine control usually is achieved in most patients.

REFERENCES

1. Van der Linden JA. De Hemicrania Menstrua. London; 1666. In Lancet; 1933.
2. Allais G, Benedetto C. Update on menstrual migraine: from clinical aspects to therapeutical strategies. Neurol Sci 2004;3:S229–31.
3. Epstein MT, Hockaday JM, Hockaday TD. Migraine and reproductive hormones throughout the menstrual cycle. Lancet 1975;1:543–8.
4. MacGregor EA. Oestrogen and attacks of migraine with and without aura. Lancet Neurol 2004;3:354–61.
5. Coururier EG, Bomhof MA, Knuistingh Neven A, et al. Menstrual migraine in a representative Dutch population sample: prevalence, disability, and treatment. Cephalalgia 2003;23:302–8.
6. Granella F, Sances G, Allais G, et al. Characteristics of menstrual and nonmenstrual attacks in women with menstrually related migraine referred to headache centers. Cephalalgia 2003;24:707–16.
7. The Headache Classification Subcommittee of the International Headache Society. The international classification of headache disorders, 2nd edition. Cephalalgia 2004;24(Suppl 1):56.
8. Silberstein SD, Merriam GR. Sex hormones and headache. J Pain Symptom Manage 1993;8:243–59.
9. MacGregor EA. "Menstrual" migraine: towards a definition. Cephalalgia 1996;16: 11–21.
10. Johnson SR. Premenstrual syndrome, premenstrual dysphoric disorder, and beyond: a clinical primer for practitioners. Obstet Gynecol 2004;104:845–59.
11. Somerville BW. The role of estradiol withdrawal in the etiology of menstrual migraine. Neurology 1972;22:355–65.
12. Somerville BW. Estrogen-withdrawal migraine. Neurology 1975;25:239–50.
13. Calhoun A, Ford S. Elimination of menstrual-related migraine beneficially impacts chronification and medication overuse. Headache 2008;48:1186–93.
14. Sargent J, Solbach P, Damasio H, et al. A comparison of naproxen sodium to propranolol hydrochloride and a placebo control for the prophylaxis of migraine headache. Headache 1985;25:320–4.
15. Al-Waili NS. Treatment of menstrual migraine with prostaglandin synthesis inhibitor mefenamic acid: double-blind study with placebo. Eur J Med Res 2000;5: 176–82.
16. Newman LC, Lipton RB, Lay CL, et al. A pilot study of oral sumatriptan as intermittent prophylaxis of menstruation-related migraine. Neurology 1998;51:307–9.
17. Newman L, Mannix LK, Landy S, et al. Naratriptan as short-term prophylaxis of menstrually associated migraine: a randomized, double-blind, placebo-controlled study. Headache 2001;41:248–56.
18. Silberstein SD, Elkin AH, Schreiber C, et al. A randomized trial of frovatriptan for the intermittent prevention of menstrual migraine. Neurology 2004;63:261–9.
19. Tuchman MM, Hee A, Emeribe U, et al. Oral zolmitriptan in the short-term prevention of menstrual migraine: a randomized, placebo-controlled study. CNS Drugs 2008;22:877–86.

20. Edelson RN. Menstrual migraine and other hormonal aspects of migraine. Headache 1985;25:376–9.
21. Silberstein SD, Bradley K. DHE-45 in the prophylaxis of menstrually related migraine. Cephalalgia 1996;16:371.
22. D'Alessandro R, Gamberini G, Lozito A, et al. Menstrual migraine: intermittent prophylaxis with a timed-release pharmacological formulation of dihydroergotamine. Cephalalgia 1983;3(Suppl 1):156–8.
23. Silberstein SD. The role of sex hormones in headache. Neurology 1992;42(Suppl 2): 37–42.
24. Dennerstein L, Morse C, Burrows G, et al. Menstrual migraine: a double-blind trial of percutaneous estradiol. Gynecol Endocrinol 1988;2:113–20.
25. de Lignieres B, Vincens M, Mauvais-Jarvis P, et al. Prevention of menstrual migraine by percutaneous oestradiol. Br Med J 1986;293:1540.
26. Calton GJ, Burnett JW. Danazol and migraine. N Engl J Med 1984;310:721–2.
27. O'Dea PK, Davis EH. Tamoxifen in the treatment of menstrual migraine. Neurology 1990;40:1470–1.
28. Herzog AG. Continuous bromocriptine therapy in menstrual migraine. Neurology 1997;48:101–2.
29. Holdaway IM, Parr CE, France J. Treatment of a patient with severe menstrual migraine using the depot LHRH analogue Zoladex. Aust N Z J Obstet Gynaecol 1991;31:164–5.
30. Murray SC, Muse KN. Effective treatment of severe menstrual migraine headaches with gonadotropin-releasing hormone agonist and add-back therapy. Fertil Steril 1997;67:390–3.
31. Neri I, Granella F, Nappi R, et al. Characteristics of headache at menopause: a clinico–epidemiologic study. Maturitas 1993;17:31–7.
32. Martin V, Wenke S, Mandell K, et al. Medical oophorectomy with and without estrogen add-back therapy in the prevention of migraine headache. Headache 2003;43:309–21.
33. Dalton K. Migraine and oral contraceptives. Headache 1976;15:247–51.
34. Davis PH. Use of oral contraceptives and postmenopusal hormone replacement: evidence on risk of stroke. Curr Treat Options Neurol 2008;10:468–74.
35. Bousser MG, Conard J, Kittner S, et al. Recommendations on the risk of ischaemic stroke associated with use of combined oral contraceptives and hormone replacement therapy in women with migraine. The International Headache Society Task Force on Combined Oral Contraceptive & Hormone Replacement Therapy. Cephalalgia 2000;20:155–6.
36. Fox AW, Davis RL. Migraine chronobiology. Headache 1998;38:436–41.
37. Sances G, Granella F, Nappi RE, et al. Course of migraine during pregnancy and postpartum: a prospective study. Cephalalgia 2003;23:197–205.
38. Silberstein SD. Headaches and women: treatment of the pregnant and lactating migraineur. Headache 1993;33:533–40.
39. Pfaffenrath V, Rehm M. Migraine in pregnancy: what are the safest treatment options? Drug Saf 1998;19:383–8.
40. Cupini LM, Matteis M, Troisi E, et al. Sex hormone related events in migrainous females. A clinical comparative study between migraine with aura and migraine without aura. Cephalalgia 1995;15:140–4.
41. Marcus DA. Managing headache during pregnancy and lactation. Expert Rev Neurother 2008;8:385–95.

42. Brandes JL. Headache related to pregnancy: management of migraine and migraine headache in pregnancy. Current Treatment Options in Neurology 2008;10:12–9.
43. Wainscot G, Volans GN, Sullivan FM, et al. The outcome of pregnancy in women suffering from migraine. Postgrad Med J 1978;54:98–102.
44. Evans EW, Lorber KC. Use of 5-HT1 agonists in pregnancy. Ann Pharmacother 2008;42:543–9.
45. Fox AW, Chambers CD, Anderson PO, et al. Evidence-based assessment of pregnancy outcome after sumatriptan exposure. Headache 2002;42:8–15.
46. MacGregor AE. Effects of oral and transdermal estrogen replacement on migraine. Cephalalgia 1999;19:124–5.
47. Facchinetti F, Nappi RE, Tirelli A, et al. Hormone supplementation differently affects migraine in postmenopausal women. Headache 2002;42:924–9.
48. Hodson J, Thompson J, al-Azzawi F. Headache at menopause and in hormone replacement therapy users. Climacteric 2000;3:119–24.
49. Nappi RE, Cagnacci A, Granella F, et al. Course of primary headaches during hormone replacement therapy. Maturitas 2001;38:157–63.

The Migraine Association with Cardiac Anomalies, Cardiovascular Disease, and Stroke

Todd J. Schwedt, MD

KEYWORDS

- Migraine • Right-to-left shunt • Patent foramen ovale
- Mitral valve prolapse • Cardiovascular disease • Stroke

Migraine has complex relations with disorders of the cerebrovasculature, the cardiovasculature, and the heart. It has been proposed that right-to-left shunt and structural cardiac anomalies may serve causal or triggering roles in the production of migraine headaches. Conversely, migraine has been identified as a risk factor for stroke and coronary artery disease. Herein, the author reviews the evidence in support of the relations of migraine to right-to-left shunt, structural cardiac anomalies, cardiovascular disease, and ischemic stroke.

MIGRAINE AND RIGHT-TO-LEFT SHUNT

Right-to-left shunt is more prevalent in patients who have migraine. Migraine is more common among those with right-to-left shunt. Although most of the focus has been on the relation between patent foramen ovale (PFO) and migraine, atrial septal defects (ASDs) and extracardiac shunts have also been associated with the occurrence of migraine.

Patent Foramen Ovale

A significant amount of attention has been recently placed on investigating the association between PFO and migraine. There have been multiple studies of PFO prevalence in migraineurs, studies of migraine prevalence in those with PFO, and

Research funding was provided by the National Institutes of Health, grant KL2 RR024994. The author has participated in industry-sponsored trials for Allergan, GSK, and AGA Medical and has provided consulting to VerusMed.

Neurology and Anesthesiology, Washington University Headache Center, Washington University School of Medicine, 660 South Euclid Avenue, Campus Box 8111, St. Louis, MO 63110, USA

E-mail address: schwedtt@neuro.wustl.edu

Neurol Clin 27 (2009) 513–523

doi:10.1016/j.ncl.2008.11.006

0733-8619/08/$ – see front matter

neurologic.theclinics.com

retrospective reports of the effect of PFO closure on migraine patterns. The large-magnitude benefit noted in these uncontrolled retrospective reports of PFO closure has created excitement in regard to a possible role for PFO closure in the treatment of intractable migraine. At this time, one prospective clinical trial of PFO closure for migraine has been completed and several others are actively enrolling.

The association between PFO and migraine has been studied bidirectionally. Several studies have examined the prevalence of PFO in subjects who have migraine, whereas others have investigated the prevalence of migraine in subjects with PFO. The odds of a patient who has migraine having PFO is 2.5 (95% confidence interval [CI]: 2.01–3.08) times greater than the odds of PFO in those who do not have migraine.[1] PFO is found in 40% to 70% of subjects who have migraine with and without aura as compared with 25% of people in the general population.[2–7] The increased risk for having PFO is attributable to migraineurs who have aura. Although migraine without aura has been studied less extensively, there is not evidence for an increased prevalence of PFO in migraineurs without aura. It is estimated that just greater than 50% of migraineurs with aura have PFO.[8] When the association between PFO and migraine is studied in the other direction, examining the prevalence of migraine among subjects with PFO, the positive association persists. The odds of a person with PFO having migraine is 5.1 times (95% CI: 4.67–5.59) that of a person without PFO.[1] Migraine prevalence ranges from 20% to 65% in subjects with PFO, compared with a point prevalence of approximately 13% for migraine in the general population.[9–21] The increased odds of migraine in the presence of PFO is attributable to migraine with aura. The odds of migraine without aura are not clearly elevated in the presence of PFO. Migraine with aura is found in 13% to 50% of subjects with PFO, a significantly higher prevalence than the expected 4% in the general population.[9–21] The odds of having migraine with aura in the presence of PFO is 3.2 (95% CI: 2.38–4.17) times the odds of migraine with aura in the absence of PFO.[1] Migraine is more prevalent among subjects with large PFO as compared with those with smaller PFO and less active right-to-left shunting.[6,12,17,19,22,23]

Multiple retrospective analyses regarding the effect of PFO closure on migraine patterns have suggested a significant benefit.[13,16,17,24,25] These retrospective noncontrolled studies serve as an important base from which prospective analyses of the effect of PFO closure on migraine patterns have been designed. The nature of the retrospective studies does not allow for conclusions to be drawn regarding the safety and efficacy of PFO closure for the treatment of migraine. Nonetheless, these studies have suggested that PFO closure results in high-magnitude benefit in a large proportion of subjects who have migraine. Despite the prevalence studies identifying an association between PFO and migraine with aura only, retrospective PFO closure studies have found similar benefits among migraineurs with and without aura. After PFO closure, approximately 50% of subjects retrospectively reported complete migraine resolution, approximately 25% reported significant reductions in headache frequency, and 25% reported no change in their headaches.[8]

The first prospective study of PFO closure for migraine was completed in late 2006. The Migraine Intervention with STARflex Technology (MIST-I) trial was a prospective, randomized, sham procedure, controlled trial conducted in Europe.[26] Subjects had migraine with aura, at least 5 migraine days per month, 7 headache-free days per month, and a moderate- or large-sized PFO. Subjects had failed standard prophylactic migraine medications from at least two different classes. Based on the results of retrospective studies of PFO closure, the primary end point was complete migraine resolution at 91 to 180 days after PFO closure. Among the 147 randomized subjects (randomized 1:1 to treatment or sham procedure), only 3 from the treatment arm and 3 from the sham procedure group had migraine resolution. Secondary end points were not met. Although the MIST-I trial was a negative study, North American trials with modestly different criteria, closure devices, and outcomes are currently enrolling.

Although there is compelling evidence for an association between PFO and migraine, the nature of the relation is not yet clear. Well-crafted hypotheses have been offered suggesting a causal relation, a triggering relation, and a coincidental association. The argument for a causal relation has focused on two main theories. First, right-to-left shunts allow for thrombi, which could develop in the PFO tunnel or elsewhere, to pass from the venous system to the arterial system, and thus reach the central nervous system. A small paradoxical embolism reaching the brain's cortical surface may trigger cortical spreading depression and migraine headache. Second, the lungs normally filter out a significant proportion of the biogenic amines from the blood before it reaches the arterial system.[27] Right-to-left shunts allow for higher concentrations of these amines, including serotonin, to reach the arterial system and potentially trigger migraine headaches. Supporters of a coincidental relation between PFO and migraine cite evidence for coinheritance of PFO and migraine. Autosomal dominant inheritance of atrial shunts linked to inheritance of migraine with aura has been demonstrated in some families.[28]

At this time, there is significant evidence supporting a positive association between PFO and migraine with aura. The nature of this association and the potential role of PFO closure for the treatment of intractable migraine are unclear, however.

Atrial Septal Defects

There is evidence that migraine is associated with ASDs. Although ASDs are most often associated with left-to-right shunting of blood, right-to-left shunting may occur during Valsalva or other activities increasing right atrial pressures.[29] Many of the studies primarily examining the relation between PFO and migraine also included small numbers of subjects with ASDs.[20,24,25] Azarbal and colleagues[25] reported migraine headache in 30% of their 23 subjects with ASD (4 with aura and 3 without aura). After ASD repair, 3 of 7 subjects had migraine resolution, 1 of 7 had improvement without resolution, and 3 had no change or worsening. Mortelmans and colleagues[29] retrospectively examined the prevalence and outcome of migraine in 75 patients who had undergone percutaneous ASD closure. Before ASD repair, 22 (29.3%) of 75 patients had migraine, 14 with and 8 without aura. There was no difference in migraine prevalence after closure (20 of 75 patients). Rather interestingly, however, this lack of difference may have been attributable to several subjects having new onset of migraine after closure as opposed to a lack of beneficial response in those with preexisting migraine. Twelve subjects with migraine before closure reported migraine resolution after ASD repair. Ten patients reported new-onset migraine after the procedure, however, 7 with aura and 3 without. Similarly, new-onset migraine has been reported after PFO closure and may be attributable to thrombi formation on the occlusion device, intra-atrial pressure imbalance, or liberation of vasoactive substances.[24,29–31]

Pulmonary Right-to-Left Shunt

If right-to-left shunt is causally associated with the production of migraine headaches, it would be expected that extracardiac shunts would also be associated with an increased prevalence of migraine. Accordingly, there is evidence that the presence of pulmonary arteriovenous malformations (AVMs) increases the risk for migraine. Pulmonary AVMs are found in one third of people with hereditary hemorrhagic telangiectasia (HHT), and HHT is the underlying disorder accounting for pulmonary AVMs in 70% of cases.[32,33] Because pulmonary AVMs result in right-to-left shunting of blood, the

HHT population is an interesting group within which to examine the association between right-to-left shunts and migraine. Thenganatt and colleagues[34] retrospectively reviewed 124 patients who had HHT and had previously been assessed for a history of migraine and pulmonary AVMs. Forty-seven (38%) of them had a history of migraine, with four fifths having migraine with aura. The presence of a pulmonary AVM was associated with migraine after adjusting for age and gender (OR = 2.4, 95% CI: 1.1–5.5). Among 14 patients who had pulmonary AVMs and migraine and underwent AVM embolization, 8 (57%) retrospectively reported migraine improvement and 6 (43%) reported no change or worsening. Post and colleagues[35] retrospectively studied 84 patients who had HHT and pulmonary AVMs to determine the baseline prevalence of migraine and the effect of AVM embolization on migraine patterns. The prevalence of migraine before AVM embolization was 45.2%, of whom 73.4% had migraine with aura. The prevalence of migraine decreased from 45.2% before embolization to 34.5% after embolization, assessed at a median follow-up time of 48 months ($P = .01$). There was a nonsignificant improvement in headache frequency and severity in those subjects who continued to have migraine after embolization. Although preliminary and inconclusive, there is suggestion that pulmonary AVMs may be associated with migraine and that treatment of these AVMs may have a beneficial effect on migraine patterns. Certainly, further investigation is required to elucidate these potential interactions.

MIGRAINE AND STRUCTURAL CARDIAC ANOMALIES UNRELATED TO RIGHT-TO-LEFT SHUNT

In addition to the positive association between migraine with aura and intracardiac right-to-left shunt, migraine may be associated with structural cardiac anomalies in the absence of shunt.

Mitral Valve Prolapse

Results from several observational studies have suggested an association between mitral valve prolapse (MVP) and migraine. A study of 230 patients who had MVP found that 27.8% had migraine, a proportion significantly larger than that expected in the general population.[36] Nearly 30% of the migraineurs had migraine with aura. Investigating the association in the converse direction, Amat and colleagues[37] found that 25% (16 of 64) of patients who had migraine had MVP as compared with 9.2% of all headache patients. MVP prevalence was equal among migraineurs with and without aura. Spence and colleagues[38] conducted a case-control study to investigate the association between MVP and migraine with aura. One hundred subjects who had migraine with aura and 100 nonheadache controls were compared. All subjects underwent transthoracic echocardiography, which was interpreted by a cardiologist blinded to the migraine status. Definite MVP was found in 15 subjects who had migraine as compared with 7 controls. Probable MVP was identified in 16 migraine subjects and 8 controls. The OR of having MVP in the presence of migraine with aura was 2.7 (95% CI: 1.17–6.29). The nature of the association between MVP and migraine is uncertain. Arguments for a causal association are based on reduced platelet survival and platelet aggregation in those who have MVP. Damaged platelets release serotonin, which has been implicated to play a role in the generation of migraine headaches.

Atrial Septal Aneurysm

The prevalence of atrial septal aneurysm (ASA) was investigated by transthoracic echocardiogram in 35 subjects who had migraine with aura, 55 subjects who had migraine without aura, and 53 nonmigraine control subjects.[39] ASA was identified in

12 (13.3%) of 90 subjects who had migraine as compared with 1 (1.9%) of 53 control subjects (P<.05). The increased frequency of ASA among migraineurs was isolated to subjects with aura. ASA was found in 28.5% of subjects who had migraine with aura and 3.6% of subjects who had migraine without aura. ASA was associated with PFO in 3 of 10 migraineurs with aura, 3 of 3 migraineurs without aura, and 1 of 1 nonmigraine control subject.

Congenital Heart Disease

A recent study found an increase in the prevalence of migraine among adults who have congenital heart disease.[40] Patients from the University of California at Los Angeles Adult Congenital Heart Disease Center were asked to complete a questionnaire to determine the presence of migraine headache. Of the 85% (395 of 466 patients) who returned the questionnaire, 45.3% were diagnosed as having migraine. Among 252 gender-matched controls who had acquired cardiovascular diseases, 11% had migraine (P<.001). Eighty percent of subjects who had congenital heart disease and migraine had aura as compared with 36% of migraineurs in the control group (P<.001). The frequency of migraine was highest among subjects who had congenital heart disease with right-to-left shunt (52%), followed by those with left-to-right shunt (44%). Of significant interest, however, the prevalence of migraine was also elevated in subjects who had congenital heart disease without shunt as compared with control subjects (38% versus 11%).

Summaries of the relation between migraine prevalence and prevalence of cardiac and vascular conditions are presented in **Tables 1** and **2**.[2–21,29,34–42]

MIGRAINE AND CARDIOVASCULAR DISEASE

Migraine has been shown to be associated with an increase in cardiovascular risk factors. This association was investigated in the Genetic Epidemiology of Migraine (GEM) study, a population-based study in The Netherlands of 5755 subjects, including 620 current migraineurs.[43] Measured cardiovascular risk factors included blood pressure, cholesterol levels, smoking, oral contraceptive use, and the Framingham risk score for death related to myocardial infarction or coronary heart disease. As compared with nonmigraine controls, migraineurs had increased odds of smoking (odds ratio [OR] = 1.43, 95% CI: 1.1–1.8), were less likely to drink alcohol (OR = 0.58, 95% CI: 0.5–0.7), and were more likely to report a parental history of early myocardial infarction. Subjects who had migraine with aura were more likely to have a total cholesterol–to–high-density lipoprotein cholesterol ratio of greater than 5, hypertension, and a history of early-onset coronary heart disease or stroke. Female

Table 1
Migraine prevalence according to cardiac or vascular risk factor.

	Migraine	No Aura	Aura
General population	13%	9%	4%
PFO	20%–65%	3%–25%	13%–50%
ASD	29.3%–30%	10.7%–13%	17.4%–18.7%
Pulmonary AVM	38%–45.2%	7.3%–11.9%	30.6%–33.3%
MVP	27.8%	19.6%	8.3%
CHD	45.3%	9.1%	36.2%

Abbreviation: CHD, congenital heart disease (without shunt).

Table 2
Prevalence of cardiac or vascular condition according to migraine status

	Patent Foramen Ovale	Mitral Valve Prolapse	Atrial Septal Aneurysm
General population	25%	2.4%	3.2%
Migraine	40%–70%	25%	13.3%
• No aura	16%–34%	25%	3.6%
• Aura	41%–72%	25%–31%	28.5%

migraineurs were more likely than controls to be using oral contraceptives (OR = 2.06, 95% CI: 1.05–4.0). The Framingham 10-year risk for coronary heart disease or myocardial infarction was higher in subjects who had migraine as compared with controls who did not have migraine. The OR of having a 1% risk was 1.51 (95% CI: 1.2–2.0), that of having a 2% to 9% risk was 1.72 (95% CI: 1.3–2.3), that of having a 10% to 20% risk was 1.43 (95% CI: 0.9–2.3), and that of having a 21% or greater risk was 2.25 (95% CI: 1.0–5.1). Although the results from this study clearly suggest that migraineurs are more likely to have cardiovascular risk factors, the direction and nature of this relation are not clear.

Migraine has been identified as a risk factor for cardiovascular disease in men and women. A large prospective cohort study by Kurth and colleagues[44] used participants in the Women's Health Study to investigate the association between migraine and cardiovascular disease. This investigation included 27,480 American women 45 years of age or older who were free of cardiovascular disease and angina at study entry and from whom data regarding migraine and lipid measurements were available. Among these women, 5125 (18.4%) reported a history of migraine and 3610 (13.1%) had migraine within the prior year. Nearly 40% (n = 1434) of women who had migraine reported migraine aura. Major cardiovascular disease occurred in 580 women during the 10-year mean follow-up period. Major cardiovascular disease was defined as the first instance of nonfatal ischemic stroke or nonfatal myocardial infarction or death attributable to ischemic cardiovascular disease. Investigators also analyzed data for first ischemic stroke, myocardial infarction, coronary revascularization, and angina. Migraine with aura increased the risk for such events after controlling for age; blood pressure; diabetes; body mass index; smoking; alcohol use; exercise; postmeno-pausal status; family history of myocardial infarction before the age of 60 years; cholesterol levels; and use of antihypertensives, hormones, oral contraceptives, and cholesterol-lowering medications. Adjusted hazard ratios in the presence of active migraine with aura were 2.15 (95% CI: 1.58–2.92; P<.001) for major cardiovascular disease, 1.91 (95% CI: 1.17–3.10; P = .01) for ischemic stroke, 2.08 (95% CI: 1.30–3.31; P = .002) for myocardial infarction, 1.74 (95% CI: 1.23–2.46; P = .002) for coronary revascularization, 1.71 (95% CI: 1.16–2.53, P = .007) for angina, and 2.33 (95% CI: 1.21–4.51; P = .01) for ischemic cardiovascular death. Migraine without aura was not associated with an increased risk for cardiovascular disease.

The association between migraine and cardiovascular disease in men was investigated using 20,084 men aged 40 to 84 years who were enrolled in the Physician's Health Study.[45] Annual questionnaires assessed for the presence of migraine and cardiovascular risk factors and the occurrence of cardiovascular end points of interest. Investigators used the following end points: first major cardiovascular event (nonfatal ischemic stroke or nonfatal myocardial infarction or death attributable to ischemic cardiovascular disease), coronary revascularization, and angina. At baseline assessment, 7.2% of the men (n = 1449) reported migraine. Information regarding the presence of aura symptoms was not collected. Just more than 11% of the total cohort had a major cardiovascular event during the mean 15.7 years of follow-up. Hazard ratios were calculated after adjusting for age, hypertension, diabetes mellitus, smoking, exercise, body mass index, alcohol use, cholesterol levels, and parental history of myocardial infarction before 60 years of age. As compared with nonmigraine controls, men who had migraine were found to have an increased risk for major cardio-vascular disease (hazard ratio = 1.24, 95% CI: 1.06–1.46; P = .008) and myocardial infarction (hazard ratio = 1.42, 95% CI: 1.15–1.77; P<.001). There were no significant increases in the risk for coronary revascularization, angina, or ischemic cardiovascular death. Because data regarding the presence of aura were not collected, it is unclear if there is an increased risk for major cardiovascular disease and myocardial infarction in migraineurs with and without aura.

The explanation for an increased risk for cardiovascular disease among migraineurs is unclear. It may be that migraineurs are at increased risk because of the migraine association with cardiac risk factors. Alternatively, the association could be explained by an increased presence of prothrombotic factors (eg, factor V Leiden, von Wille-brand factor), increased inflammatory response related to neurogenic inflammation, vascular endothelial damage or dysfunction, shared underlying genetic predisposi-tion, or use of antimigraine medications.[46–48] Regardless of the biologic explanation, the increased risk for cardiovascular disease among migraineurs has led to the recom-mendation that clinicians carefully assess their patients who have migraine for cardiovascular risk factors and treat modifiable risk factors when present.[49]

MIGRAINE AND STROKE

Migraine is a risk factor for ischemic stroke. This increased risk is greatest among young women who have frequent migraine with aura, especially if they smoke or use oral contraceptive pills. Nonetheless, studies suggest that male and female migraineurs, whether young or old, are at increased risk for ischemic stroke.

A meta-analysis of 14 studies examining the association between migraine and ischemic stroke included studies published before 2004.[50] Increased stroke risk was found for migraineurs with and without aura. Overall, migraine was associated with a relative risk for stroke of 2.16 (95% CI: 1.89–2.48). Migraineurs without aura had a relative risk of 1.83 (95% CI: 1.06–3.15), whereas those with aura had a relative risk of 2.27 (95% CI: 1.61–3.19). Studies suggest that the risk for ischemic stroke in migraineurs is more than tripled in smokers and is quadrupled in migraineurs using oral contraceptive pills.[47,51,52] Migraineurs should be counseled about not smoking, and the risks and benefits of oral contraceptive use must be carefully discussed.

Studies published since the time of the meta-analysis further support the associa-tion between migraine and ischemic stroke. Investigation of migraineurs in the Women's Health Study found that migraineurs with aura had a relative risk of 1.7 (95% CI: 1.11–2.66) for ischemic stroke as compared with controls who did not have migraine.[44] The increased risk was highest among the youngest group in the cohort, 45 to 55 years of age (only women 45 years of age and older were included), for whom the relative risk was 2.25 (95% CI: 1.30–3.91). There was not an increased risk for ischemic stroke in migraineurs without aura. A nonsignificant increase in the risk for ischemic stroke in migraineurs was found in the Atherosclerosis Risk in Communities Study.[53] In this study of men and women 55 years of age and older, migraineurs had a relative risk for ischemic stroke of 1.84 (95% CI: 0.89–3.82). The Stroke Prevention in Young Women Study found that women aged 15 to 49 years with probable migraine with aura had an OR of 1.5 (95% CI: 1.1–2.0) for ischemic stroke.[54] Migraineurs with aura who smoked cigarettes and used oral contraceptives had a 7.0-fold increased odds of stroke (95% CI: 1.3–22.8) as compared with migraineurs with aura who did not smoke and use oral contraceptives. Women without aura were not at increased stroke risk.

Kruit and colleagues[55] performed a cross-sectional population study of Dutch adults 30 to 60 years of age to investigate the prevalence of stroke and white matter lesions in subjects who had migraine. None of the 295 migraineurs (161 had migraine with aura) or the 140 age- and gender-matched controls reported symptoms of stroke. Brain MRI evidence for stroke was found in 8.1% of those with migraine and 5.0% of controls, however, which was a nonsignificant difference. The adjusted OR for cerebellar strokes in migraineurs as compared with nonmigraine controls was 7.1 (95% CI: 0.9–55; P = .02). Posterior circulation strokes were found in 0.7% of controls as compared with 5.4% of migraineurs. This risk was even higher for migraineurs with aura and for those who had frequent migraine attacks. Migraineurs with aura with one or more migraine attacks per month had an adjusted OR for ischemic stroke in the posterior circulation (cerebellum) of 15.8 (95% CI: 1.8–140). Just more than 10% (7 of 69) of migraineurs with aura with at least one attack per month had MRI evidence of a posterior circulation stroke. More than 80% of strokes found in migraineurs were located in areas of the brain perfused by the posterior circulation.[56] Ninety percent of these were located in arterial watershed (border zone) areas of the cerebellum. Strokes were small and often multiple.

The exact cause of the increased risk for symptomatic and asymptomatic stroke in the presence of migraine is not known. Embolism and hypoperfusion are hypothesized, given the location and pattern of many of these strokes (cerebellar watershed distribution). Other possibilities relate to endothelial dysfunction, an increase in vascular risk factors among migraineurs, the increased prevalence of PFO, the use of migraine-specific medications, and a genetic link between migraine and ischemic stroke.[47,48]

SUMMARY

Migraine is associated with cardiac and pulmonary right-to-left shunt and with structural cardiac anomalies in the absence of shunt. Furthermore, migraine presence elevates the risk for cardiovascular disease and ischemic stroke. Further investigation is required to determine the nature and mechanisms of the migraine association with these conditions.

REFERENCES

1. Schwedt TJ, Demaerschalk BM, Dodick DW. Patent foramen ovale and migraine: a quantitative systematic review. Cephalalgia 2008;28:531–40.
2. Hagen PT, Scholz DG, Edwards WD. Incidence and size of patent foramen ovale during the first 10 decades of life: an autopsy study of 965 normal hearts. Mayo Clin Proc 1984;59:17–20.
3. Anzola GP, Magoni MD, Guindani M, et al. Potential source of cerebral embolism in migraine with aura. A transcranial Doppler study. Neurology 1999;52:1622–5.
4. Dalla Volta G, Guindani M, Zavarise P, et al. Prevalence of patent foramen ovale in a large series of patients with migraine with aura, migraine without aura and cluster headache, and relationship with clinical phenotype. J Headache Pain. 2005;6:328–30.
5. Ferrarini G, Malferrari G, Zucco R, et al. High prevalence of patent foramen ovale in migraine with aura. J Headache Pain. 2005;6:71–6.

6. Carod-Artal FJ, Da Silveira Ribeiro L, Braga H, et al. Prevalence of patent foramen ovale in migraine patients with and without aura compared with stroke patients. A transcranial Doppler study. Cephalalgia 2006;26:934–9.

7. Tembl J, Lago A, Sevilla T, et al. Migraine, patent foramen ovale and migraine triggers. J Headache Pain 2007;8:7–12.

8. Schwedt TJ, Dodick DW. Patent foramen ovale and migraine—bringing closure to the subject. Headache 2006;46:663–71.

9. Stewart WF, Lipton RB, Celentano DO, et al. Prevalence of migraine headache in the United States: relation to age, income, race, and other socioeconomic factors. JAMA 1992;267:64–9.

10. Lipton RB, Stewart WF, Diamond S, et al. Prevalence and burden of migraine in the United States: data from the American Migraine Study II. Headache 2001; 41:646–57.

11. Sztajzel R, Genoud D, Roth S, et al. Patent foramen ovale, a possible cause of symptomatic migraine: a study of 74 patients with acute ischemic stroke. Cerebrovasc Dis 2002;13:102–6.

12. Wilmshurst P, Pearson M, Nightingale S. Re-evaluation of the relationship between migraine and persistent foramen ovale and other right-to-left shunts. Clin Sci (Lond) 2005;108:365–7.

13. Reisman M, Christofferson RD, Jesurum J, et al. Migraine headache relief after transcatheter closure of patent foramen ovale. J Am Coll Cardiol 2005;45:493–5.

14. Post MC, Thijs V, Herroelen L, et al. Closure of a patent foramen ovale is associated with a decrease in prevalence of migraine. Neurology 2004;62:1439–40.

15. Schwerzmann M, Wiher S, Nedeltchev K, et al. Percutaneous closure of patent foramen ovale reduces the frequency of migraine attacks. Neurology 2004;62: 1399–401.

16. Morandi E, Anzola GP, Angeli S, et al. Transcatheter closure of patent foramen ovale: a new migraine treatment? J Interv Cardiol 2003;16:39–42.

17. Wilmshurst P, Nightingale S. Relationship between migraine and cardiac and pulmonary right-to-left shunts. Clin Sci (Lond) 2001;100:215–20.

18. Anzola GP, Frisoni GB, Morandi E, et al. Shunt-associated migraine responds favorably to atrial septal repair: a case-control study. Stroke 2006;37:430–4.

19. Anzola GP, Morandi E, Casilli F, et al. Different degrees of right-to-left shunting predict migraine and stroke: data from 420 patients. Neurology 2006;66: 765–7.

20. Wilmshurst P, Nightingale S, Pearson M, et al. Relation of atrial shunts to migraine in patients with ischemic stroke and peripheral emboli. Am J Cardiol 2006;98: 831–3.

21. Kimmelstiel C, Gange C, Thaler D. Is patent foramen ovale closure effective in reducing migraine symptoms? A controlled study. Catheter Cardiovasc Interv 2007;69:740–6.

22. Schwerzmann M, Nedeltchev K, Lagger F, et al. Prevalence and size of directly detected patent foramen ovale in migraine with aura. Neurology 2005;65:1415–8.

23. Jesurum JT, Fuller CJ, Velez CA, et al. Migraineurs with patent foramen ovale have larger right-to-left shunt despite similar atrial septal characteristics. J Headache Pain 2007;8:209–16.

24. Wilmshurst PT, Nightingale S, Walsh KP, et al. Effect on migraine of closure of cardiac right-to-left shunts to prevent recurrence of decompression illness or stroke for haemodynamic reasons. Lancet 2000;356:1648–51.

25. Azarbal B, Tobis J, Suh W, et al. Association of interatrial shunts and migraine headaches. J Am Coll Cardiol 2005;45:489–92.

26. Dowson A, Mullen MJ, Peatfield R, et al. Migraine intervention with STARFlex technology (MIST) trial: a prospective, multicenter, double-blind, sham-controlled trial to evaluate the effectiveness of patent foramen ovale closure with STARFlex septal repair implant to resolve refractory migraine headache. Circulation 2008; 117:1397–404.

27. Gillis CN, Pitt BR. The fate of circulating amines within the pulmonary circulation. Annu Rev Physiol 1982;44:269–81.

28. Wilmshurst PT, Pearson MJ, Nightingale S, et al. Inheritance of persistent foramen ovale and atrial septal defects and the relation to familial migraine with aura. Heart 2004;90:1315–20.

29. Mortelmans K, Post M, Thijs V, et al. The influence of percutaneous atrial septal defect closure on the occurrence of migraine. Eur Heart J 2005;26:1533–7.

30. Yankovsky AE, Kuritzky A. Transformation into daily migraine with aura following transcutaneous atrial septal defect closure. Headache 2003;43:496–8.

31. Wilmshurst PT, Nightingale S, Walsh KP, et al. Clopidogrel reduces migraine with aura after transcatheter closure of persistent foramen ovale and atrial septal defects. Heart 2005;91:1173–5.

32. Gossage JR, Kanj G. State of the art: pulmonary arteriovenous malformations. Am J Respir Crit Care Med 1998;158:643–61.

33. Nanthakumar K, Hyland RH, Graham AT, et al. Contrast echocardiography for detection of pulmonary arteriovenous malformations. Am Heart J 2001;141: 243–6.

34. Thenganatt J, Schneiderman J, Hyland RH, et al. Migraines linked to intrapulmonary right-to-left shunt. Headache 2006;46:439–43.

35. Post MC, Thijs V, Schonewille WJ, et al. Embolization of pulmonary arteriovenous malformations and decrease in prevalence of migraine. Neurology 2006;66: 202–5.

36. Litman GI, Friedman HM. Migraine and the mitral valve prolapse syndrome. Am Heart J 1978;96:610–4.

37. Amat G, Jean Louis P, Loisy C, et al. Migraine and the mitral valve prolapse syndrome. Adv Neurol 1982;33:27–9.

38. Spence JD, Wong DG, Melendez LJ, et al. Increased prevalence of mitral valve prolapse in patients with migraine. Can Med Assoc J 1984;131:1457–60.

39. Carerj S, Narbone MC, Zito C, et al. Prevalence of atrial septal aneurysm in patients with migraine: an echocardiographic study. Headache 2003;43:725–8.

40. Truong T, Slavin L, Kashani R, et al. Prevalence of migraine headaches in patients with congenital heart disease. Am J Cardiol 2008;101:396–400.

41. Freed LA, Levy D, Levine RA, et al. Prevalence and clinical outcome of mitral-valve prolapse. N Engl J Med 1999;341:1–7.

42. Serafini O, Misuraca G, Siniscalchi A, et al. Prevalence of aneurysm of the interatrial septum in the general population and in patients with a recent episode of cryptogenic ischemic stroke: a tissue harmonic imaging transthoracic echocardiography study in 5,631 patients. Monaldi Arch Chest Dis 2006;66:264–9.

43. Scher AI, Terwindt GM, Picavet HSJ, et al. Cardiovascular risk factors and migraine. The GEM population-based study. Neurology 2005;64:614–20.

44. Kurth T, Gaziano JM, Cook NR, et al. Migraine and risk of cardiovascular disease in women. JAMA 2006;296:283–91.

45. Kurth T, Gaziano M, Cook NR, et al. Migraine and risk of cardiovascular disease in men. Arch Intern Med 2007;167:795–801.

46. Tietjen GE. Migraine and ischaemic heart disease and stroke: potential mechanisms and treatment implications. Cephalalgia 2007;27:981–7.

47. Kurth T. Migraine and ischaemic vascular events. Cephalalgia 2007;27:967–75.
48. Lee ST, Chu K, Jung KH, et al. Decreased number and function of endothelial progenitor cells in patients with migraine. Neurology 2008;70:1510–7.
49. Bigal ME, Lipton RB. Migraine as a risk factor for deep brain lesions and cardiovascular disease. Cephalalgia 2007;27:976–80.
50. Etminan M, Takkouche B, Isorna FC, et al. Risk of ischaemic stroke in people with migraine: systematic review and meta-analysis of observational studies. Br Med J 2005;330:63–5.
51. Tzourio C, Tehindrazanarivelo A, Iglesias S, et al. Case-control study of migraine and risk of ischaemic stroke in young women. Br Med J 1995;310:830–3.
52. Chang CL, Donaghy M, Poulter N. Migraine and stroke in young women: case-control study. The World Health Organisation Collaborative Study of Cardiovascular Disease and Steroid Hormone Contraception. Br Med J 1999;318:13–8.
53. Stang PE, Carson AP, Rose KM, et al. Headache, cerebrovascular symptoms, and stroke: the Atherosclerosis Risk in Communities study. Neurology 2005;64: 1573–7.
54. MacClellan LR, Giles W, Cole J, et al. Probable migraine with visual aura and risk of ischemic stroke. The Stroke Prevention in Young Women study. Stroke 2007;38: 2438–45.
55. Kruit MC, van Buchem MA, Hofman PAM, et al. Migraine as a risk factor for subclinical brain lesions. JAMA 2004;291:427–34.
56. Kruit MC, Launer LJ, Ferrari MD, et al. Infarcts in the posterior circulation territory in migraine. The population-based MRI CAMERA study. Brain 2005;128:2068–77.

Tension-Type Headache

Lars Bendtsen, MD, PhD*, Rigmor Jensen, MD, PhD

KEYWORDS

- Tension-type headache • Diagnosis • Disability
- Mechanisms • Treatment

Tension-type headache (TTH) is the most costly and common form of headache and what many people consider a normal headache, in contrast to migraine. At the same time, it is the least studied type of headache, although scientific acceptance and interest have amplified within the past decade. Although TTH previously was considered primarily psychogenic, a neurobiologic basis has been demonstrated.[1–3] Current epidemiologic and pathophysiologic knowledge and treatment strategies for TTH are reviewed.

DEFINITION

The recent second version of the International Headache Society classification[4] distinguishes between three forms of TTH mainly on basis of headache frequency: (1) infrequent episodic TTH (fewer than 12 headache days per year), (2) frequent episodic TTH (between 12 and 180 days per year), and (3) chronic TTH (at least 180 days per year).

Chronic TTH differs from the episodic forms not only in frequency but also with respect to pathophysiology, lack of effect to most treatment strategies, more medication overuse, more disability, and higher personal and socioeconomic costs.[5] The infrequent episodic form has little impact on individuals and can be regarded as trivial and without need for medical attention. Patients who have frequent episodic or chronic TTH encounter considerable disability and warrant specific intervention.

DIAGNOSIS

TTH is characterized by a bilateral, pressing, tightening pain of mild to moderate intensity, occurring in short episodes of variable duration (episodic forms) or continuously (chronic form). The headache is not associated with the typical migraine features, such as vomiting, severe photophobia, and phonophobia. In the chronic form, only one of these accompanying symptoms is allowed and only mild nausea is accepted.[4] Because of lack of accompanying symptoms and milder pain intensity, patients rarely are severely incapacitated by their pain. TTH is the most featureless of the primary

Danish Headache Center, Department of Neurology, University of Copenhagen, Glostrup Hospital, DK-2600 Glostrup, Denmark
* Corresponding author.
E-mail address: larben01@glo.regionh.dk (L. Bendtsen).

Neurol Clin 27 (2009) 525–535
doi:10.1016/j.ncl.2008.11.010
0733-8619/08/$ – see front matter © 2009 Elsevier Inc. All rights reserved.

neurologic.theclinics.com

headaches and, because many secondary headaches may mimic TTH, a diagnosis of TTH requires exclusion of other organic disorders.

A general and neurologic examination and prospective follow-up using diagnostic headache diaries[6] with registration of all consumed drugs are, therefore, of utmost importance to reach a diagnosis. There are no reliable specific paraclinical tests that are useful in differential diagnosis. Manual palpation of the pericranial muscles and their insertions should be done[2,3] to demonstrate a possible muscular factor for patients and to plan treatment strategy, where physical training and relaxation therapy are important components.

EPIDEMIOLOGY

TTH varies considerably in frequency and duration, from rare, short-lasting episodes of discomfort to frequent, long-lasting, or even continuous disabling headaches. Pooling these extremes in an overall prevalence, therefore, may be misleading. The lifetime prevalence of TTH was as high as 78% in a population-based study in Denmark, but the majority had episodic infrequent TTH (1 day a month or less) without specific need for medical attention.[7] Nevertheless, 24% to 37% had TTH several times a month, 10% had it weekly, and 2% to 3% of the population had chronic TTH, usually lasting for the greater part of a lifetime.[7,8]

The female-to-male ratio of TTH is 5:4 indicating that, unlike migraine, women are affected only slightly more than men.[9,10] The average age of onset of TTH is higher than in migraine, namely 25 to 30 years in cross-sectional epidemiologic studies.[8] The prevalence peaks between ages 30 to 39 and decreases slightly with age.

The incidence of developing headache de novo has been estimated only rarely. In a Danish epidemiologic follow-up study, the annual incidence for TTH was 14.2 per 1000 person years for frequent TTH (female-to-male 3:1),[11] decreasing with age. Risk factors for developing TTH were poor self-rated health, inability to relax after work, and sleeping few hours per night.[11]

A recent review of the global prevalence and burden of headaches[10] showed that the disability of TTH was greater than that of migraine, indicating that the overall cost of TTH is greater than that of migraine. Two Danish studies have shown that the number of workdays missed in the population was 3 times higher for TTH than for migraine[8,12] and a United States study also found that absenteeism resulting from TTH is considerable.[13] Also, indirect costs of all headaches are several times higher than those of migraine alone, indicating that the cost of nonmigraine headaches (mainly TTH) is higher than that of migraine.[14] The burden is particularly high for the minority who have substantial and complicating comorbidities.[15]

The prognosis of TTH has not been analyzed extensively. In a 12-year longitudinal epidemiologic study from Denmark, 549 persons participated in the follow-up study. Among 146 subjects who had frequent episodic TTH and 15 who had chronic TTH at baseline, 45% experienced remission, 39% had unchanged frequent episodic TTH, and 16% had unchanged or newly developed chronic TTH at follow-up. Poor outcome was associated with baseline chronic TTH, coexisting migraine, not being married, and sleeping problems.[11]

PATHOPHYSIOLOGY

Headaches generally are reported to occur in relation to emotional conflict and psychosocial stress, but the cause-and-effect relationship is not clear. A recent review[16] concluded that there is no increase in anxiety or depression in patients who had infrequent TTH whereas frequent TTH was associated with higher rates of anxiety and depression. As in other chronic pain disorders, psychologic abnormalities in TTH may be viewed as secondary rather than primary. Maladaptive coping strategies (eg, catastrophizing and avoidance) seem to be common in TTH.[16] In addition, it recently was demonstrated that depression increases vulnerability to TTH in patients who have frequent headaches during and after a laboratory stress test and that the induced headache was associated with elevated pericranial muscle tenderness.[17] The investigators suggested that depression may aggravate existing central sensitization (discussed later) in patients who have frequent headaches.[17] Thus, there may be a bidirectional relationship between depression and frequent TTH.

The origin of pain in TTH traditionally has been attributed to increased contraction and ischemia of head and neck muscles. Many laboratory-based electromyographic (EMG) studies, however, have reported normal or only slightly increased muscle activity in TTH,[3] and it has been demonstrated that muscle lactate levels are normal during static muscle exercise in patients who have chronic TTH, ruling out muscle ischemia as a cause of the pain.[18] Many studies have consistently shown that the pericranial myofascial tissues are considerably more tender in patients who have TTH than in healthy subjects, and that the tenderness is positively associated with the intensity and the frequency of TTH.[3,19-21] It also has been demonstrated that the consistency of pericranial muscles is increased[22] and that patients who have TTH are more liable to develop shoulder and neck pain in response to static exercise than healthy controls.[23] Moreover, infusion of hypertonic saline into various pericranial muscles elicits referred pain that is perceived as head pain in healthy subjects,[24] and recent studies reported an increased number of active trigger points in pericranial muscles in patients who have frequent episodic TTH and in patients who have chronic TTH.[25]

The increased myofascial pain sensitivity in TTH could be the result of release of inflammatory mediators resulting in excitation and sensitization of peripheral sensory afferents,[2] but this hypothesis was challenged by a study demonstrating normal interstitial concentrations of inflammatory mediators and metabolites in a tender point of patients who had chronic TTH.[26] EMG activity has been reported increased in myofascial trigger points,[27] and it is possible that continuous activity in a few motor units over a long time could be sufficient for excitation or sensitization of peripheral nociceptors.[2] Mork and colleagues[28] infused a combination of endogenous substances into the trapezius muscle and reported that patients who had frequent episodic TTH developed more pain than healthy controls. Concomitant psychophysical measures indicated that a peripheral sensitization of myofascial sensory afferents was responsible for the muscular hypersensitivity in these patients.

To summarize, pericranial myofascial pain sensitivity is increased in patients who have TTH and peripheral mechanisms most likely play a role in the pathophysiology of TTH. Peripheral sensitization of myofascial nociceptors could play a role in increased pain sensitivity but firm evidence for a peripheral abnormality is lacking.

The increased myofascial pain sensitivity in TTH also could be caused by central factors, such as sensitization of second-order neurons at the level of the spinal dorsal horn/trigeminal nucleus, sensitization of supraspinal neurons, and decreased antinociceptive activity from supraspinal structures.[2] Pain detection thresholds have been reported normal in patients who have episodic TTH in studies performed before the separation between the infrequent and frequent form was made.[2] In contrast, pain detection thresholds have been reported decreased in patients who have frequent episodic TTH,[29,30] and pain detection and tolerance thresholds are found decreased in patients who had chronic TTH in all studies performed with sufficient sample size.[2,20,30-32] The nociceptive hypersensitivity has been consistently found in response to different stimulus modalities in various tissues at cephalic and extracephalic locations. These data from clinical studies recently were confirmed in a population-based study demonstrating a close relation between altered pain perception and chronification of headache.[19] In addition, a previously reported increase in TTH prevalence over a 12-year period was related to increased pain sensitivity.[33]

The fact that chronic TTH patients are hypersensitive to stimuli applied at cephalic and at extracephalic, nonsymptomatic locations strongly indicates that synaptic transmission of nociceptive input within the central nervous system is increased in this group of patients, because peripheral sensitization would have more localized effects.[34,35] The expansion of hypersensitivity to other tissues, such as skin, is consistent with referred hyperalgesia, which may be explained by convergence of multiple peripheral sensory afferents onto sensitized spinal cord neurons. The widespread and unspecific nature of the hypersensitivity, however, suggests that the central sensitization also involves supraspinal neurons.[2] Thus, it can be concluded that nociceptive processing in the central nervous system is increased in patients who have chronic TTH, whereas central nociceptive processing seems to be normal in patients who have infrequent episodic TTH.

It has been hypothesized that the central sensitization could be caused by prolonged nociceptive input from tender pericranial myofascial tissues.[2] This hypothesis is supported further by a recent study demonstrating decrease in volume of gray matter brain structures involved in pain processing in patients who had chronic TTH.[36] This decrease was correlated positively with duration of headache and most likely a consequence of central sensitization generated by prolonged input from pericranial myofascial structures.[5,36,37] Decreased antinociceptive activity from supraspinal structures (ie, deficient descending inhibition) also may contribute to the increased pain sensitivity in chronic TTH.[2,32]

Final evidence for the cause-and-effect relationship between frequent headache and central sensitization has to come from longitudinal studies. This recently was provided in a 12-year follow-up study demonstrating that patients who developed episodic TTH had increased pericranial myofascial tenderness but normal general pain sensitivity at follow-up, whereas subjects who developed chronic TTH had normal pain sensitivity at baseline but developed increased central pain sensitivity at follow- up.[38] The investigators concluded that increased pain sensitivity is a consequence of frequent TTH, not a risk factor, and that the results support that central sensitization plays an important role for the chronification of TTH.[38]

The hypothesis of central sensitization in TTH is supported further by clinical pharmacologic studies.[39] Thus, amitriptyline reduces headache and pericranial myofascial tenderness in patients who have chronic TTH.[40] The reduction of myofascial tenderness during treatment with amitriptyline may be caused by a segmental reduction of central sensitization in combination with an enhanced efficacy of noradrenergic or serotonergic descending inhibition.[40] Moreover, nitric oxide synthase inhibitors that reduce central sensitization in animal models of persistent pain also reduce headache and pericranial myofascial tenderness and hardness in patients who have chronic TTH.[41]

To summarize, pericranial myofascial mechanisms probably are of importance in episodic TTH, whereas sensitization of pain pathways in the central nervous system resulting from prolonged nociceptive stimuli from pericranial myofascial tissues seems to be responsible for the conversion of episodic to chronic TTH (**Fig. 1**). This delineates two major targets for future treatment strategies: (1) identifying the source of peripheral nociception in order to prevent the development of central sensitization and thereby the conversion of episodic into chronic TTH and (2) reducing established central sensitization.[1–3]

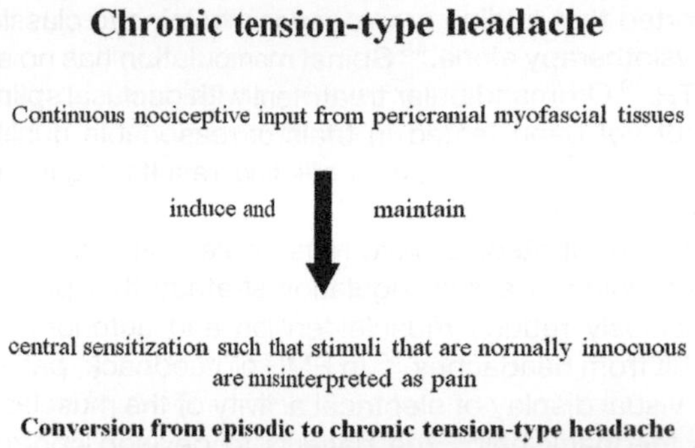

Chronic tension-type headache

Continuous nociceptive input from pericranial myofascial tissues

induce and | maintain

central sensitization such that stimuli that are normally innocuous
are misinterpreted as pain

Conversion from episodic to chronic tension-type headache

Fig. 1. The proposed pathophysiologic model of chronic TTH delineates two major aims for future research: (1) identifying the source of peripheral nociception in order to prevent the development of central sensitization in patients who have episodic TTH and thereby the conversion of episodic into chronic TTH and (2) reducing established central sensitization in patients who have chronic TTH.

TREATMENT

A correct diagnosis should be assured by means of a headache diary[6] recorded over at least 4 weeks. The diagnostic problem encountered most often is discriminating between TTH and mild migraines. The diary also may reveal triggers and medication overuse, and it establishes a baseline against which to measure the efficacy of treatments. Identification of a high intake of analgesics is essential as other treatments largely are ineffective in the presence of medication overuse.[42] Significant comorbidities (eg, anxiety or depression) should be identified and treated concomitantly.

Information about the nature of the disease is important. Muscle pain can lead to a disturbance of the brain's pain-modulating mechanisms,[2,38] so that normally innocuous stimuli are perceived as painful, with secondary perpetuation of muscle pain and risk for anxiety and depression. Physicians taking this problem seriously may have a therapeutic effect, particularly if are patients are concerned about serious disease (eg, brain tumor) and can be reassured by thorough examination. A detailed analysis of trigger factors should be performed, because avoidance of trigger factors may have a long-lasting effect. The triggers reported most frequently for TTH are stress (mental or physical), irregular or inappropriate meals, high intake of coffee and other caffeine-containing drinks, dehydration, sleep disorders, too much or too little sleep, reduced or inappropriate physical exercise, psychologic problems, and variations during the female menstrual cycle and hormonal substitution.[43,44] Most of triggers are self-reported and so far none of the triggers has been systematically tested. It should be explained to patients that frequent TTH only seldom can be cured but a meaningful improvement can be obtained with the combination of nonpharmacologic and pharmacologic treatments. These treatments are described separately but should go hand in hand.

Nonpharmacologic management should be considered for all patients who have TTH and is used widely. Scientific evidence for efficacy of most treatment modalities, however, is sparse.[45] Physical therapy is the most used nonpharmacologic treatment of TTH and includes improvement of posture, relaxation, exercise programs, hot and cold packs, ultrasound, and electrical stimulation.[46] Active treatment strategies generally are recommended.[46] A controlled study[47] combined various techniques, such as massage, relaxation, and home-based exercises, and found a modest effect.

It recently was reported that adding craniocervical training to classical physiotherapy was better than physiotherapy alone.[48] Spinal manipulation has no effect on the treatment of episodic TTH.[49] Oromandibular treatment with occlusal splints often is recommended but has not yet been tested in trials of reasonable quality and cannot be recommended in general.[50] There are conflicting results regarding the efficacy of acupuncture for the treatment of TTH.[51–53]

Psychologic treatment strategies have reasonable scientific support for effectiveness.[54] Relaxation training is a self-regulation strategy that provides patients with the ability to consciously reduce muscle tension and autonomic arousal that can precipitate and result from headaches.[54] In EMG biofeedback, patients are presented with an auditory or visual display of electrical activity of the muscles in the face, neck, or shoulders. This feedback helps the patients to develop control over pericranial muscle tension. It is most likely that cognitive changes (ie, self-efficacy) rather than reductions in muscle tension account for the improvement in TTH with EMG biofeedback. Cognitive-behavioral therapy (stress management) aims to teach patients to identify thoughts and beliefs that generate stress and aggravate headaches.[54] The exact degree of effect of psychologic treatment strategies is difficult to estimate, but cognitive-behavioral therapy has been found comparable with treatment with tricyclic antidepressants, whereas a combination of the two treatments seemed more effective than either treatment alone.[55]

Acute pharmacologic therapy refers to the treatment of individual attacks of headache in patients who have episodic and chronic TTH. Most headaches in patients who have episodic TTH are mild to moderate and the patients often can self-manage with simple analgesics. The efficacy of the simple analgesics tends to decrease with increasing frequency of the headaches. In patients who have chronic TTH, the headaches often are associated with stress, anxiety, and depression; simple analgesics usually are ineffective but should be used with caution because of the risk for medication-overuse headache with a regular intake of simple analgesics more than 14 days a month or triptans or combination analgesics more than 9 days a month.[42] Other interventions, such as nondrug treatments and prophylactic pharmacotherapy, should be considered.

Most randomized placebo-controlled trials have demonstrated that aspirin (in doses of 500 mg and 1000 mg)[56] and acetaminophen (1000 mg)[56] are effective in the acute therapy for TTH. There is no consistent difference in efficacy between aspirin and acetaminophen. The nonsteroidal anti-inflammatory drugs (NSAIDs), ibuprofen (200–400 mg), naproxen sodium (375–550 mg), ketoprofen (25–50 mg), and diclofenac potassium (50–100 mg) all have been demonstrated more effective than placebo in acute TTH.[57] Most, but not all, comparative studies report that these NSAIDs are more effective than acetaminophen and aspirin.[57]

The combination of analgesics with caffeine, codeine, sedatives, or tranquilizers frequently is used and increased efficacy when adding caffeine to aspirin or ibuprofen has been reported.[57] Combination analgesics, however, generally should be avoided because of the risk for dependency, abuse, and chronification of the headache.[42] Triptans do not have a clinically relevant effect, and muscle relaxants have not been demonstrated effective in TTH.[57]

To summarize, simple analgesics are the mainstays in the acute therapy for TTH (**Fig. 2**). Acetaminophen (1000 mg) may be recommended as drug of first choice because of better gastric side-effect profile.[58] If acetaminophen is not effective, Ibuprofen (400 mg) may be recommended because of a favorable gastrointestinal side-effect profile compared with other NSAIDs.[58] Physicians should be aware of the risk for developing medication-overuse headache as a result of frequent and

Pharmacotherapy

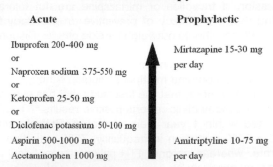

Acute	Prophylactic
Ibuprofen 200-400 mg or Naproxen sodium 375-550 mg or Ketoprofen 25-50 mg or Diclofenac potassium 50-100 mg	Mirtazapine 15-30 mg per day
Aspirin 500-1000 mg Acetaminophen 1000 mg	Amitriptyline 10-75 mg per day

Fig. 2. Pharmacologic treatment paradigm for TTH.

excessive use of analgesics in acute therapy.[42] Triptans, muscle relaxants, and opioids do not have a role in the treatment of TTH.

Prophylactic pharmacotherapy should be considered in patients who have chronic TTH who do not respond to nonpharmacologic treatment. The tricyclic antidepressant, amitriptyline, is the only drug proved effective in several controlled trials in TTH.[59] The two most recent studies reported that amitriptyline (75 mg per day) reduced headache index (duration × intensity) by 30% compared with placebo.[55,60] The effect is long lasting (at least 6 months)[55] and not related to the presence of depression.[60] It is important that patients be informed that this is an antidepressant agent but has an independent action on pain. Amitriptyline should be started at low dosages (10 mg/day) and titrated by 10 mg weekly until patients have good therapeutic effect or side effects are encountered. The maintenance dose usually is 30 to 70 mg daily administered 1 to 2 hours before bedtime to help circumvent any sedative adverse effects. A significant effect of amitriptyline may be observed in the first week on the therapeutic dose.[60] It is advisable, therefore, to change to other prophylactic therapy if patients do not respond after 4 weeks on maintenance dose. The side effects of amitriptyline include dry mouth, drowsiness, dizziness, obstipation, and weight gain.

The tricyclic antidepressant, clomipramine, and the tetracyclic antidepressants, maprotiline and mianserin, are reported as more effective than placebo, whereas the selective serotonin reuptake inhibitors (SSRIs) are not found effective.[59] Antidepressants with action on serotonin and noradrenaline seem as effective as amitriptyline with the advantage that they are tolerated in doses needed for the treatment of concomitant depression. Thus, the noradrenergic and specific serotonergic antidepressant, mirtazapine (30 mg/day), reduced headache index by 34% more than placebo in difficult-to-treat patients, including patients who had not responded to amitriptyline.[61] The serotonin and noradrenaline reuptake inhibitor, venlafaxine (150 mg/day),[62] reduced headache days from 15 to 12 per month. The latter study[62] is difficult to compare with the other studies discussed,[55,60,61] however, because it was a small parallel group study performed in a mixed group of patients who had frequent episodic or chronic TTH. Tizanidine, botulinum toxin, propranolol or valproic acid can not be recommended at present for the prophylactic treatment of TTH.[59]

To summarize, the initial approach to prophylactic pharmacotherapy for chronic TTH is through the use of amitriptyline (see Fig. 2). Concomitant use of daily analgesics should be avoided. If patients do not respond to amitriptyline, mirtazapine could be attempted. Venlafaxine or SSRIs could be considered in patients who have concomitant depression, if tricyclics or mirtazapine are not tolerated. Physicians should keep in mind that the efficacy of preventive drug therapy for TTH often is modest and that the efficacy should outweigh the side effects. Discontinuation should be attempted every 6 to 12 months.

As neither nonpharmacologic nor pharmacologic management is highly efficient, it usually is recommended to combine multiple strategies although proper evidence is lacking. It is reassuring, therefore, that the first study that has evaluated the efficacy of a multidisciplinary headache clinic reports positive results.[63] Treatment results for all patients discharged within 1 year were evaluated. Patients who had episodic TTH demonstrated a 50% reduction in frequency, 75% reduction in intensity, and 33% in absence rate, whereas chronic TTH patients responded with 32%, 30%, and 40% reductions, respectively.[63]

REFERENCES

1. Ashina M. Neurobiology of chronic tension-type headache. Cephalalgia 2004; 24(3):161–72.
2. Bendtsen L. Central sensitization in tension-type headache—possible pathophysiological mechanisms. Cephalalgia 2000;20(5):486–508.
3. Jensen R. Pathophysiological mechanisms of tension-type headache: a review of epidemiological and experimental studies. Cephalalgia 1999;19(6):602–21.
4. Headache Classification Subcommittee of the International Headache Society. The international classification of headache disorders. 2nd edition. Cephalalgia 2004;24(Suppl 1):1–160.
5. Bendtsen L, Jensen R. Tension-type headache: the most common, but also the most neglected, headache disorder. Curr Opin Neurol 2006;19(3):305–9.
6. Russell MB, Rasmussen BK, Brennum J, et al. Presentation of a new instrument: the diagnostic headache diary. Cephalalgia 1992;12(6):369–74.
7. Lyngberg AC, Rasmussen BK, Jorgensen T, et al. Has the prevalence of migraine and tension-type headache changed over a 12-year period? A Danish population survey. Eur J Epidemiol 2005;20(3):243–9.
8. Rasmussen BK. Epidemiology of headache. Cephalalgia 1995;15(1):45–68.
9. Andlin-Sobocki P, Jonsson B, Wittchen HU, et al. Cost of disorders of the brain in Europe. Eur J Neurol 2005;12(Suppl 1):1–27.
10. Stovner L, Hagen K, Jensen R, et al. The global burden of headache: a documentation of headache prevalence and disability worldwide. Cephalalgia 2007;27(3): 193–210.
11. Lyngberg AC, Rasmussen BK, Jorgensen T, et al. Prognosis of migraine and tension-type headache: a population-based follow-up study. Neurology 2005; 65(4):580–5.
12. Lyngberg AC, Rasmussen BK, Jorgensen T, et al. Secular changes in health care utilization and work absence for migraine and tension-type headache: a population based study. Eur J Epidemiol 2005;20(12):1007–14.
13. Schwartz BS, Stewart WF, Lipton RB. Lost workdays and decreased work effectiveness associated with headache in the workplace. J Occup Environ Med 1997; 39(4):320–7.
14. Berg J, Stovner LJ. Cost of migraine and other headaches in Europe. Eur J Neurol 2005; 12(Suppl 1):59–62.
15. Jensen R, Stovner LJ. Epidemiology and comorbidity of headache. Lancet Neurol 2008;7(4):354–61.

16. Heckman BD, Holroyd KA. Tension-type headache and psychiatric comorbidity. Curr Pain Headache Rep 2006;10(6):439–47.
17. Janke EA, Holroyd KA, Romanek K. Depression increases onset of tension-type headache following laboratory stress. Pain 2004;111(3):230–8.
18. Ashina M, Stallknecht B, Bendtsen L, et al. In vivo evidence of altered skeletal muscle blood flow in chronic tension-type headache. Brain 2002;125:320–6.
19. Buchgreitz L, Lyngberg AC, Bendtsen L, et al. Frequency of headache is related to sensitization: a population study. Pain 2006;123(1–2):19–27.
20. Fernandez-De-LAS-Penas C, Cuadrado ML, Arendt-Nielsen L, et al. Increased pericranial tenderness, decreased pressure pain threshold, and headache clinical parameters in chronic tension-type headache patients. Clin J Pain 2007;23(4):346–52.
21. Lipchik GL, Holroyd KA, O'Donnell FJ, et al. Exteroceptive suppression periods and pericranial muscle tenderness in chronic tension-type headache: effects of psychopathology, chronicity and disability. Cephalalgia 2000;20(7):638–46.
22. Ashina M, Bendtsen L, Jensen R, et al. Muscle hardness in patients with chronic tension-type headache: relation to actual headache state. Pain 1999;79(2–3): 201–5.
23. Christensen M, Bendtsen L, Ashina M, et al. Experimental induction of muscle tenderness and headache in tension-type headache patients. Cephalalgia 2005;25(11):1061–7.
24. Schmidt-Hansen PT, Svensson P, Jensen TS, et al. Patterns of experimentally induced pain in pericranial muscles. Cephalalgia 2006;26(5):568–77.
25. Fernandez-De-Las-Penas C, Cuadrado ML, Arendt-Nielsen L, et al. Myofascial trigger points and sensitization: an updated pain model for tension-type headache. Cephalalgia 2007;27(5):383–93.
26. Ashina M, Stallknecht B, Bendtsen L, et al. Tender points are not sites of ongoing inflammation - in vivo evidence in patients with chronic tension-type headache. Cephalalgia 2003;23(2):109–16.
27. Hubbard DR, Berkoff GM. Myofascial trigger points show spontaneous needle EMG activity. Spine 1993;18(13):1803–7.
28. Mork H, Ashina M, Bendtsen L, et al. Possible mechanisms of pain perception in patients with episodic tension-type headache. A new experimental model of myofascial pain. Cephalalgia 2004;24(6):466–75.
29. Mork H, Ashina M, Bendtsen L, et al. Induction of prolonged tenderness in patients with tension-type headache by means of a new experimental model of myofascial pain. Eur J Neurol 2003;10(3):249–56.
30. Schmidt-Hansen PT, Svensson P, Bendtsen L, et al. Increased muscle pain sensitivity in patients with tension-type headache. Pain 2007;129(1–2):113–21.
31. Ashina S, Bendtsen L, Ashina M, et al. Generalized hyperalgesia in patients with chronic tension-type headache. Cephalalgia 2006;26(8):940–8.
32. Sandrini G, Rossi P, Milanov I, et al. Abnormal modulatory influence of diffuse noxious inhibitory controls in migraine and chronic tension-type headache patients. Cephalalgia 2006;26(7):782–9.
33. Buchgreitz L, Lyngberg A, Bendtsen L, et al. Increased prevalence of tension-type headache over a 12-year period is related to increased pain sensitivity. A population study. Cephalalgia 2007;27(2):145–52.
34. Milanov I, Bogdanova D. Pain and tension-type headache: a review of the possible pathophysiological mechanisms. J Headache Pain 2004;5:4–11.
35. Treede RD, Meyer RA, Raja SN, et al. Peripheral and central mechanisms of cutaneous hyperalgesia. Prog Neurobiol 1992;38(4):397–421.

36. Schmidt-Wilcke T, Leinisch E, Straube A, et al. Gray matter decrease in patients with chronic tension type headache. Neurology 2005;65(9):1483–6.
37. Mathew NT. Tension-type headache. Curr Neurol Neurosci Rep 2006;6(2):100–5.
38. Buchgreitz L, Lyngberg AC, Bendtsen L, et al. Increased pain sensitivity is not a risk factor but a consequence of frequent headache: a population-based follow-up study. Pain 2007 [-E-pub ahead of print].
39. Bendtsen L. Sensitization: its role in primary headache. Curr Opin Investig Drugs 2002;3(3):449–53.
40. Bendtsen L, Jensen R. Amitriptyline reduces myofascial tenderness in patients with chronic tension-type headache. Cephalalgia 2000;20(6):603–10.
41. Ashina M, Bendtsen L, Jensen R, et al. Possible mechanisms of action of nitric oxide synthase inhibitors in chronic tension-type headache. Brain 1999;122(9):1629–35.
42. Katsarava Z, Jensen R. Medication-overuse headache: where are we now? Curr Opin Neurol 2007;20(3):326–30.
43. Rasmussen BK, Jensen R, Schroll M, et al. Interrelations between migraine and tension-type headache in the general population. Arch Neurol 1992;49:914–8.
44. Ulrich V, Russell MB, Jensen R, et al. A comparison of tension-type headache in migraineurs and in non-migraineurs: a population-based study. Pain 1996; 67(2–3):501–6.
45. Jensen R. Tension-type headache. Curr Treat Options Neurol 2001;3(2):169–80.
46. Jensen R, Roth JM. Psysiotherapy of tension-type headaches. In: Olesen J, Goadsby PJ, Ramadan N, et al, editors. The headaches. 3rd edition. Philadelphia: Lippincott Williams Wilkins; 2005. p. 721–6.
47. Torelli P, Jensen R, Olesen J. Physiotherapy for tension-type headache: a controlled study. Cephalalgia 2004;24(1):29–36.
48. van Ettekoven H, Lucas C. Efficacy of physiotherapy including a craniocervical training programme for tension-type headache; a randomized clinical trial. Cephalalgia 2006;26(8):983–91.
49. Bove G, Nilsson N. Spinal manipulation in the treatment of episodic tension-type headache: a randomized controlled trial. JAMA 1998;280(18):1576–9.
50. Graff-Radford SB, Canavan DW. Headache attributed to orofacial/temporomandibular pathology. In: Olesen J, Goadsby PJ, Ramadan N, et al, editors. The headaches. 3rd edition. Philadelphia: Lippincott Williams Wilkins; 2005. p. 1029–35.
51. Davis MA, Kononowech RW, Rolin SA, et al. Acupuncture for tension-type headache: a meta-analysis of randomized, controlled trials. J Pain 2008;9(8):667–77.
52. Endres HG, Bowing G, Diener HC, et al. Acupuncture for tension-type headache: a multicentre, sham-controlled, patient-and observer-blinded, randomised trial. J Headache Pain 2007;8(5):306–14.
53. Melchart D, Streng A, Hoppe A, et al. Acupuncture in patients with tension-type headache: randomised controlled trial. BMJ 2005;331(7513):376–82.
54. Holroyd KA, Martin PR, Nash JM. Psychological treatments of tension-type headache. In: Olesen J, Goadsby PJ, Ramadan N, et al, editors. The headaches. 3rd edition. Philadelphia: Lippincott Williams Wilkins; 2005. p. 711–9.
55. Holroyd KA, O'Donnell FJ, Stensland M, et al. Management of chronic tension-type headache with tricyclic antidepressant medication, stress management therapy, and their combination: a randomized controlled trial. JAMA 2001; 285(17):2208–15.
56. Steiner TJ, Lange R, Voelker M. Aspirin in episodic tension-type headache: placebo-controlled dose-ranging comparison with paracetamol. Cephalalgia 2003;23(1):59–66.

57. Ashina S, Ashina M. Current and potential future drug therapies for tension-type headache. Curr Pain Headache Rep 2003;7(6):466–74.
58. Langman MJ, Weil J, Wainwright P, et al. Risks of bleeding peptic ulcer associated with individual non-steroidal anti-inflammatory drugs. Lancet 1994; 343(8905):1075–8.
59. Bendtsen L, Mathew NT. Prophylactic pharmacotherapy of tension-type headache. In: Olesen J, Goadsby PJ, Ramadan N, et al, editors. The headaches. 3rd edition. Philadelphia: Lippincott Williams Wilkins; 2005. p. 735–41.
60. Bendtsen L, Jensen R, Olesen J. A non-selective (amitriptyline), but not a selective (citalopram), serotonin reuptake inhibitor is effective in the prophylactic treatment of chronic tension-type headache. J Neurol Neurosurg Psychiatr 1996; 61(3):285–90.
61. Bendtsen L, Jensen R. Mirtazapine is effective in the prophylactic treatment of chronic tension-type headache. Neurology 2004;62(10):1706–11.
62. Zissis N, Harmoussi S, Vlaikidis N, et al. A randomized, double-blind, placebo-controlled study of venlafaxine XR in out-patients with tension-type headache. Cephalalgia 2007;27(4):315–24.
63. Zeeberg P, Olesen J, Jensen R. Efficacy of multidisciplinary treatment in a tertiary referral headache centre. Cephalalgia 2005;25(12):1159–67.

Trigeminal Autonomic Cephalalgias

Todd D. Rozen, MD[a,b]

KEYWORDS

- Trigeminal autonomic cephalalgias • Cluster headache
- SUNCT syndrome • Paroxysmal hemicrania
- Hemicrania continua • Indomethacin

The trigeminal autonomic cephalalgias (TACs) are a group of primary headache syndromes all marked by headache and associated autonomic features, including lacrimation, eyelid ptosis, nasal rhinorrhea or congestion, and the presence of a Horner's syndrome (ptosis with miotic pupil). The brain stem connection between the trigeminal system and the parasympathetic autonomic nervous system allows us to understand how trigeminal-based pain can be associated with autonomic symptomatology. The TACs include cluster headache, paroxysmal hemicrania, short-lasting unilateral neuralgiform headache attacks with conjunctival injection and tearing (SUNCT) syndrome, and hemicrania continua (HC).

CLUSTER HEADACHE

Cluster headache is a stereotypic episodic headache disorder marked by frequent attacks of short-lasting, severe, unilateral head pain with associated autonomic symptoms. A cluster headache is defined as an individual attack of head pain, whereas a cluster period or cycle is the time during which a patient is having daily cluster headaches. Most patients who have cluster headache have episodic cluster headache, indicating that they have remission periods between cluster cycles, whereas a few unfortunate individuals have chronic cluster headache, in which cycles occur for more than 1 year without remission or with remission periods lasting less than 1 month.

Typical cluster headache location is retro-orbital, periorbital, and occipitonuchal. Maximum pain is normally retro-orbital in more than 70% of patients. Pain quality is described as boring, stabbing, burning, or squeezing. Cluster headache intensity is always severe and never mild, although headache pain intensity may be less at the beginning and end of cluster periods. Cluster headaches that awaken a patient from sleep are more severe than those occurring during the day. The one-sided nature of cluster headaches is a trademark. Patients who have cluster headache normally

[a] Michigan Head-Pain and Neurological Institute, 3120 Professional Drive, Ann Arbor, MI 48104, USA
[b] Department of Neurology, Wayne State University, Detroit, MI 48201, USA
E-mail address: tdrozmigraine@yahoo.com

Neurol Clin 27 (2009) 537–556
doi:10.1016/j.ncl.2008.11.005
0733-8619/08/$ – see front matter © 2009 Elsevier Inc. All rights reserved.

neurologic.theclinics.com

experience cluster headaches on the same side of the head their entire life. Only in 15% of patients do the headaches shift to the other side of the head at the next cluster period, and side shifting during the same cluster cycle only occurs in 5% of patients. The duration of individual cluster headaches is between 15 minutes and 180 minutes, with more than 75% attacks lasting less than 60 minutes. Attack frequency is between one and three attacks per day, with most patients experiencing two or fewer headaches in a day. Peak time periods for daily cluster headache onset are 1:00 to 2:00 AM, 1:00 to 3:00 PM, and after 9:00 PM; thus, most patients who have cluster headache can complete their occupation requirements without experiencing headaches during the work day. The headaches have a predilection for the first rapid eye movement sleep phase; thus, the patient who has cluster headache awakens with a severe headache 60 to 90 minutes after falling asleep. The duration of the cluster period normally lasts between 2 and 12 weeks, and patients generally experience one or two cluster periods per year. Remission periods (headache-free time between cluster cycles) average 6 months to 2 years. Cluster headache is marked by its associated autonomic symptoms that typically occur on the same side as the head pain but can be bilateral. Lacrimation is the most common associated symptom, occurring in 73% of patients, followed by conjunctival injection in 60%, nasal congestion in 42%, nasal rhinorrhea in 22%, and a partial Horner's syndrome in 16% to 84%. Symptoms generally attributed to migraine can also occur during a cluster headache, including nausea, vomiting, photophobia, and phonophobia. During an individual cluster headache, patients are unable to sit or stand completely still. Cluster is really a state of agitation, because remaining still seems to make the pain worse. Some patients who have cluster headache state that they lie down with a cluster headache, but when questioning them, they do not lie still but roll around on the bed in agony. Many patients develop their own routine during a cluster attack, including banging their heads against the wall, crawling on the floor, taking hot showers, or just screaming out in pain. Only approximately 3% can lie still during an attack.[1] Many patients develop suicidal ideations during a headache.

Treatment

All patients who have cluster headache require treatment. Other primary headache syndromes can sometimes be managed nonmedicinally, but in regard to cluster headache, medication, sometimes even polypharmacy, is indicated. Cluster headache treatment can be divided into three classes. Abortive therapy is treatment given at the time of an attack to provide therapy for that individual attack alone. Transitional therapy can be considered to be an intermittent or short-term preventive treatment. An agent is started at the same time as the patient's true maintenance preventive medication. The transitional therapy provides attack relief for the patient who has cluster headache while the maintenance preventive medication is being built up to a therapeutic dosage. Preventive therapy consists of daily medication, which is supposed to reduce the frequency of headache attacks, lower attack intensity, and lessen attack duration. The main goal of cluster headache preventive therapy should be to make a patient cluster headache–free on preventives, even though the patient is still in the midst of a cluster cycle. Because most patients who have cluster headache have episodic cluster headache, medications are only used while a patient is in cycle and are stopped during remission periods.

Abortive therapy

The goal of abortive therapy for cluster headache is fast, effective, and consistent relief. There is no role for over-the-counter agents or butalbital-containing compounds in cluster headache and little if any need for opiates. Abortives need to show effect usually within 20 minutes, because the attacks are short in duration. Typical cluster headache abortive options are as follows:

1. Sumatriptan injection or nasal spray (>90% effective)
2. Oxygen: 100% oxygen administered by means of a face mask at 8–15 L/min (70% of patients obtain relief)
3. Dihydroergotamine: intramuscular, subcutaneous, or intravenous
4. Ergotamine: oral or suppository
5. Zolmitriptan nasal spray or administered orally: 10 mg or 5 mg
6. Intranasal lidocaine (fewer than one third of patients respond)
7. Greater occipital nerve (GON) blockade

Sumatriptan Subcutaneous sumatriptan is the most effective medication for the symptomatic relief of cluster headache. In a placebo-controlled study, injectable sumatriptan at a dose of 6 mg was significantly more effective than placebo, with 74% of patients having complete relief by 15 minutes compared with 26% of placebo-treated patients.[2] In long-term open-label studies, sumatriptan is effective in 76% to 100% of all attacks within 15 minutes, even after repetitive daily use for several months.[3] Interestingly, sumatriptan seems to be 8% less effective in chronic cluster headache than in episodic cluster headache. Sumatriptan is contraindicated in patients who have uncontrolled hypertension and a past history of myocardial infarction or stroke. As almost all patients who have cluster headache have a strong history of cigarette smoking; the physician must closely monitor cardiovascular risk factors in these patients.

Sumatriptan nasal spray (20 mg) has been shown to be more effective than placebo in the acute treatment of cluster attacks. In more than 80 patients tested, intranasal sumatriptan reduced cluster headache pain from extremely severe, severe, or moderate to mild or no pain at 30 minutes in 58% of sumatriptan users versus 30% of patients given placebo on the first attack treated, whereas the rates were 50% (sumatriptan) versus 33% (placebo) after the second treated attack.[1] Sumatriptan nasal spray seems to be efficacious for cluster headache but less effective than subcutaneous injection. Sumatriptan nasal spray should be considered as a cluster headache abortive in patients who cannot tolerate injections or when, situationally (eg, an office setting), injections would be considered socially unacceptable.

In many instances, patients who have cluster headache may need to use sumatriptan more than once a day for days to weeks at a time. There is still controversy as to whether patients who have cluster headache can develop analgesic rebound headache. Hering-Hanit[4] noted that the use of daily injectable sumatriptan in four patients who had cluster headache led to a marked increase in the frequency of cluster attacks 3 to 4 weeks after initiating treatment. In three patients, the character of the cluster headache changed, whereas two patients experienced prolongation of their cluster headache period. Withdrawal of sumatriptan reduced the frequency of headaches. Even though daily sumatriptan may be benefiting a patient who has cluster headache, the goal should be to have the patient cluster headache–free on preventive medication not using abortives to achieve a cluster headache–free status.

Oxygen Oxygen inhalation is an excellent abortive therapy for cluster headache. Typical dosing is 100% oxygen given by means of a non-rebreather face mask at 7 to 10 L/min for 20 minutes. In some patients, oxygen is completely effective at aborting an attack if taken when the pain is at maximal intensity, whereas in others, the attack is only delayed for minutes to hours rather than completely alleviated. It is not uncommon for a patient who has cluster headache to be headache-free while on oxygen but to redevelop pain immediately after the oxygen is removed. Overall, oxygen is an attractive therapy because it is completely safe and can be used multiple times during the day. Large home oxygen tanks are prescribed for patients who have cluster headache, whereas portable tanks can be taken to the workplace. In Kudrow's landmark study using oxygen,[5] 75% of patients responded to 100% oxygen at 7 L/min, although only 57% of older patients who had chronic cluster headache obtained relief. A recent study[6] documented a gender difference in response to oxygen, because only 59% of female patients responded to oxygen, whereas 87% of men did. In almost every textbook and article written on the subject of cluster headache treatment, patients are instructed to use 100% oxygen by means of a non-rebreather face mask at a rate of 7 to 10 L/min. The rationale behind this prescribed oxygen flow rate is unknown, but it has become doctrine since the study by Kudrow.[5] Prescribing higher flow rates of oxygen up to 12 L/min has recently been suggested, but there is no documentation that this may improve efficacy. The abortive effect of higher oxygen flow rates (up to 15 L/min) in patients who have cluster headache and are refractory to standard oxygen therapy is unknown. Rozen[7] recently documented three patients who had cluster headache and demonstrated no response to standard oxygen therapy but had complete cluster headache relief when exposed to higher oxygen flow rates of 15 L/min. From this clinical observation, it seems that patients who have cluster headache should not be deemed refractory to oxygen therapy unless flow rates up to 15 L/min have been used.

Zolmitriptan Zolmitriptan is one of the second-generation triptan compounds that has shown good efficacy in migraine. In a double-blind controlled trial, the efficacy of 5 and 10 mg of oral zolmitriptan was tested versus placebo in the treatment of individual cluster headache attacks.[8] A two-point reduction on a five-point pain intensity scale at 30 minutes was used as a positive response end point. Forty-seven percent of patients taking zolmitriptan at a dose of 10 mg had a positive response versus 40% receiving 5 mg and 29% receiving placebo. The difference reached statistical significance for zolmitriptan, 10 mg, versus placebo. Significantly more patients reported mild or no pain 30 minutes after treatment with zolmitriptan at doses of 5 and 10 mg (57% and 60%, respectively) than after placebo (42%). The response rates for zolmitriptan are not as dramatic as those seen with oxygen or injectable sumatriptan, but this is the first oral triptan shown to have efficacy as a cluster abortive and is an alternative treatment option in patients who cannot tolerate injections or intranasal preparations and have failed oxygen or find it difficult to use in acute situations. Zolmitriptan nasal spray has also shown efficacy for treating individual cluster attacks in two recent studies using 10-mg dosing.[9]

Other possible effective abortives for the patient who has intractable cluster headache

1. Intranasal lidocaine, 4% (may need to be compounded), given as one spray in the nostril on the side of the headache, can be repeated in 10 to 15 minutes, and the patient may use up to four sprays per day.
2. Olanzapine, 2.5 to 10 mg administered orally per headache, can be quite sedating and not only seems to take away the pain but can reduce the agitation along with the headaches. This is a useful choice if the patient cannot use triptans and has failed oxygen therapy.[10]
3. Chlorpromazine suppository, 25 mg: 1 to 2 supp (25–50 mg) to abort a headache
4. Indomethacin supp, 50 mg: 1 supp every 30 minutes up to 150 mg total
5. GON blockade if patient is in the office or emergency department and is having a cluster headache attack and does not respond to triptans or oxygen; a large-volume

suboccipital nerve block can typically abort a cluster headache within 10 minutes of administration.
6. Subcutaneous octreotide (somatostatin analogue), 100 μg, was significantly superior to placebo (P<.01) in the acute treatment of a cluster headache.[11] It is not yet readily used in headache clinics.
7. Dihydroergotamine nasal spray or intramuscular injection

Transitional therapy

Transitional cluster therapy is a short-term preventive treatment that bridges the time between cluster diagnosis and the time when the true traditional maintenance preventive agent becomes efficacious. Transitional preventives are started at the same time the maintenance preventive is begun. The transitional preventive should provide the patient who has cluster headache with almost immediate pain relief and allow the patient to be headache-free or near headache-free while the maintenance preventive medication dose is being tapered up to an effective level. When the transitional agent is tapered off, the maintenance preventive should have kicked in; thus, the patient should have no gap in headache preventive coverage. Transitional treatment options are as follows:

1. Corticosteroids: prednisone taper; start at 60–80 mg, taper over 10–12 days
2. Naratriptan: (2.5 mg) one tablet twice daily for 7 days or frovatriptan (2.5 mg) administered orally one to two times daily
3. Dihydroergotamine (DHE): daily intramuscular injections (1 mg once or twice daily) for 1 week or intravenous infusion of DHE (1 mg BID or TID) for 3 days
4. Occipital nerve blockade

Corticosteroids A short course of corticosteroids is the best-known transitional therapy for cluster headache. Typically, within 24 to 48 hours of administration, patients become headache-free, and by the time the steroid taper has ended, the patient's main preventive agent has started to become effective. Prednisone and dexamethasone are the most typically used corticosteroids in cluster headache. A typical taper would be prednisone, 80 mg, for the first 2 days, followed by 60 mg for 2 days, 40 mg for 2 days, 20 mg for 2 days, 10 mg for 2 days, and then stopping the agent. There is no set manner in which to dose corticosteroids in cluster headache. Kudrow[5] noted that prednisone provided substantial cluster pain relief in 77% of 77 patients who had episodic cluster headache and partial improvement in another 12%. Patients who have chronic cluster headache did not fare as well, with only 40% of 15 patients treated showing marked improvement.

Dexamethasone at a dose of 4 mg twice a day for 2 weeks followed by 4 mg/d for 1 week has also been shown to be effective.[12] When dexamethasone or prednisone is tapered, however, the cluster attacks frequently recur. Therefore, corticosteroids are primarily useful for inducing rapid remission in patients who have episodic cluster headache, although they may provide a brief respite for patients who have chronic cluster headache. Long-term use of corticosteroids in these patients must be resisted.

A typical dosing schedule is as follows: prednisone, 80 mg, on days 1 and 2; 60 mg on days 3 and 4; 60 mg on days 5 and 6; 40 mg on days 7 and 8; 20 mg on days 8 and 9; and 10 mg on days 10 and 11.

Dihydroergotamine Intravenous DHE is an attractive transitional treatment but is more labor-intensive, because patients need to be admitted or brought to an outpatient infusion center for therapy. Typically, within 1 or 2 days of repetitive DHE treatment, cluster headache attacks stop and do not return for days to months. This allows time for a maintenance preventive agent to be started, and when the effects of the DHE wear off, the true maintenance preventive medication's effects have already kicked in. Mather and collegues[13] reported the use of repetitive intravenous DHE in 54 patients who had cluster headache (23 episodic and 31 chronic). At the same time that DHE was initiated, a preventive agent was also started. One hundred percent of patients had complete relief of attacks with DHE. At a 3-month follow-up, 93% of the patients who had episodic cluster headache remained cluster headache–free and 7% demonstrated a 50% to 74% improvement. For the patients who had chronic cluster headache, 44% were chronic headache–free at 3 months and another 52% showed at least a 50% improvement. While on DHE therapy, sumatriptan and other vasoconstrictive agents cannot be used concomitantly.

Occipital nerve blockade Anthony[14] was the first to report the use of occipital nerve blockade to arrest cluster headache attacks. Mitsias and collegues[15] recently treated 12 patients with GON blocks; a total of 24 blocks were performed on 24 attacks. Twenty-three (96%) were successful in completely aborting a cluster headache cycle within 7 days. Peres and collegues[16] treated 14 patients who had cluster headache with GON blockade as transitional therapy. The mean number of headache-free days was 13.1. Four patients (28.5%) had a good response, 5 (35.7%) had a moderate response, and 5 (35.7%) had no response. The GON block was well tolerated, with no adverse events. Headache intensity, frequency, and duration were significantly decreased comparing the week before with the week after the nerve block ($P < .003$, $P = .003$, and $P < .005$, respectively). Anecdotally, occipital nerve blockade using a combination of an anesthetic (eg, lidocaine) and steroid (eg, triamcinolone) not only breaks an ongoing single attack of cluster headache but, when used interictally, can prevent cluster headache attacks from coming on for at least 1 to 2 days but sometimes for up to 6 weeks. There are isolated instances in which nerve blockade has terminated an ongoing cluster headache period. Nerve blockade seems to work in cluster headache even in the absence of defined neck trigger points. Some newer European studies suggest that occipital nerve blockade can provide pain relief for up to 4 weeks.

Preventive therapy

Preventive agents are absolutely necessary in patients who have cluster headache unless the cluster headache periods last for less than 2 weeks. Preventive medications are only used while the patient is in cycle, and they are tapered off once a cluster headache period has ended. If a patient decides to remain on a preventive agent even after he or she has gone out of cycle, this does not seem to prevent a subsequent cluster headache period from starting. The maintenance preventive should be started at the time a transitional agent is given. Most physicians treating cluster headache increase the dosages of the preventive agents quickly to get a desired response. Large dosages, much higher than that suggested in the Physician's Desk Reference, are sometimes necessary when treating cluster headache. A well-recognized trait of patients who have cluster headache is that they can tolerate medications much better than patients who do not have cluster headache. Most of the recognized cluster headache preventives can be used in episodic and chronic cluster headache. Polypharmacy is not discouraged in cluster headache prevention. If a patient has a partial response on one agent, another preventive can be added to this rather than starting over from scratch. Not unlike the multiple preventive regimen used in trigeminal neuralgia, cluster attacks are so severe that add-on therapy is encouraged. Preventive agents include the following:

1. Verapamil (80 mg): dose range: 80-960 mg; quick taper up, can push to high levels (>480 mg); electrocardiogram with every dose change greater than 480 mg and serial electrocardiograms every 3–6 months even with stable dosing
2. Lithium carbonate (300 mg): dose range: 300–900 mg
3. Divalproex sodium extended release (500 mg): dose range: 500–3000 mg
4. Topiramate (25 mg): dose range: 50–400 mg (typical dose is 75 mg or less)
5. Melatonin (3 mg): 9 mg at bedtime

Verapamil Verapamil seems to be the best first-line preventive therapy for episodic and chronic cluster headache. It can be used safely in conjunction with sumatriptan, ergotamine, corticosteroids, and other preventive agents. Leone and collegues[17] compared the efficacy of verapamil with placebo in the prophylaxis of episodic cluster headache. After 5 days of run-in, 15 patients received verapamil (120 mg three times daily) and 15 received placebo (three times daily) for 14 days. These researchers found a significant reduction in attack frequency and abortive agent consumption in the group receiving verapamil.

The initial starting daily dosage of verapamil is 80 mg given three times a day or getting up to this dosage within 3 to 5 days. The non–sustained-release formulation seems to work better than the sustained-release preparation, but there is no literature proving this. Doses are typically increased by 80 mg every 3 to 7 days. If a patient needs more than 480 mg/d, an electrocardiogram is necessary before each dose change thereafter to guard against heart block. It is not uncommon for patients who have cluster headache to need doses as high as 900 mg to gain cluster remission. Recent data suggest that even on a stable dose of verapamil for months to years, electrocardiographic changes may occur; thus, serial electrocardiograms on a 3- to 6-month basis are required while on verapamil. A study by Cohen and collegues[18] showed that of 108 study patients, 19% had abnormalities in atrioventricular conduction while on verapamil at a mean dose of 567 ± 290 mg/d; 12% had first-degree heart block (PR >0.2 seconds), with 1 requiring a permanent pacemaker; and 8% had other arrhythmias, including junctional rhythm (complete heart block) in 4 patients, second-degree heart block in 1 patient, and right bundle branch block in 4 patients. Thirty-six percent of patients exhibited bradycardia, although verapamil needed to be discontinued only in four cases.

Lithium carbonate Lithium carbonate therapy is still considered a mainstay of cluster prevention, but its narrow therapeutic window and high side-effect profile make it less desirable than other newer preventives. As of 2001, there have been 28 clinical trials looking at the efficacy of lithium in cluster headache therapy. For chronic cluster headache, 78% of patients treated (in 25 trials) have improved on lithium, whereas 63% of patients who have episodic headache have gained cluster headache remission on lithium. When lithium was compared with verapamil in a single trial, both agents were found to be effective but verapamil caused fewer side effects and had a more rapid onset of action.[19] A single double-blind placebo-controlled trial failed to show superiority of lithium (800 mg sustained release) over placebo. This study was stopped 1 week after treatment began, however, and there was an unexpectedly high placebo response rate of 31%.[20] The treatment period was therefore too short to be conclusive.

The initial starting dosage of lithium is 300 mg at bedtime, with dose adjustments usually not higher than 900 mg/d. Lithium is often effective at serum concentrations (0.3–0.8 mM) lower than those usually required for the treatment of bipolar disorder. Most patients who have cluster headache benefit from dosages between 600 and

900 mg/d. During the initial treatment stages, lithium serum concentrations should be checked repeatedly to guard against toxicity. Serum lithium concentrations should be measured in the morning 12 hours after the last dose. In addition, before starting lithium, renal and thyroid functions need to be checked. Adverse events related to lithium include tremor, diarrhea, and polyuria.

Valproic acid In an open-label investigation, 26 patients (21 with chronic cluster headache and 5 with episodic cluster headache) were treated with divalproex sodium.[21] The mean decrease in headache frequency was 53.9% for the patients who had chronic cluster headache and 58.6% for the patients who had episodic cluster headache. The mean dose of divalproex sodium used was 838 mg, which could be considered a low dose by cluster headache standards. Recently, a double-blind placebo-controlled study of sodium valproate (1000–2000 mg/d) in cluster headache was completed. Ninety-six patients were included: 50 in the sodium valproate group and 46 in the placebo group. After a 7-day run-in period, patients were treated for 2 weeks. Primary efficacy was the percentage of patients having an at least 50% reduction in the average number of attacks per week between the run-in period and the last week of treatment. Fifty percent of subjects in the sodium valproate group and 62% in the placebo group had significant improvement ($P = .23$). Because of the high success rate in the placebo group, the investigators thought that they could make no conclusion about the efficacy of sodium valproate in cluster headache.[22] Divalproex sodium is still considered an effective therapy for cluster headache. Suggested dosing is extended-release divalproex sodium starting at 500 mg at bedtime and increasing by 500 mg every 5 to 7 days up to 3000 mg.

Topiramate Topiramate is a newer antiepileptic agent that maybe efficacious in migraine and cluster headache prevention. Lainez and collegues[23] treated 26 patients (12 who had episodic cluster headache and 14 who had chronic cluster headache) with topiramate to a maximum dose of 200 mg. Topiramate rapidly induced cluster headache remission in 15 patients, reduced the number of attacks more than 50% in 6 patients, and reduced the cluster headache period duration in 12 patients. The mean time to remission was 14 days, but remission was obtained within the first days of treatment with extremely low doses (25–75 mg/d) in 7 patients. Six patients discontinued treatment because of side effects (all with daily doses greater than 100 mg) or lack of efficacy. Topiramate should be initiated at a dose of 25 mg/d and increased in 25-mg increments every 5 days up to 75 mg. The patient should be monitored at this dose for several weeks before deciding if the dose needs to be increased.

Melatonin Serum melatonin levels are reduced in patients who have cluster headache, particularly during a cluster headache period. This loss of melatonin may be the inciting event necessary to produce at least nocturnal cluster headache attacks. The efficacy of oral melatonin at a dose of 10 mg was evaluated in a double-blind placebo-controlled trial.[24] Cluster headache remission within 3 to 5 days occurred in 5 of 10 patients who received melatonin compared with none of 10 patients who received placebo. Melatonin only seemed to work in patients who had episodic cluster headache. Recently, melatonin has also been shown to be an effective preventive in chronic cluster headache.[25] A negative study was published using melatonin for cluster headache prevention, but the dosing was lower than that of the other studies and a sustained preparation was given.[26] Anecdotally, it is the author's belief that melatonin should be initiated in all patients who have cluster headache as a first-line preventive, sometimes even before verapamil. It has minimal side effects, and it can turn off nocturnal cluster headaches (typically the most severe attacks) in a substantial number of patients within 24 hours. Melatonin also seems to prevent daytime attacks. In addition, even when melatonin does not completely resolve all the attacks, it seems to lower the dose necessary of the other add-on preventives. For example, a patient who had long-standing cluster headache and was seen at an academic headache clinic always became cluster headache–free on valproic acid at a dose of 1500 mg. After being placed on melatonin, he only needed a valproic acid dose of 500 mg to become cluster headache–free. Melatonin in the clinic seems to work as well in chronic cluster headache as in episodic headache, and some patients who have chronic cluster headache become cluster headache–free on melatonin monotherapy. The typical dose of melatonin used is 9 mg given at bedtime (three 3-mg tablets), but higher doses may be necessary. If one brand of commercial melatonin does not work, another should be tried, because the true amount of melatonin in various over-the-counter brands varies widely. The positive effects of lithium may depend on its ability to increase serum melatonin levels.

Other less well-documented but effective preventive treatments

1. Daily triptans (naratriptan and frovatriptan)[27]
2. Gabapentin. There are recent data to suggest that gabapentin may work in patients who have chronic cluster headache. Schuh-Hofer and collegues[28] noted that gabapentin was effective as an add-on therapy in patients who had chronic cluster headache and had failed a first-line cluster headache preventive.
3. Baclofen showed a response in an open-label investigation.[29] A dosing suggestion is 10 to 20 mg administered orally three to four times daily.
4. Clonidine patch
5. Mycophenolate mofetil[30] is a steroid-sparing immunosuppressive agent and can be used as a possible preventive strategy in patients who only respond to corticosteroids. Serial blood work is required when mycophenolate mofetil is prescribed.
6. Neuro-hormonal modulation therapy
   a. Clomiphene citrate is a synthetic nonsteroidal ovulatory stimulant that can increase testosterone levels in men by competing with endogenous estrogen at hypothalamic estrogen receptors. In essence, clomiphene citrate blocks the endogenous estrogen feedback inhibition of luteinizing hormone (LH)–releasing hormone, thus leading to an increase in LH and follicle-stimulating hormone levels, with subsequent Leydig cell stimulation and testosterone production. The manner by which clomiphene citrate prevents cluster headache can only be speculated on, possibly by increasing testosterone levels, modulating hypothalamic estrogen receptors, or modulating prostaglandin E_2 levels. The author has reported on the effectiveness of this agent in chronic treatment of refractory cluster headache and SUNCT syndrome.[31,32]
   b. Testosterone supplementation. Low testosterone levels documented in patients who had cluster headache led Nicolodi and colleagues[33] to give testosterone supplementation to patients who had chronic cluster headache in the early 1990s. Most of the treated patients showed no change in headache intensity or attack frequency, but all subjects had a dramatic increase in sexual activity. A more recent investigation, however, did demonstrate a positive influence of testosterone administration for treatment-resistant cluster headache, with some treated patients having total remission of attacks.[34] The conflicting treatment response to testosterone may reflect the fact that testosterone levels are not always low in patients who have cluster headache, and testosterone levels have been found to be normal in some studies.

c. Leuprolide. A gonadotropin-releasing hormone analogue was looked at in a single-dose study and led to a decrease in cluster headache pain intensity and attack frequency in 26 of 30 patients studied who had chronic cluster headache.[35] Twelve patients had complete resolution of their headaches 17 days after leuprolide administration. Before treatment, all patients had normal testosterone and LH levels, with an initial increase in serum LH and testosterone levels (days 1–5) after leuprolide injection, followed by a marked reduction in both. The testosterone levels remained low for 30 days, whereas the duration of headache improvement lasted for 3.25 months. This study, in which testosterone levels were actually persistently lowered rather than increased, gives more credence to the thought that altering testosterone levels alone may not be the prime effect of hormonal manipulation therapy for cluster headache. This investigation was the first to suggest that giving a medication that can directly alter the hypothalamic-pituitary-gonadal axis can suppress cluster headache. Based on these promising results, it is somewhat surprising that leuprolide has not been looked at further for cluster headache prevention.

d. Psilocybin or lysergic acid diethylamide (LSD). This is absolutely something that the author would never recommend; however, the potential benefits of psilocybin or LSD are plastered throughout the Internet, and the report of an interview-based trial was published in Neurology.[36] These are ergot-based compounds.

Surgical Treatment of Cluster Headache

Surgical treatment of cluster headache should only be considered after a patient has exhausted all medicinal options or when a patient's medical history precludes the use of typical cluster headache abortive and preventive medications. Patients who have episodic cluster headache should rarely, if ever, be referred for surgery because of the presence of remission periods. Once medical therapy has been deemed a failure in patients who have cluster headache, only those patients who have strictly side-fixed headaches should be considered for surgery. If a patient has had past episodes in which cluster headache attacks have alternated sides, there is a high risk after surgery for having attack recurrence on the side opposite to the side on which surgery was performed. This can be truly devastating for a patient who has cluster headache. Other criteria for cluster surgery include pain mainly localizing to the ophthalmic division of the trigeminal nerve, a psychologically stable individual, and an individual without an addicting personality. Patients who have cluster headache must understand that, in most instances, to alleviate their cluster pain, the trigeminal nerve has to be injured, leaving them not only with facial analgesia but with a risk for developing severe adverse events, including corneal anesthesia and anesthesia dolorosa.

Past surgical therapies for cluster headache are discussed in this section. It is suggested that anything that may damage the trigeminal nerve should not be suggested as treatment for cluster headache. Newer procedures, such as hypothalamic or GON stimulation, or possibly radiofrequency (RF) procedures directed at the trigeminal nerve, are suggested. Nerve cutting is not suggested, and even decompression surgery seems to be drastic and not extremely successful.

Surgical Techniques for Cluster Headache

Anatomically, it makes sense that to turn off the cluster headache and its associated autonomic symptoms, and surgery should be directed toward the sensory trigeminal nerve and the cranial parasympathetic system. Changing the firing pattern of the hypothalamus, the possible "cluster generator" would also be an intriguing technique to abort cluster headache.

Surgery on the Cranial Parasympathetic System

The parasympathetic autonomic pathway can be interrupted by sectioning the greater superficial petrosal nerve, the nervus intermedius, or the sphenopalatine ganglion. Based on the trigeminal autonomic (TAC) reflex pathway hypothesis for cluster headache pathogenesis, this technique should obliterate the autonomic symptoms associated with a cluster headache but would not seem likely to affect the cluster-associated pain, because this is a trigeminal nerve–driven response, although the nervus intermedius may have nociceptive fibers. From reports in the literature, techniques targeting the autonomic system in cluster headache have provided inconsistent pain relief in patients and, even when deemed initially effective, have had high recurrence rates.

Surgery on the Sensory Trigeminal Nerve

Procedures directed toward the sensory trigeminal nerve include alcohol injection into supraorbital and infraorbital nerves, alcohol injection into the Gasserian (trigeminal) ganglion, avulsion of infraorbital/supraorbital/supratrochlear nerves, retrogasserian glycerol injection, RF trigeminal gangliorhizolysis, and trigeminal root section. Overall, these techniques have been the most successful at alleviating cluster headache pain; however, with some of the procedures, there is the possibility of severe adverse events.

Radiofrequency thermocoagulation

RF thermocoagulation is the most commonly used surgical technique for cluster headache, and it provides one of the best options for pain relief. The results of RF rhizotomies in cluster headache are encouraging, although there are only a few studies in the literature. Maxwell[37] treated 8 patients who had chronic cluster headache with RF, all of whom had initial pain relief. In 5 of 8 patients, pain relief lasted for a mean of 32 months. Mathew and Hurt[38] treated 27 patients who had chronic cluster headache, with a mean follow-up of 28 months. Twenty of the patients did "good to excellent." Sweet[39] treated 20 patients with RF, and 11 of them had continuous pain relief for up to 20 years. Taha and Tew[40] recently reviewed the charts of 7 patients who had chronic cluster headache and received RF gangliorhizolysis. All patients had immediate pain relief; at follow-up, 2 patients remained pain-free 7 and 20 years later. Three patients had mild pain recurrence that was controlled with medication 6 to 12 months after surgery, and 2 patients did poorly, with complete pain recurrence within 2 months of surgery. There was no association between patient age, gender, attack duration, preoperative response to lidocaine blockade, and relief with RF. Overall, with RF, approximately 50% of patients have done well, 20% have done fair to good, and approximately 30% have failed the procedure. Adverse events with RF include moderate facial dysesthesia, severe facial dysesthesias, corneal sensory loss, and anesthesia dolorosa. The surgeon can reduce side effects by making the end point hypoalgesia rather than analgesia. Other less common but devastating side effects include intracranial hemorrhage, stroke, infection, and motor weakness, which typically resolves over 1 to 6 months.

Advantages of RF include a highly specific technique, safety in the elderly, low recurrence rates, low mortality, and the fact that the surgeon can vary the amount of sensory loss. Disadvantages of RF include its being an expensive technique, its being a tedious skilled procedure, corneal anesthesia, sensory loss beyond the area affected, possible anesthesia dolorosa, and keratitis. Anesthesia dolorosa or painful numbness has been described by some patients who have cluster headache as a much worse sensation than the cluster headaches themselves, especially because it is a constant sensation.

New Strategies

Hypothalamic stimulation

There has always been a suggestion that there is a hypothalamic influence over cluster headache based on the circadian rhythmicity of the syndrome and the neurohormonal changes identified in patients who have cluster headache. Functional imaging has been able to strengthen this theory. May and collegues[41] studied 9 patients who had cluster headache with positron emission tomography (PET). Cluster headaches were triggered with nitroglycerin. During a cluster headache attack, areas that were activated on PET included the anterior cingulate cortex (B/L), posterior thalamus, insula cortex, and basal ganglia regions, which are all known to be involved in pain processing or response to pain. Unique to cluster headache was activation in the ipsilateral inferior posterior hypothalamic gray matter. Whether the hypothalamus was acting as a cluster headache generator or modulator of cluster pain could not be determined from this study and, at present, is still a major question in cluster headache pathogenesis. Based on the PET findings, Leone and colleagues[42] began to look at the role of hypothalamic stimulation in the treatment of refractory cluster headache. These researchers have now treated more than 14 treatment-refractory patients who had chronic cluster headache with electrode implantation into the posterior inferior hypothalamus. Almost every patient has had a tremendous reduction in cluster headache frequency, and some have become pain-free. The response is not immediate but can take weeks to months. There have been no major adverse events from the Italian group, but a recent pilot study from Belgium reported one death.[43] The relation to the stimulator surgery is unknown. What is exciting about this new surgical technique is that knowledge of pathogenesis helped in the discovery of a therapy for cluster headache. The fact that it may take weeks to months to see a positive effect suggests that the neuromodulation of cluster headache is by complex pathways and not just a manifestation of acute stimulation of the posterior hypothalamus.

Greater occipital nerve stimulation

There have been three investigations[44] looking at the efficacy of GON stimulation in chronic refractory cluster headache. The essence is that this can be quite effective in a subset of patients; however, unlike an occipital nerve block that can work in seconds, the stimulator may not start to show any effect for weeks to upward of 5 months after stimulator placement, suggesting more central neuromodulation rather than a direct effect of stimulating the nerve. It does not seem that response to a GON block predicts response to an implantable stimulator.

INDOMETHACIN-RESPONSIVE TRIGEMINAL AUTONOMIC CEPHALALGIAS

Chronic paroxysmal hemicrania (CPH) and HC are defined by their response to indomethacin. A short discussion on these two syndromes is followed by treatment suggestions.

Chronic Paroxysmal Hemicrania

CPH is a rare syndrome marked by headaches of short duration, high frequency of attacks, and associated autonomic symptoms. It was first described by Sjaastad and Dale in 1974[45] and has now been diagnosed all over the world. CPH pain location is normally orbital, temporal, and above or behind the ear, and it is one-sided. The pain is severe in intensity and may radiate to the neck or ipsilateral shoulder. The pain has been described as boring, claw-like, or pulsatile. Residual mild pain may remain between attacks. Normal headache duration is between 2 and 30 minutes. Unlike cluster headache, there is no predilection for nocturnal attacks in CPH, although attacks can certainly awaken a patient from sleep. Associated symptoms are marked by autonomic phenomena. Most patients who have CPH exhibit lacrimation (62%), followed by nasal congestion (42%), conjunctival injection and rhinorrhea (36%), and ptosis (33%).[46] CPH attacks can sometimes be triggered by rotating the neck or flexing the head to the side of the headaches or by applying external pressure to the transverse processes of C4 to C5 or the C2 nerve root on the symptomatic side.

Hemicrania Continua

The term hemicrania continua was first introduced in 1984 by Sjaastad and Spierings.[47] Initially, HC was thought to be a rare syndrome, although it is now believed to be more common and probably routinely misdiagnosed. There are more than 90 reported cases in the literature. HC, like migraine and CPH, has a female predominance. There are two recognized forms of HC: the nonremitting form, which occurs in approximately 85% of patients (no remission periods), and the remitting form. The nonremitting form can be continuous from onset or evolve from the remitting form. In regard to the clinical characteristics of HC, there are two patterns of headache. Patients who have HC experience a continuous daily head pain that is present 24 hours per day 7 days per week and pain exacerbation periods that occur with varying frequency from multiple times per week to every third month or less. The daily continuous pain of HC is usually of mild to moderate intensity, affecting the temple or periorbital region. It is always present on the same side of the head. There are some reports of the pain of HC switching sides or being bilateral, but in those cases, a true diagnosis of HC comes into question. The pain exacerbation periods are marked by moderate to severe pain lasting hours to days in duration with associated symptoms that are seen in patients who have migraine and cluster headache. Migrainous symptoms include nausea, vomiting, photophobia, and phonophobia. Autonomic symptoms include unilateral lacrimation, ptosis, nasal congestion, and rhinorrhea. Other key symptoms that are commonly seen during a pain exacerbation period include eyelid swelling, eyelid twitching, and "ice pick" headaches. Some patients who have HC also complain of a foreign body sensation in the eye on the same side as their headache, such as a feeling as though there is a piece of sand in the eye or an eyelash. Patients who have HC can also experience auras typically occurring just before a pain exacerbation period. On indomethacin, the headache and aura alleviate. One of the best descriptions of the clinical features of HC has come from an observational study from the Jefferson Headache Center in Philadelphia.[48] Thirty-four new cases of HC were identified. The baseline continuous headache was mild to moderate in intensity with no headache-related disability and rare associated symptoms. During the headache exacerbation period, pain was normally severe. Associated symptoms included migrainous photophobia in 59% of patients, phonophobia in 59% of patients, nausea in 53% of patients, and vomiting in 24% of patients. Autonomic symptoms consisted of lacrimation in 53% of patients, nasal congestion in 21% of patients, and ptosis in 18% of patients. Seventy-four percent of the patients experienced at least one autonomic symptom during the pain exacerbation period. The presence of jab or jolt headaches was noted in 41% of patients. Interestingly, the exacerbation headache met the IHS criteria for migraine in 71% of patients. The most common form of HC was the continuous pattern from onset (53%), followed by continuous evolving from remitting (35%) and remitting (12%) forms.

Indomethacin treatment

The normal starting dosage of indomethacin for CPH and HC is one 25-mg tablet given three times a day for 3 days; this dosage can be increased to two tablets (50 mg) given three times a day if there is not total relief of pain. Most individuals respond with a dosage of 150 mg/d, and the response can be dramatic, with quick dissipation of headache symptoms. A beneficial effect is normally seen within 48 hours after the correct dosage has been found. Some individuals need indomethacin at a dosage as high as 300 mg/d, but safety concerns prevent sustaining such a high dose. If there is no response at 150 mg/d and the physician still suspects CPH or HC, an extra 25-mg dose can be added every 3 days, to a total of 225 mg/d or the onset of side effects. If the patient does not respond at 75 mg given three times a day, one should consider an alternative diagnosis. Sjaastad and colleagues[49] found that individuals requiring high doses of indomethacin (200–250 mg/d) are more apt to have underlying secondary causes of CPH. Side effects of indomethacin therapy are mainly gastrointestinal disturbances with dyspepsia or ulcer development. The gastrointestinal side effects can normally be controlled with histamine type 2 receptor antagonists, proton pump inhibitors, or prostaglandins. Misoprostol at a dose of 100 to 200 mg given four times a day is successful in preventing nonsteroidal-induced ulcers. This agent is not well tolerated by patients, however, because of its side effects of diarrhea and abdominal pain. There are also renal implications to long-term indomethacin use, including the development of renal papillary necrosis. Individuals normally require continuous dosing, which may be lifelong dosing. Symptoms usually recur as soon as 12 hours or up to several days after discontinuing indomethacin.

Other nonindomethacin treatments

1. Cyclooxygenase (COX)-2 inhibitors: CPH and HC have shown some positive response to celecoxib. The dosage is typically high, ranging from 200 mg two to four times daily. At these doses, the gastrointestinal protection these agents afford may be lost. In addition, the safety of COX-2 inhibitors, when used on a continuous basis, has come into question.[50–52]
2. Melatonin: melatonin has a similar chemical structure to indomethacin and has been shown to have anti-inflammatory and antinociceptive properties.[53] The pain-relieving mechanisms of melatonin are not completely understood, but recent reports have suggested that melatonin can increase the release of endogenous β-endorphins, and its antihyperalgesic effect seems to involve nitric oxide and opiate pathways. Melatonin has now been shown to help alleviate the pain of HC[54] and primary stabbing headache,[55] and patients become pain-free on melatonin in some cases. Melatonin should be tried on all patients with indomethacin-sensitive headache, including those who are doing well on indomethacin to try to lower the indomethacin dose or to come off indomethacin entirely or in those who have contraindications to indomethacin.
3. Topiramate: there are recent case reports of HC and CPH responding to topiramate.[56]
4. Occipital nerve stimulation: a positive response was reported in a patient who had HC, although the author questions whether this was a posttraumatic headache syndrome and not HC.
5. CPH-specific treatments: in 1996, Evers and colleagues[57] presented alternative drug treatments for CPH. Twenty-two other agents have been studied in

CPH;[57] the most successful alternative preventative drug is verapamil at a dose of 240 to 320 mg/d. Acetylsalicylic acid, naproxen, and a piroxicam derivative have demonstrated some effect in a small number of cases. Acetazolamide was effective in a single case report. Prednisone is effective at high doses for controlling CPH but is not considered to be an adequate chronic therapy regimen because of its side-effect profile. CPH shows a poor response to carbamazepine and oxygen. Sumatriptan has been a good abortive agent in several case reports, although it is not uncommon to see it not work on CPH attacks.

SHORT-LASTING UNILATERAL NEURALGIFORM HEADACHE ATTACKS WITH CONJUNCTIVAL INJECTION AND TEARING SYNDROME

The SUNCT syndrome was first described by Sjaastad and colleagues[58] in 1978. The description of the complete syndrome came in 1989.[59] SUNCT syndrome is one of the rarest of the primary headache disorders. Many headache specialists have stated that they have never seen SUNCT syndrome.

SUNCT syndrome is composed of brief attacks of moderate to severe head pain with associated autonomic disturbances of conjunctival injection, tearing, rhinorrhea, or nasal obstruction. The typical age of onset is between 40 and 70 years; the mean age of onset is 51 years. The pain of SUNCT syndrome is normally localized to an orbital or periorbital distribution, although the forehead and temple can be the main sites of pain. Head pain can radiate to the temple, nose, cheek, ear, and palate. The pain is normally side-locked and remains unilateral throughout an entire attack. In rare instances, the pain of SUNCT syndrome can be bilateral. Pain severity is normally moderate to severe, unlike, for example, cluster headache pain, which is always severe. The character of pain is described most often as a stabbing, burning, pricking, or electric shock-like sensation. Pain duration is extremely short, lasting between 5 and 240 seconds, with an average duration of 10 to 60 seconds. This extremely brief pain duration sets SUNCT syndrome apart from other primary headache syndromes (eg, cluster headache, CPH, migraine). Pain onset is abrupt, with maximum intensity being reached in 2 to 3 seconds. The pain of SUNCT syndrome normally plateaus at a maximum intensity for several seconds and then quickly abates. Some individuals experience a "sawtooth-like" pattern, with rapid changes in maximum intensity levels.[60] SUNCT syndrome can occur at any time of the day and does not show a tendency toward nocturnal attacks; only 1.2% of reported sufferers have nighttime episodes. Attack frequency varies greatly between sufferers and within an individual sufferer. The usual attack frequency ranges anywhere from 1 to more than 80 episodes a day. Individuals can experience from less than 1 attack an hour to more than 30 an hour. Mean attack frequency is 28 attacks per day. Most patients who have SUNCT syndrome are pain-free between attacks, although there are isolated reports of patients experiencing low background pain interictally. SUNCT syndrome is an episodic disorder that presents in a relapsing or remitting pattern. Each symptomatic period can last from several days to several months, and a person who has SUNCT syndrome typically has one to two symptomatic periods a year. The longest documented symptomatic period has been 5 years, and the highest number of reported SUNCT episodes in 1 year is 22. Remissions typically last months but can last years. Symptomatic periods seem to increase in frequency and duration over time.

All documented patients who have SUNCT syndrome experience conjunctival injection and lacrimation (ipsilateral to the side of the head pain) with each attack. Ipsilateral rhinorrhea or nasal obstruction occurs in 67% of individuals. Less frequent associated symptoms include eyelid edema, a decreased palpebral fissure, facial redness, photophobia, and blepharospasm. Typically, conjunctival injection and eye tearing start within 1 to 2 seconds of pain onset and remain until the head pain ceases, sometimes outlasting the pain by up to 30 seconds. Rhinorrhea, conversely, starts in the middle to late part of an attack. Nausea, vomiting, photophobia, and phonophobia are not normally associated with SUNCT syndrome. SUNCT syndrome can occur spontaneously, but many sufferers have identified triggering maneuvers, including mastication, nose blowing, coughing, forehead touching, eyelid squeezing, neck movements (rotation, extension, and flexion), and ice-cream eating. In SUNCT syndrome, there is no refractory period between pain attacks; thus, if a trigger zone is stimulated during the ending phase of a previous attack, a new one can begin immediately. This is unlike the refractory period of trigeminal neuralgia. General and neurologic examinations are normal in patients who have SUNCT syndrome during and between attacks, except for the documented autonomic signs, which quickly abate when the attack ends. Individuals may have tenderness to palpation over the supraorbital and infraorbital nerves but little else.

Treatment

In many instances, SUNCT syndrome is refractory to medical therapy, and there were really no effective treatments until recently. The extremely short duration of head pain would seem to preclude the use of abortive treatment in patients who have SUNCT syndrome. By the time a patient who has SUNCT syndrome would take an abortive medication for an individual headache, the attack would theoretically already be completed. There are isolated cases reporting sumatriptan alleviation of the pain of SUNCT syndrome, but these probably reflect spontaneous attack remissions rather than drug-induced remissions. Preventive agents that have previously been tried include aspirin, paracetamol, indomethacin, naproxen, ergotamine, DHE, sumatriptan, prednisone, methysergide, verapamil, valproate, lithium, propranolol, amitriptyline, and carbamazepine.[61] Carbamazepine has shown a partial effect in some patients. Combining carbamazepine and a short course of corticosteroids at the onset may be more efficacious than starting with carbamazepine alone. Azathioprine was shown to be somewhat effective in one patient. Greater occipital and supraorbital nerve blockade has been unsuccessful.

Suggested treatments that have shown efficacy in SUNCT syndrome include the following:

1. Lamotrigine[62]
2. Gabapentin[63]
3. Topiramate[64]

For the more intractable patient who has SUNCT syndrome, suggested treatments include the following:

1. Clomiphene citrate (see the description in the section on cluster headache)[32]
2. Intravenous lidocaine[65] is not used often in the United States but is a common treatment in Europe.
3. Hypothalamic stimulation was shown to be efficacious in a single case of refractory SUNCT.[66]
4. Other surgical procedures that have been tried in SUNCT syndrome and have produced mixed results include glycerol rhizotomy, gamma-knife surgery, microvascular decompression of the trigeminal nerve, and balloon compression of retroganglionic fibers.

SUMMARY

The TACs are a unique group of primary headache conditions marked by head pain and autonomic symptoms. These conditions are unique in their attack duration, attack frequency, and attack intensity. Accurate diagnosis of a TAC subtype needs to be made, because treatment response depends on the condition.

REFERENCES

1. van Vliet JA, Bahra A, Martin V, et al. Intranasal sumatriptan is effective in the treatment of acute cluster headache—a double-blind placebo-controlled crossover study. Cephalalgia 2001;21:267–72.
2. Ekbom K. Treatment of acute cluster headache with sumatriptan. N Engl J Med 1991;325:322–6.
3. Ekbom K, Krabbe A, Micieli G, et al. Cluster headache attacks treated for up to three months with subcutaneous sumatriptan (6 mg) (Sumatriptan Long-Term Study Group). Cephalalgia 1995;15:230–6.
4. Hering-Hanit R. Alteration in nature of cluster headache during subcutaneous administration of sumatriptan. Headache 2000;40:41–4.
5. Kudrow L. Response of cluster headache attacks to oxygen inhalation. Headache 1981;21:1–4.
6. Rozen TD, Niknam R, Shechter AL, et al. Gender differences in clinical characteristics and treatment response in cluster headache patients. Cephalalgia 1999;19: 323.
7. Rozen TD. High oxygen flow rates for cluster headache. Neurology 2004;63:593.
8. Bahra A, Gawel MJ, Hardebo JE, et al. Oral zolmitriptan is effective in the acute treatment of cluster headache. Neurology 2000;54:1832–9, 22.
9. Rapoport AM, Mathew NT, Silberstein SD, et al. Zolmitriptan nasal spray in the acute treatment of cluster headache: a double-blind study. Neurology 2007; 69(9):821–6.
10. Rozen TD. Olanzapine as an abortive agent for cluster headache. Headache 2001;41:813–6.
11. Mathura MS, Levy MJ, Meeran K, et al. Subcutaneous octreotide in cluster headache: randomized placebo-controlled double-blind crossover study. Ann Neurol 2004;56(4):488–94.
12. Anthony M, Daher BN. Mechanisms of action of steroids in cluster headache. In: Rose FC, editor. New advances in headache research 2. London: Smith Gordon; 1992. p. 271–4.
13. Mather PJ, Silberstein SD, Schulman EA, et al. The treatment of cluster headache with repetitive intravenous dihydroergotamine. Headache 1991;31:525–32.
14. Anthony M. Arrest of attacks of cluster headache by local steroid injection of the occipital nerve. In: Clifford Rose F, editor. Migraine. Basel: Karger; 1985. p. 169–73.
15. Mitsias PD, Norris L, Junn F, et al. Greater occipital nerve block for intractable cluster headache. Cephalalgia 2001;21:502.
16. Peres MF, Stiles MA, Siow HC, et al. Greater occipital nerve blockade for cluster headache. Cephalalgia 2002;22:520–2.
17. Leone M, D'Amico D, Attanasio A, et al. Verapamil is an effective prophylactic for cluster headache: results of a double blind multicenter study versus placebo. In: Olesen J, Goadsby PJ, editors. Cluster: headache and related conditions. Oxford: Oxford University Press; 1999. p. 296–9.

18. Cohen AS, Mathura MS, Goadsby PJ, et al. Electrocardiographic abnormalities in patients with cluster headache on verapamil therapy. Neurology 2007;69(7): 668–75.

19. Bussone G, Leone M, Peccarisi C, et al. Double blind comparison of lithium and verapamil in cluster headache prophylaxis. Headache 1990;30:411–7.

20. Steiner TJ, Hering R, Couturier EG, et al. Double-blind placebo-controlled trial of lithium in episodic cluster headache. Cephalalgia 1997;17:673–5.

21. Freitag FG, Diamond S, Diamond ML, et al. Divalproex sodium in the preventative treatment of cluster headache. Headache 2000;40:408.

22. El Amrani M, Massiou H, Bousser MG. A negative trial of sodium valproate in cluster headache: methodological issues. Cephalalgia 2002;22:205–8.

23. Lainez MJ, Pascual J, Pascual AM, et al. Topiramate in the prophylactic treatment of cluster headache. Headache 2003;43:784–9.

24. Leone M, Damico D, Moschiano F, et al. Melatonin versus placebo in the prophylaxis of cluster headache: a double blind pilot study with parallel groups. Cephalalgia 1996;16:494–6.

25. Peres MF, Rozen TD. Melatonin in the preventive treatment of chronic cluster headache. Cephalalgia 2001;21:993–5.

26. Pringsheim T, Magnoux E, Dobson CF, et al. Melatonin as adjunctive therapy in the prophylaxis of cluster headache: a pilot study. Headache 2002;42:787–92.

27. Siow HC, Pozo-Rosich P, Silberstein SD. Frovatriptan for the treatment of cluster headaches. Cephalalgia 2004;24(12):1045–8.

28. Schuh-Hofer S, Israel H, Neeb L, et al. The use of gabapentin in chronic cluster headache patients refractory to first-line therapy. Eur J Neurol 2007;14(6):694–6.

29. Hering-Hanit R, Gadoth N. The use of baclofen in cluster headache. Curr Pain Headache Rep 2001;5(1):79–82.

30. Rozen TD. Complete but transient relief of chronic cluster headache with mycophenolate mofetil. Headache 2004;44:818–20.

31. Rozen T. Clomiphene citrate for treatment refractory chronic cluster headache. Headache 2008;48:286–90.

32. Rozen TD, Saper JR, Sheftell FD, et al. Clomiphene citrate as a new treatment for SUNCT (hormonal manipulation for hypothalamic influenced trigeminal autonomic cephalalgias). Headache 2005;45:754–6.

33. Nicolodi M, Sicuteri F, Poggioni M, et al. Hypothalamic modulation of nociception and reproduction in cluster headache. II. Testosterone-induced increase of sexual activity in males with cluster headache. Cephalalgia 1993;13:258–60.

34. Stillman MJ. Testosterone replacement therapy for treatment refractory cluster headache. Headache 2006;46:925–33.

35. Nicolodi M, Sicuteri F, Poggioni M, et al. Hypothalamic modulation of nociception and reproduction in cluster headache. I. Therapeutic trials of leuprolide. Cephalalgia 1993;13:253–7.

36. Sewell RA, Halpern JH, Pope HG Jr. Response of cluster headache to psilocybin and LSD. Neurology 2006;66(12):1920–2.

37. Maxwell RE. Surgical control of chronic migrainous neuralgia by trigeminal gangliorhizolysis. J Neurosurg 1982;57:459–66.

38. Mathew NT, Hurt W. Percutaneous radiofrequency trigeminal gangliorhizolysis in intractable cluster headache. Headache 1988;28:328–31.

39. Sweet WH. Surgical treatment of chronic cluster headache. Headache 1988;28: 660 70.

40. Taha JM, Tew JM. Long-term results of radiofrequency rhizotomy in the treatment of cluster headache. Headache 1995;35:193–6.

41. May A, Bahra A, Buchel C, et al. Hypothalamic activation in cluster headache attacks. Lancet 2001;352:275–8.
42. Leone M, Franzini A, D'Amico D, et al. Long-term follow-up of hypothalamic stimulation to relieve intractable chronic cluster headache. Neurology 2004;62(suppl 5):A355–6.
43. Schoenen J, Di Clemente L, Vandenheede M, et al. Hypothalamic stimulation in chronic cluster headache: a pilot study of efficacy and mode of action. Brain 2005;128:940–7.
44. Burns B, Watkins L, Goadsby PJ, et al. Treatment of medically intractable cluster headache by occipital nerve stimulation: long-term follow-up of eight patients. Lancet 2007;369(9567):1099–106.
45. Sjaastad O, Dale I. Evidence for a new (?) treatable headache entity. Headache 1974;14:105–8.
46. Antonaci F, Sjaastad O. Chronic paroxysmal hemicrania (CPH): a review of the clinical manifestations. Headache 1989;29:648–56.
47. Sjaastad O, Spierings EL. Hemicrania continua: another headache absolutely responsive to indomethacin. Cephalalgia 1984;4:65–70.
48. Peres MFP, Silberstein SD, Nahamias S, et al. Hemicrania continua is not that rare. Neurology 2001;57:948–51.
49. Sjaastad O, Stovner LJ, Stolt-Nielsen A, et al. CPH and hemicrania continua: requirements of high indomethacin dosages—an ominous sign? Headache 1995;35:363–7.
50. Mathew NT, Kailasam J, Fischer A, et al. Responsiveness to celecoxib in chronic paroxysmal hemicrania. Neurology 2000;55:316.
51. Peres MF, Silberstein SD. Hemicrania continua responds to cyclooxygenase-2 inhibitors. Headache 2002;42:530–1.
52. Rozen T.D. High dose celecoxib and rofecoxib in the treatment of hemicrania continua. Neurology 2002;58(suppl 3):A471.
53. Peres MFP, Stiles MA, Oshinsky M, et al. Remitting form of hemicrania continua with seasonal pattern. Headache 2001;41:592–4.
54. Rozen TD. Melatonin responsive hemicrania continua. Headache 2006;46:1203–4.
55. Rozen TD. Melatonin as treatment for idiopathic stabbing headache. Neurology 2003;61:865–6.
56. Camarda C, Camarda R, Monastero R, et al. Chronic paroxysmal hemicrania and hemicrania continua responding to topiramate: two case reports. Clin Neurol Neurosurg 2008;110(1):88–91.
57. Evers S, Husstedt IW. Alternatives in drug treatment of chronic paroxysmal hemicrania. Headache 1996;36:429–32.
58. Sjaastad O, Russell. D, Horven I, et al. Multiple neuralgiform unilateral headache attacks associated with conjunctival injection and appearing in clusters. A nosological problem. Proceedings of the Scandinavian Migraine Society 1978, 31.
59. Sjaastad O, Saunte C, Salvesen R, et al. Short-lasting unilateral neuralgiform headache attacks with conjunctival injection, tearing, sweating, and rhinorrhea. Cephalalgia 1989;9:147–56.
60. Pareja JA, Sjaastad O. SUNCT syndrome in the female. Headache 1994;34:217–20.
61. Goadsby PJ, Lipton RB. A review of paroxysmal hemicranias, SUNCT syndrome and other short-lasting headaches with autonomic features, including new cases. Brain 1997;120:193–209.
62. D'Andrea G, Granella F, Ghiotto N, et al. Lamotrigine in the treatment of SUNCT syndrome. Neurology 2001;57:1723–5.

63. Porta-Etessam J, Martinez-Salio A, Berbel A, et al. Gabapentin (Neurontin) in the treatment of SUNCT syndrome. Cephalalgia 2002;22:249–50.
64. Rossi P, Cesarino F, Faroni J, et al. SUNCT syndrome successfully treated with topiramate: case reports. Cephalalgia 2003;23:998–1000.
65. Mathura MS, Cohen AS, Goadsby PJ, et al. SUNCT syndrome responsive to intravenous lidocaine. Cephalalgia 2004;24(11):985–92.
66. Leone M, Franzini A, D'Andrea G, et al. Deep brain stimulation to relieve drug-resistant SUNCT. Ann Neurol 2005;57(6):924–7.

Other Primary Headaches

Julio Pascual, MD, PhD

KEYWORDS

- Stabbing headache • Cough headache • Exertional headache
- Sexual headache • Hypnic headache
- Primary thunderclap headache • Hemicrania continua
- New daily persistent headache

Within the umbrella of "other primary headaches," the classification of the International Headache Society (IHS) includes a variety of clinically heterogeneous headaches: primary stabbing headaches, primary cough headache, primary exertional headache, primary headache associated with sexual activity, hypnic headache, primary thunderclap headache, and new daily persistent headache (NDPH).[1] All are reviewed here, except for hemicrania continua, which is discussed elsewhere in this issue of the *Neurologic Clinics of North America*. The pathogenesis of these headaches is poorly understood, and their treatment is based on uncontrolled trials. One important issue to keep in mind when confronting these headaches is that they may be symptomatic to structural lesions and therefore usually need careful neuroimaging evaluation.

PRIMARY STABBING HEADACHE

This headache—previously known as ice-pick pain, jabs and jolts, or ophthalmodynia periodica—consists of unilateral, ultrashort, and localized stabs of pain in the distribution of the first division of the trigeminal nerve and occurs in the absence of organic disease. The IHS diagnostic criteria for stabbing headache appear in **Box 1**.[1,2]

The prevalence of stabbing headache is difficult to estimate because many individuals only suffer a few stabs throughout their lives, which are easily forgotten. In different studies, prevalence has ranged from 1% to 35% of the general population.[2,3] Stabbing headache is more frequent in migraineurs (~40%) and in cluster headache patients (~30%). Stabbing headache is more frequent in women (3:1) and usually occurs after adolescence. This headache is characterized by ultrashort, severe jabbing pains that occur as single episodes or as brief repeated volleys. The pain is very frequently unilateral and unifocal in the distribution of the trigeminal nerve, usually in the orbital region, but multifocal, even bilateral, patterns have been described. Stabbing headaches have the shortest duration of all known headaches, lasting 1 to 2

Service of Neurology, University Hospital Marqués de Valdecilla, 39008 Santander, Spain
E-mail address: juliopascual@telefonica.net

Neurol Clin 27 (2009) 557–571
doi:10.1016/j.ncl.2009.01.005
0733-8619/09/$ – see front matter © 2009 Elsevier Inc. All rights reserved.

neurologic.theclinics.com

Box 1

Diagnostic criteria for primary stabbing headache

A. Head pain occurring as a single stab or a series of stabs fulfilling criteria B and C

B. Exclusively or predominantly felt in the distribution of the first division of the trigeminal nerve (orbit, temple, and parietal area)

C. Stabs last for up to a few seconds and recur with irregular frequency, ranging from one to many per day

D. No accompanying symptoms

E. Not attributed to another disorder

---

seconds in more than two thirds of cases; rarely, pain can last up to 10 seconds. The frequency of attacks ranges from fewer than once to more than 50 times per day. In the vast majority of patients, there are no trigger factors, autonomic symptoms, or migrainelike associated symptoms. Even though the clinical picture suggests a trigeminal nerve hyperexcitability, the mechanism of idiopathic stabbing headache is unknown.[2,4]

Primary headache disorders presenting with short-lived pains as the primary symptom include trigeminal neuralgia, short-lasting unilateral neuralgiform headache attacks with conjunctival injection and tearing (SUNCT syndrome), and chronic paroxysmal hemicrania. Trigeminal neuralgia involving the first division of the trigeminal nerve is a differential diagnostic possibility. The existence of trigger points and the response to carbamazepine in trigeminal neuralgia are important clues. The ultrashort duration and the lack of autonomic features distinguish stabbing headache from SUNCT syndrome and from chronic paroxysmal hemicrania.[2,4]

Adult patients who have new-onset primary stabbing headache should undergo a diagnostic evaluation to exclude secondary causes, although most cases are idiopathic. Ice pick–like pains have been described with ocular or cranial trauma, with acute glaucoma, and with intracranial lesions such as pituitary tumors or meningioma at the onset of cerebrovascular disease or herpes zoster.[2–6]

Pharmacologic treatment of patients who have occasional jabs is not necessary. For patients who have frequent attacks, indomethacin is the medication of choice (grade C recommendation).[1,2,4,7] Duration of treatment must be individualized. Melatonin, gabapentin, and celecoxib have been useful in a few cases and can be given in patients who are intolerant or show a partial response to indomethacin.

PRIMARY COUGH HEADACHE

Primary cough headache, that is, headache precipitated by coughing or straining in the absence of any intracranial disorder, is considered a rare entity. Rasmussen and Olesen[8] showed that the lifetime prevalence of cough headache is 1% (95% confidence interval: 0–2). In the last 10 years, of the 6412 patients attending the author's neurology department due to headache, 68 (1.1%) consulted because of cough headache.[9]

Cough headache can be a primary benign condition or secondary to structural cranial disease. The diagnostic criteria for primary cough headache appear in **Box 2**. From series previous to CT and MRI availability, it was concluded that only around 20% of patients who had cough headache had structural lesions, most of them

---

Box 2
Diagnostic criteria for primary cough headache

A. Headache fulfilling criteria B and C

B. Sudden onset, lasting from 1 second to 30 minutes

C. Brought on by and occurring only in association with coughing, straining, or Valsalva maneuver

D. Not attributed to another disorder

---

a type I Chiari's malformation (**Fig. 1**).[10–13] More than half of cough headache patients studied with modern neuroradiologic techniques, however, have symptomatic cough headache due to tonsillar descent or, very rarely, to other space-occupying lesions in the posterior fossa/foramen magnum area (**Fig. 2**).[9,14] Around 30% of patients who have type I Chiari's malformation experience headache aggravated by Valsalva maneuvers, mainly cough.[15] In summary, it can be concluded that about half of patients who have cough headache show no demonstrable etiology, whereas in the remaining patients, cough headache is secondary to structural lesions, mostly at the foramen magnum level.[2,9,14]

The clinical picture of primary cough headache is very characteristic, which allows differentiation from secondary cases (see **Box 2**).[2,14,16,17] Primary cough headache

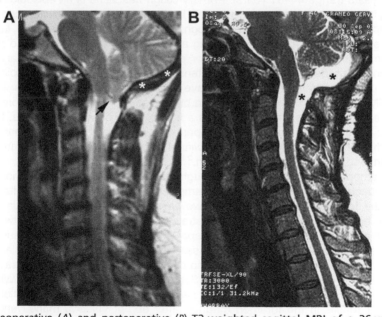

Fig. 1. Preoperative (*A*) and postoperative (*B*) T2-weighted sagittal MRI of a 36-year-old woman who had cough headache. (*A*) Note the presence of tonsillar descent (*arrow*) and flattening of posterior fossa (*asterisks*) and the absence of cisterna magna. (*B*) After posterior fossa reconstruction, notice the appearance of cisterna magna with restitution of cerebrospinal fluid transit (*asterisks*) with upward migration of the tonsils. *From* Pascual J. Activity-related headache. In: Gilman S, editor. MedLink neurology. San Diego (CA): MedLink Corporation. Available at: www.medlink.com/. Accessed July 13, 2008; with permission.

Posterior fossa occupying lesions presenting as cough headache

| arachnoid cyst | dermoid tumor | meningioma |

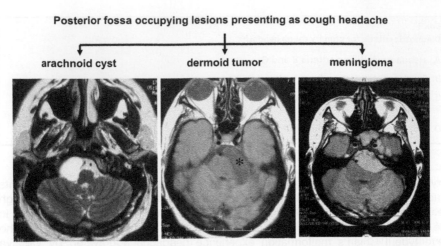

Fig. 2. Examples of patients consulting due to secondary cough headache who were not diagnosed with type I Chiari's malformation. Notice the identical location of the three tumors. *From* Pascual J, González-Mandly A, Martin R, et al. Headaches precipitated by cough, prolonged exercise or sexual activity: a prospective etiological and clinical study. J Headache Pain 2008;9:259–66; with permission.

does not begin earlier than age 40 years—its mean age of onset in the modern series was 67 years (range 44–81 years). Primary cough headache is an episodic disease, ranging from 2 months to 2 years. The pain begins immediately or within seconds after a precipitant. Precipitants include cough, sneezing, blowing the nose, laughing, crying, singing, lifting a burden, straining at stool, and stooping. Sustained physical exercise is not a precipitating factor for primary cough headache. Primary cough headache is moderate to severe in intensity, with a sharp, stabbing, splitting, or even explosive quality. Most patients have bilateral headaches all the time. The pain is usually maximal in the occipital region but is also in the frontal or temporal region or at the vertex. The pain typically lasts a few seconds or several minutes. In a few patients, a dull, aching pain follows the paroxysm for several hours.[18] Primary cough headache is not associated with other clinical manifestations, even with nausea and vomiting, and responds to indomethacin.[2,9,14,16,17]

The pathophysiology of secondary cough headache is reasonably well understood. The headache seems to be due to a temporary impaction of the cerebellar tonsils below the foramen magnum.[19–22] In two patients who had cough headache and tonsillar herniation, Williams[19] demonstrated a pressure difference between the ventricle and the lumbar subarachnoid space during coughing.[5] The pressure difference, named craniospinal pressure dissociation, displaced the cerebellar tonsils into the foramen magnum. Williams also observed that the headache disappeared after decompressive craniectomy.[20] Subsequently, Nightingale and Williams[21] described four more patients who had headache due to episodic impaction of the cerebellar tonsils in the foramen magnum after abrupt Valsalva maneuvers. In the author's series, not only it was demonstrated that tonsillar descent is the cause of cough headache but it also was shown that the presence of cough headache in type I Chiari's malformation patients correlated only with the degree of tonsillar descent.[14] Pujol and colleagues,[23] using cine phase-contrast MRI, were able to detect this abnormal pulsatile motion of the cerebellar tonsils in type I Chiari's malformation patients but not in control subjects. This movement produced a selective obstruction of the cerebrospinal fluid flow from the cranial cavity to the spine (**Fig. 3**). The amplitude of the tonsillar pulsation and the severity of the arachnoid space reduction were associated with cough headache.[23] All these data confirm that symptomatic cough headache is secondary to type I Chiari's malformation and that this pain is due to compression or traction of the causally displaced cerebellar tonsils on pain-sensitive dura and other anchoring structures around the foramen magnum innervated by the first cervical roots.

The pathophysiology of primary cough headache is not known. The possibility of a sudden increase in venous pressure being sufficient to cause headache due to an increase in brain volumen has been proposed.[24] There should be other contributing factors, however, such as a hypersensitivity of some receptors (to pressure) hypothetically localized on the venous vessels.[25] One of the potential etiologies for this transient receptor sensitization could be a hidden or previous infection.[17] Finally, Chen and co-workers[26] recently found that patients who have primary cough headache are associated with a more crowded posterior cranial fossa, which may be a further contributing factor for the pathogenesis of this headache syndrome.

The presence of a type I Chiari's malformation or any other lesions causing obstruction of cerebrospinal fluid pathways or displacing cerebral structures must be excluded before cough headache is assumed to benign. Cough headache can be the only clinical manifestation of type I Chiari's malformation for several years in about one fifth of symptomatic patients. In the author's experience, however, most if not all patients who have symptomatic cough headache finally develop posterior fossa symptoms or signs, mainly dizziness/vertigo, unsteadiness, and syncopes.[9,14] Symptomatic cough headache begins, on average, 3 decades earlier than primary cough headache, does not show a clear male predominance, and does not respond to indomethacin.[9,14]

Migraine, cluster headache, postlumbar puncture headache, and idiopathic intracranial hypertension can be aggravated but not elicited by cough. Given the differential diagnosis outlined previously, every patient who has cough headache should

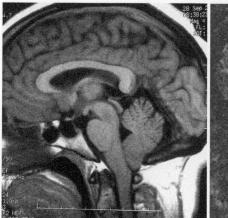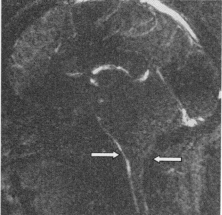

Fig. 3. Cine phase-contrast MRI (*right panel*) of a 33-year-old woman who had type I Chiari's malformation (*left panel*) presenting as cough headache showing difficulties in cerebrospinal fluid circulation anteriorly and posteriorly in the foramen magnum region (*arrows*). *From* Pascual J, González-Mandly A, Martin R, et al. Headaches precipitated by cough, prolonged exercise or sexual activity: a prospective etiological and clinical study. J Headache Pain 2008;9:259–66; with permission.

undergo MRI of the brain to rule out a posterior fossa lesion. Despite scattered reports, there is not enough scientific background to support unruptured aneurysms,[27] carotid stenosis,[28,29] or vertebrobasilar disease[30] as specific causes for cough headache. Therefore, a magnetic resonance angiography (MRA) study is not mandatory in these patients (**Fig. 4**).

Acute treatment is impractical because of the short duration and multiplicity of cough headaches. Primary cough headache responds to indomethacin given prophylactically at doses usually ranging from 25 to 150 mg daily.[31,32] The mechanism of action of this drug is unknown but could include a decrease in intracranial pressure,[33,34] which would explain the benefits seen with lumbar puncture or acetazolamide in patients who have primary cough headache.[24,35,36]

Patients who have symptomatic cough headache do not consistently respond to any known pharmacologic treatment (including indomethacin) and need specific surgical treatment. It has been shown that suboccipital craniectomy relieves cough headache in type I Chiari's malformation patients.[9,14]

PRIMARY EXERTIONAL HEADACHE

This headache is brought on by prolonged physical exercise. Contrary to primary cough headache, primary exertional headache is typical of young people (age range 10–48 years in the author's series), with a male predominance. In terms of consultation, exertional headache is less common than cough headache. Most cases occur in patients who have a personal or family history of migraine.[2,9,14] This headache may be triggered by any kind of prolonged physical exercise,[37–39] at least enough

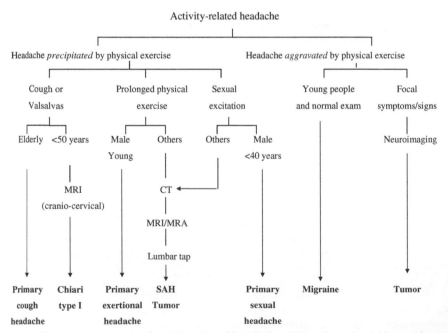

Fig. 4. Differential diagnosis of activity-related headache. SAH, subarachnoid hemorrhage. *Adapted from* Pascual J. Activity-related headache. In: Gilman S, editor. MedLink neurology. San Diego (CA): MedLink Corporation. Available at: www.medlink.com/. Accessed July 13, 2008; with permission.

exercise sufficient to double the resting pulse for over 10 seconds but ordinarily for minutes or even hours. Headache usually occurs at the peak of the exercise and subsides when the activity ceases, although on some occasions, headache can last up to 2 days. Exertional headache is described as aching, pounding, or throbbing and has many migraine characteristics, with associated nausea, vomiting, and photophobia, and some phonophobia. It may be bilateral (~60% of the cases) or unilateral.[2,9,14] Diagnostic criteria are shown in **Box 3**.

Even in the presence of a typical clinical picture, the diagnosis of primary exertional headache can be made only after an extensive investigation. Contrary to cough headache, however, more than 80% of patients consulting due to exertional headache are primary cases (see **Fig. 4**). For typical patients (middle-aged men who have a normal examination), it is mandatory to exclude any kind of intracranial space-occupying lesion and sentinel hemorrhage due to vascular malformations.[2,9,14] Very rarely, exertional headache is a symptom of middle cerebral artery dissection or pheochromocytoma.[40–45] MRI followed by MRA should be the screening procedure. In equivocal cases, a lumbar tap could also be considered. A number of articles have documented exertional[46,47]—and recently nonexertional[48]—vascular headaches as the presenting symptoms of cardiac ischemia ("cardiac cephalgia"). In these rare cases, assessment of cardiac enzymes and an ECG are indicated.

The etiology of benign exertional headache is presumed to be related to cerebral vasodilation that is extracranial and intracranial in nature. In these patients, cerebral blood flow velocity increases and the pulsatility index decreases compared with control subjects. In this respect, exertional headache may resemble the headaches associated with high altitude and fever.

For nonincapacitating cases or for patients who have a low exercise frequency, the first, and sometimes only, recommendation should be transient exercise moderation or abstinence. Lambert and Burnett[49] described how a prescribed warm-up period prevented swimmer's headache. Leaving exercise abstinence aside, there is no absolute evidence of the value of pharmacologic treatments in the management of primary exertional headache. In general, antimigraine preventive medications show some benefit. For most patients, β-blockers at the usual antimigraine doses seem useful.[2,9,14] There are well-documented cases in which exertional headache did not improve or β-blockers could not be tolerated. Some of these patients seemed to improve on indomethacin in doses varying from 25 to 150 mg per day.[31] There is no consensus on the treatment duration in these cases. Primary exertional headache is usually a transient clinical picture, usually lasting less than 3 months and rarely longer than 6 months. Therefore, the author recommends stopping the preventive treatment after 3 to 6 months to check for headache reappearance.

Acute therapy immediately before physical exercise could theoretically be a good alternative for some patients. Simple analgesics and nonsteroidal anti-inflammatory

---

Box 3
Diagnostic criteria for primary exertional headache

A. Pulsating headache fulfilling criteria B and C

B. Lasting from 5 minutes to 48 hours

C. Brought on by and occurring only during or after physical exertion

D. Not attributed to another disorder

drugs do not seem to prevent the development of exertional headaches. Ergotamine seems to be useful. Triptans could theoretically be an alternative treatment to ergotamine but, again, there is no definite scientific evidence on the possible value of triptans in the acute treatment of exertional headache.

PRIMARY SEXUAL HEADACHE

Headaches may occur during sexual activities associated with intercourse or independent of intercourse (eg, masturbation) or orgasm. There are three types of sexual headaches. The dull type resembles tension-type headache. Postural sexual headache is a low–cerebrospinal fluid pressure type of headache resulting from a tear of the dura during sexual intercourse.[50,51] The most common is the explosive type, now called orgasmic headache. Patients who have orgasmic headache often also suffer exertional headache and rarely cough headache.[9,14,51,52] As occurs in exertional headache, there is a bilateral comorbidity between sexual headache and migraine.[53] These similarities seem logical because sexual intercourse combines prolonged physical exercise and the Valsalva maneuver. Primary orgasmic headache occurs typically in young middle-aged people (average age of 40 years in the author's series) and is most common in men (4:1). Pain location is bilateral ("over the temples") in 75% of patients. In the author's experience, all cases showed a pulsating component. Pain duration ranges from 1 minute to 4 days (median 10 minutes). Nausea and phono/photophobia are not uncommon. The median duration of symptomatic period is 2 months. The diagnostic criteria for orgasmic headache appear in **Box 4**.

The pathophysiology of orgasmic headache is unknown, although sudden hemodynamic changes have been proposed as an explanation.[51,52] The etiologies for secondary cases comprise subarachnoid bleeding and, more rarely, intracranial masses.[9,14] Therefore, diagnostic investigation in these headaches must begin with a neuroimaging study (CT or MRI) to rule out subarachnoid bleeding, followed by an angioMRI. Conventional angiography, a lumbar tap, or both would be indicated in punctual cases in which there is a high suspicion of bleeding despite a negative angioMRI, but are not as routine (see **Fig. 4**).

Management is identical to that of prolonged exertional headache.

HYPNIC HEADACHE

Hypnic headache is a recurrent, sleep-related, primary headache condition. Hypnic headache was described by Raskin[25] in 1988. Its epidemiology is unknown, but in terms of clinical practice, hypnic headache is rare, accounting for fewer than 1% of patients attending a specialized headache clinic. Diagnostic criteria appear in **Box 5**. Hypnic headache usually begins after age 50 years (mean ~60 years, range 30–83 years) and is more prevalent in women (65%) than in men. By definition, the attack occurs at night when sleeping (or during a nap in 10% of cases), waking

---

Box 4
Diagnostic criteria for primary orgasmic headache

A. Sudden severe ("explosive") headache fulfilling criterion B

B. Occurs at orgasm

C. Not attributed to another disorder

Box 5
Diagnostic criteria for hypnic headache

A. Dull headache fulfilling criteria B–D

B. Develops only during sleep and awakens patient

C. Has at least two of the following characteristics:

    Occurs more than15 times per month

    Lasts less than 15 minutes after waking

    First occurs after age 50 years

D. No autonomic symptoms and no more than one of nausea, photophobia, or phonophobia

E. Not attributed to another disorder

---

the patient at a constant time interval ("alarm clock headache"). Headache is usually mild to moderate, being severe in 20% of the cases, and lasts 15 to 180 minutes, but longer attacks of up to 10 hours have also been described. Pain location is not characteristic, being bilateral in approximately two thirds of cases. Regarding frequency, half of the patients have daily attacks (range one per week to six per night). Triggers or autonomic phenomena are not part of the clinical picture of hypnic headache. Contrary to stabbing headache, a history of the most common primary headaches is not associated with the development of hypnic headache.[54–60]

Pathophysiologic mechanisms of hypnic headache are speculative. It has been hypothesized that hypnic headache is the result of dysfunction within the suprachiasmatic nucleus in the hypothalamus, which is considered the brain pacemaker. Supporting this hypothesis, connections between the suprachiasmatic nucleus and pain-modulating brainstem nuclei (raphe and periaqueductal gray matter) are well demonstrated. Melatonin is secreted by the pineal gland and is also a marker of circadian rhythms. A decrease in nocturnal secretion of melatonin has also been suggested as a potential mechanism for hypnic headache. Finally, because this syndrome occurs only during sleep and usually coincides with a dream, an abnormal regulation of rapid eye movement sleep has been postulated as an explanation for hypnic headache.[60–62]

The diagnosis of hypnic headache relies on its clinical picture and normal physical examination. Due to its rarity, it is necessary to rule out structural intracranial disorders and trigeminal autonomic cephalgias (see the article on this topic elsewhere in this issue), which may almost exclusively or only occur as nocturnal attacks. In the author's experience, the most common confounding diagnoses for patients consulting due to a suspicion of hypnic headache are (1) nocturnal peaks of arterial hypertension, frequently in hypertensive patients who receive treatment early in the morning; and (2) rebound phenomenon in migraineurs with analgesic overuse.

There are no controlled trials for the treatment of hypnic headache. Lithium interacts with the pain-modulating systems possibly involved in this syndrome, indirectly increases nocturnal production of melatonin, and remains the most popular treatment for hypnic headache (grade C recommendation). Lithium carbonate can be initiated at 300 mg at night and increased to 600 mg after 1 or 2 weeks if necessary. Poor tolerability to lithium is not rare, mainly in elderly patients. Melatonin has been shown to be useful in some cases, as has nocturnal caffeine (although it induces insomnia). There are scattered case reports communicating the usefulness of flunarizine, verapamil, prednisone, indomethacin, acetazolamide, gabapentin, and pizotifen.[60,63]

PRIMARY THUNDERCLAP HEADACHE

This headache is of high intensity with abrupt onset, mimicking that seen in the case of a ruptured cerebral aneurysm. The diagnostic criteria for primary thunderclap headache appear in **Box 6**. The recognition that thunderclap headache can be a primary headache disorder has only recently been considered, and the IHS argues that this evidence is preliminary.[1] The prevalence of primary thunderclap headache is not known. This syndrome predominantly affects individuals between ages 20 and 50 years and has a female predominance.[2]

Thunderclap headache may occur as a benign and recurring headache disorder in the absence of structural intracranial lesions. The clinical picture is very characteristic. Headache appears suddenly and reaches a maximum within 30 seconds and usually lasts for several hours but may persist for weeks. Headache can be diffuse but is often occipital in location and can be accompanied by migrainous symptoms such as nausea and vomiting. In approximately two thirds of patients, headache repeats over a period of 2 weeks, whereas the remaining patients experience headache attacks for up to several years. Headache may appear spontaneously or may be triggered by exercise, bathing in hot water, hyperventilation, or by sexual intercourse. By definition, there are no focal symptoms/signs, and neuroimaging (CT and MRI) and cerebrospinal examinations are normal.[2,64–67]

The pathophysiology of primary thunderclap headache is unclear, but hypersensitivity of the cranial autonomic system has been proposed as an explanation. An excessive sympathethic activity, an abnormal vascular response to circulating cathecolamines, or an aberrant central sympathetic neurogenic reflex could explain the occurrence of thunderclap headache in patients who have pheochromocytoma, with acute hypertensive crisis in patients who take amphetamine or cocaine or foods containing tyramine while concurrently using monoaminoxidase inhibitors.[2]

Thunderclap headache is frequently associated with secondary causes; therefore, the search for an underlying cause should be quick and exhaustive. Distinguishing between primary and secondary thunderclap headache is not possible on the basis of clinical data alone. The differential diagnosis must include serious vascular intracranial disorders, particularly subarachnoid hemorrhage, but also intracerebral hemorrhage, cerebral venous thrombosis, unruptured vascular malformations, arterial dissection (intra and extracranial), pheochromocytoma, central nervous system angeitis, colloid cyst of the third ventricle, cerebrospinal hypotension, acute sinusitis with

---

Box 6
Diagnostic criteria for primary thunderclap headache

A. Severe pain fulfilling criteria B and C

B. Both of the following characteristics:

   Sudden onset, reaching a maximum intensity within 1 minute

   Lasting from 1 hour to 10 days

C. Does not recur regularly over subsequent weeks or months

D. Not attributed to another disorder

barotraumas, and consumption of sympathomimetic drugs, especially amphetamine and cocaine. It is possible that most patients diagnosed with primary thunderclap headache suffer from the syndrome of reversible cerebral vasculitis/vasoconstriction of unknown etiology.[64–66] This benign angiopathy of the central nervous system can be diagnosed solely on the basis of angiographic abnormalities, without supporting evidence for inflammation on tests such as cerebrospinal examination or brain biopsy. This syndrome include entities such as the Call-Fleming syndrome, thunderclap headache with reversible vasospasm, benign angiopathy of the central nervous system, postpartum angiopathy, migrainous vasospasm or migraine angeitis, and drug-induced cerebral arteritis or angiopathy. These clinicoradiologic syndromes are usually self-limited to 3 months and are characterized by recurrent acute and severe headaches that require differentiation from subarachnoid hemorrhage and by reversible multifocal cerebral vasoconstriction (or vasospasm). In a few patients, this condition is complicated by reversible posterior leukoencephalopathy syndrome. There is no confirmatory test for the diagnosis of the syndrome of reversible cerebral vasoconstriction. In patients presenting with thunderclap headache, the usual presenting symptom of this condition, the initial focus should be to rule out other conditions by performing CT, MRI, and laboratory tests including vasculitis and toxicologic screening. Transcranial Doppler can show diffusely elevated blood velocities, which typically normalize over a period of days to weeks. The characteristic angiographic pattern of multifocal narrowing and dilatation of the intracerebral arteries is best seen by conventional angiography or with less-invasive tests like MRA. This technique is particularly useful to document reversal of the vasoconstriction.[2,64–66]

There is no established treatment. A short course of steroids can be justified to cover for cerebral vasculitis while awaiting the results of serial angiography. In a recent article, nimodipine was demonstrated to prevent further attacks of thunderclap headaches in most patients and should be recommended for 2 to 3 months. It is also important to avoid vasoconstrictors such as triptans, ergot derivatives, or cocaine and similar drugs.[2,64–66]

NEW DAILY PERSISTENT HEADACHE

NDPH has been recognized by the second edition of the IHS classification as a separate entity from chronic tension-type headache.[1] NDPH is daily and unremitting from (or almost from) the moment of onset, typically in individuals who do not have a prior history of headache. As stated by the IHS, NDPH may take one of two subforms: self-limiting, which typically resolves without therapy within several months; and refractory, which is resistant to aggressive treatment. The prevalence of chronic daily headache in population-based studies is approximately 4% to 5%. The prevalence of NDPH is approximately 0.1% of the general population.[6] In specialty headache clinics, approximately 10% of patients who have chronic daily headache meet the criteria for NDPH.

NDPH has a female predominance (2.5:1). Diagnosed at all ages, NDPH usually begins in the second and third decade in women and in the fifth decade in men. Typically, patients are able to pinpoint the exact date their headache started. In at least half the cases, headache begins in relation to an infection or flulike illness or a stressful life event. Pain is described as fairly constant and moderate to severe. Location is heterogeneous and not characteristic, and more than half of patients complain of migrainous-associated symptoms (in this order: nausea, phono/photophobia, vomiting). The current diagnostic criteria for NDPH appear in **Box 7**.[68–70]

Box 7
Diagnostic criteria for primary new daily persistent headache

A. Headache for longer than 3 months fulfilling criteria B–D

B. Headache is daily and unremitting from onset or from less than 3 days from onset

C. At least two of the following pain characteristics:

  Bilateral location

  Pressing/tightening (nonpulsating) quality

  Mild or moderate intensity

  Not aggravated by routine physical activity such as walking or climbing stairs

D. Both of the following:

  No more than one: photophobia, phonophobia, or mild nausea

  Neither moderate or severe nausea nor vomiting

E. Not attributed to another disorder

The etiology of NDPH usually remains unknown. Because NDPH begins simultaneously with a viral-like syndrome in some patients, an infectious cause has been proposed. Reactivation of Epstein-Barr virus or other infectious agents has been hypothesized as the trigger for the development of NDPH due to an activated immune response, setting up a state of continuous neurogenic inflammation. This hypothesis is far from being proved, and in about half of NDPH cases, there is no recognized trigger.[68]

Diagnosis of NDPH is one of exclusion. Secondary causes of NDPH appear in **Box 8**. Low–cerebrospinal fluid pressure headache due to spontaneous cerebrospinal fluid pressure leak, cerebral vein thrombosis, headache attributed to infection (particularly viral), and medication overuse headache can mimic NDPH presentation and should always be carefully ruled out with appropriate investigations.

NDPH is difficult to manage. These patients commonly receive preventive medications used to treat migraine, such as β-blockers, topiramate, valproic acid, or

---

Box 8
Secondary causes of new daily persistent headache

Cerebral vein thrombosis

Low–cerebrospinal fluid pressure headache

High–cerebrospinal fluid pressure headache

Medication overuse headache

Carotid or vertebral artery dissection

Giant cell arteritis

Meningitis

Sphenoid sinusitis

Cervical facet syndrome

Posttraumatic headache

gabapentin, with very low efficacy. Tricyclics, selective serotonin reuptake inhibitors, and muscle relaxants are usually inefficacious.[68–70]

REFERENCES

1. Headache Classification Committee of the International Headache Society. The international classification of headache disorders. 2nd edition. Cephalalgia 2004;24(Suppl 1):1–160.
2. Dodick D, Pascual J. Primary stabbing, cough, exertional, and thunderclap headaches. In: Olesen J, Goadsby PJ, Ramadan NM, et al, editors. The headaches. 3rd edition. Philadelphia: Lippincott Williams & Wilkins; 2006. p. 831–9.
3. Sjaastad O, Pettersen H, Bakketeig LS. The Vaga study; epidemiology of headache I: the prevalence of ultrashort paroxysms. Cephalalgia 2001;21:207–15.
4. Pareja JA, Ruiz J, de Isla C, et al. Idiopathic stabbing headache (jabs and jolts syndrome). Cephalalgia 1996;16:93–6.
5. Levy MJ, Matharu MS, Goadsby PJ. Prolactinomas, dopamine agonists and headache: two case reports. Eur J Neurol 2003;10:169–71.
6. Mascellino AM, Lay CL, Newman LC. Stabbing headache as the presenting manifestation of intracranial meningioma: a report of two patients. Headache 2001;41:599–601.
7. Dodick D. Indomethacin responsive headache syndromes. Curr Pain Headache Rep 2004;8:19–28.
8. Rasmussen BK, Olesen J. Symptomatic and nonsymptomatic headaches in a general population. Neurology 1992;42:1225–31.
9. Pascual J, González-Mandly A, Martín R, et al. Headaches precipitated by cough, prolonged exercise or sexual activity: a prospective etiological and clinical study. J Headache Pain 2008;9:259–66.
10. Symonds C. Cough headache. Brain 1956;79:557–68.
11. Nick J. Exertional Headache. A series of 43 cases. Sem Hop Paris 1980;56:525–31 [In French].
12. Rooke ED. Benign exertional headache. Med Clin North Am 1968;52:801–8.
13. Sands GH, Newman L, Lipton R. Cough, exertional and other miscellaneous headaches. Med Clin North Am 1991;75:733–47.
14. Pascual J, Iglesias F, Oterino A, et al. Cough, exertional, and sexual headaches: an analysis of 72 benign and symptomatic cases. Neurology 1996;46:1520–4.
15. Pascual J, Oterino A, Berciano J. Headache in type I Chiari malformation. Neurology 1992;42:1519–21.
16. Boes CJ, Matharu MS, Goadsby PJ. Benign cough headache. Cephalalgia 2002;22:772–9.
17. Pascual J. Activity-related headache. In: Gilman S, editor. MedLink neurology. San Diego (CA): MedLink Corporation. Available at: www.medlink.com. Accessed July 13, 2008.
18. Diamond S. Prolonged benign exertional headache: its clinical characteristics and response to indomethacin. Headache 1982;22:96–8.
19. Williams B. Cerebrospinal fluid pressure changes in response to coughing. Brain 1976;99:331–46.
20. Williams B. Cough headache due to craniospinal pressure dissociation. Arch Neurol 1980;37:226–30.
21. Nightingale S, Williams B. Hindbrain hernia headache. Lancet 1987;1:731–4.
22. Sansur CA, Heiss JD, DeVroom HL, et al. Pathophysiology of headache associated with cough in patients with Chiari I malformation. J Neurosurg 2003;98:453–8.

23. Pujol J, Roig C, Capdevilla A, et al. Motion of the cerebellar tonsils in Chiari type I malformation studied by cine-phase constrast MRI. Neurology 1995;45:1746–53.
24. Wang SJ, Fuh JL, Lu SR. Benign cough headache is responsive to acetazolamide. Neurology 2000;55:149–50.
25. Raskin NH. Short-lived head pains. Neurol Clin 1997;15:143–52.
26. Chen YY, Lirng JF, Fuh JL, et al. Primary cough headache is associated with posterior fossa crowdedness: a morphometric MRI study. Cephalalgia 2004;24: 694–9.
27. Smith WS, Messing RO. Cerebral aneurysm presenting as cough headache. Headache 1993;33:203–4.
28. Britton TC, Guiloff RJ. Carotid artery disease presenting as cough headache. Lancet 1988;1:1406–7.
29. Rivera M, del Real MA, Teruel JL, et al. Carotid artery disease presenting as cough headache in a patient with haemodialysis. Postgrad Med J 1991;67:702.
30. Satikov IN, Mattle HP. Vertebrobasilar dolicoectasia and exertional headache. J Neurol Neurosurg Psychiatry 1978;41:930–3.
31. Diamond S, Medina JL. Benign exertional headache: successful treatment with indomethacin. Headache 1979;19:249.
32. Mathew NT. Indomethacin-responsive headache syndromes. Headache 1981;21: 147–50.
33. Slavik RS, Rhoney DH. Indomethacin: a review of its cerebral blood flow effects and potential use for controlling intracranial pressure in traumatic brain injury patients. Neurol Res 1999;21:491–9.
34. Rasmussen M. Treatment of elevated intracranial pressure with indomethacin: friend or foe? Acta Anaesthesiol Scand 2005;49:1577–8.
35. Raskin NH. The cough headache syndrome: treatment. Neurology 1995;45:1784.
36. Chalaupka FD. Therapeutic effectiveness of acetazolamide in hindbrain hernia headache. Neurol Sci 2000;21:117–9.
37. Dalessio DJ. Effort migraine. Headache 1974;14:53.
38. Indo T, Takahashi A. Swimmer's headache. Headache 1990;30:485–7.
39. Paulson GW. Weightlifter's headache. Headache 1983;23:193–4.
40. Paulson GW, Zipf RE, Beekman JF. Pheochromocytoma causing exercise-related headache and pulmonary edema. Ann Neurol 1979;5:96–9.
41. Fleetcroft R, Maddocks JL. Headache due to ischaemic heart disease. J R Soc Med 1985;78:676.
42. Blacky RA, Rittlemeyer JT, Wallace MR. Headache angina. Am J Cardiol 1987;60: 730.
43. Lefkowitz D, Biller J. Bregmatic headache as a manifestation of myocardial ischemia. Arch Neurol 1982;39:120.
44. Vernay D, Deffond D, Fraysse P, et al. Walk headache: an unusual manifestation of ischemic heart disease. Headache 1993;29:350–1.
45. Bowen J, Oppenheimer G. Headache as presentation of angina: reproduction of symptoms during angioplasty. Headache 1993;33:238–9.
46. Lipton RB, Lowenkopf T, Leckie RS, et al. Cardiac cephalgia: a treatable form of exertional headache. Neurology 1997;49:813–6.
47. Lance JW, Lambros J. Unilateral exertional headache as a symptom of cardiac ischemia. Headache 1998;38:315–6.
48. Gutiérrez-Morlote J, Pascual J. Cardiac cephalgia is not necessarily an exertional headache. Cephalalgia 2002;22:765–6.
49. Lambert RW, Burnet DL. Prevention of exercise induced migraine by quantitative warm-up. Headache 1985;25:317–9.

50. Frese A, Eikerman A, Frese K, et al. Headache associated with sexual activity. Demography, clinical features, and comorbidity. Neurology 2003;61:796–800.
51. Evers S, Lance JW. Primary headache attributed to sexual activity. In: Olesen J, Goadsby PJ, Ramadan NM, et al, editors. The headaches. 3rd edition. Philadelphia: Lippincott Williams & Wilkins; 2006. p. 841–5.
52. Silbert PL, Edis RH, Stewart-Wynne EG, et al. Benign vascular sexual headache and exertional headache: interrelationships and long term prognosis. J Neurol Neurosurg Psychiatry 1991;54:417–21.
53. Biehl K, Evers S, Frese A. Comorbidity of migraine and headache associated with sexual activity. Cephalalgia 2007;27:1271–3.
54. Rains JC, Poceta JS. Sleep-related headache syndromes. Semin Neurol 2005;25:69–80.
55. Dodick DW, Eross EJ, Parish JM, et al. Clinical, anatomical, and physiologic relationship between sleep and headache. Headache 2003;43:282–92.
56. Paiva T, Farinha A, Martins A, et al. Chronic headaches and sleep disorders. Arch Intern Med 1997;157:1701–5.
57. Evans RW, Dodick DW, Schwedt TJ. The headaches that awake us. Headache 2006;46:678–81.
58. Ohayon MM. Prevalence and risk factors of morning headaches in the general population. Arch Intern Med 2004;164:97–102.
59. Paiva T, Batista A, Martins P, et al. The relationship between headaches and sleep disturbances. Headache 1995;35:590–6.
60. Newman LC, Mosek A. Hypnic headaches. In: Olesen J, Goadsby PJ, Ramadan NM, et al, editors. The headaches. 3rd edition. Philadelphia: Lippincott Williams & Wilkins; 2006. p. 847–9.
61. Ralph MR, Foster RG, Davis FC, et al. Transplanted suprachiasmatic nucleus determines circadian period. Science 1990;247:975–8.
62. Iguichi H, Kato KI, Ibayashi H. Age-dependent reduction in serum melatonin concentrations in healthy human subjects. J Clin Endocrinol Metab 1982;55:27–9.
63. Evers S, Goadsby PJ. Hypnic headache: clinical features, pathophysiology and treatment. Cephalalgia 2003;23:20–3.
64. Calabrese LH, Dodick DW, Schwedt TJ, et al. Narrative review: reversible cerebral vasoconstriction syndromes. Ann Intern Med 2007;146:34–44.
65. Dodcik DW, Brown RD Jr, Britton JW, et al. Non-aneurysmal thunderclap headache with diffuse, multifocal, segmental and reversible vasospasm. Cephalalgia 1999;19:118–23.
66. Chen SP, Fuh JL, Lirng JF, et al. Recurrent primary thunderclap headache and benign CNS angiopathy: spectra of the same disorder? Neurology 2006;67:2164–9.
67. Castillo J, Muñoz P, Guitera V, et al. Epidemiology of chronic daily headache in the general population. Headache 1999;38:497–506.
68. Evans RW, Rozen TD. Etiology and treatment of new daily persistent headache. Headache 2001;4:830–2.
69. Li D, Rozen TD. The clinical characterisation of new daily persistent headache. Cephalalgia 2002;22:66–9.
70. Rozen TD, Jensen R. New daily persistent headache. In: Olesen J, Goadsby PJ, Ramadan NM, et al, editors. The headaches. 3rd edition. Philadelphia: Lippincott Williams & Wilkins; 2006. p. 855–7.

Index

Note: Page numbers of article titles are in **boldface** type.

Neurol Clin 27 (2009) 573–582
doi:10.1016/S0733-8619(09)00014-0
0733-8619/09/$ – see front matter © 2009 Elsevier Inc. All rights reserved.

Moving?

Make sure your subscription moves with you!

To notify us of your new address, find your **Clinics Account Number** (located on your mailing label above your name), and contact customer service at:

E-mail: elspcs@elsevier.com

800-654-2452 (subscribers in the U.S. & Canada)
314-453-7041 (subscribers outside of the U.S. & Canada)

Fax number: 314-523-5170

Elsevier Periodicals Customer Service
11830 Westline Industrial Drive
St. Louis, MO 63146

*To ensure uninterrupted delivery of your subscription, please notify us at least 4 weeks in advance of move.

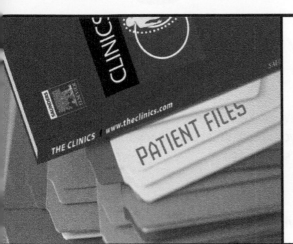
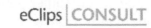
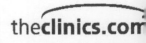

Printed and bound by CPI Group (UK) Ltd, Croydon, CR0 4YY

03/10/2024

01040452-0013